NUCLEAR MEDICINE
TECHNOLOGY

Procedures and Quick Reference

NUCLEAR MEDICINE
TECHNOLOGY

Procedures

and

Quick Reference

PETE SHACKETT, BA, ARRT(N), CNMT

LIPPINCOTT WILLIAMS & WILKINS

A **Wolters Kluwer** Company

Philadelphia · Baltimore · New York · London
Buenos Aires · Hong Kong · Sydney · Tokyo

Editor: Lawrence McGrew
Managing Editor: Angela Heubeck
Marketing Manager: Christen DeMarco
Project Editor: Shannon Benner

530 Walnut Street
Philadelphia, PA 19106-3780 USA

351 West Camden Street
Baltimore, MD 21201-2436 USA

Printed in the United States of America

Library of Congress Cataloging-in-Publication Data

Shackett, Pete.
    Nuclear medicine technology : procedures and quick reference / by Pete Shackett.
       p.   cm.
    Includes bibliographical references and index.
    ISBN 0-7817-1981-X
    1. Radioisotope scanning—Handbooks, manuals, etc. I. Title.
RC78.7.R4 S48 1999
616.07'575—dc21
                                            99-052131

The publishers have made every effort to trace the copyright holders for borrowed material. If they have inadvertently overlooked any, they will be pleased to make the necessary arrangements at the first opportunity.

To purchase additional copies of this book, call our customer service department at **(800) 638-3030** or fax orders to **(301) 824-7390.** For other book services, including chapter reprints and large quantity sales, ask for the Special Sales department.

Canadian customers should call **(800) 665-1148,** or fax **(800) 665-0103.** For all other calls originating outside of the United States, please call **(301) 714-2300** or fax us at **(301) 824-7390.**

Visit Lippincott Williams & Wilkins on the Internet: **http://www.lww.com** or contact our customer service department at **custserv@wwilkins.com**. Lippincott Williams & Wilkins customer service representatives are available from 8:30 am to 6:00 pm, EST, Monday through Friday, for telephone access.

00 01 02 03 04

1 2 3 4 5 6 7 8 9 10

Dedication

I would like to dedicate this work to my lovely wife, Carolyn, and our canine gatekeeper and life-mate, Brandy.

In loving memory of my parents, Bertha and Wilfard Shackett.

Many thanks to Dr. Max H. Lombardi, Director of Nuclear Medicine Technology (Retired), Hillsborough Community College, Tampa, FL, for the opportunity of knowledge and his encouragement and inspiration. I would also like to thank Mr. Bud Rogers, CNMT, Chief Technologist, Bayfront Medical Center, St. Petersburg, FL, along with the many technologists, students, nurses, and physicians who contributed opinions and were consulted for information during the development of this manual.

Disclaimer

This manual is intended to be a technologist's book. It is an amalgamation of protocols from many institutions, technologists' experiences, and written resources. It is to serve only as a guide in the performance of the procedures listed. Specific department protocols should always be followed as written when available. The manual is *not* intended to be the consummate and quintessential encyclopedia of nuclear medicine. The scope of the manual covers the basic data needed for most routine imaging and includes a reference section of peripheral material used on a daily basis by many personnel (not only nuclear medicine) within the hospital setting. Tables, charts, and data are incorporated that are usually difficult to find quickly or in one source. These may be of use to departments, students, physicians' reading rooms, various diagnostic technicians, and nursing stations. A list of references is included that were used in the collation of this material in hopes that the readers will pursue them for more specific information. If there is ever a question, without question, discuss it with your radiologist or nuclear physician. Thank you.

TABLE OF **CONTENTS**

SCANS

1.   Adrenocortical Scan **3**

2.   Adrenal Medulla: Pheochromocytoma Scan (mIBG) **9**

3.   Angiography **16**

4.   Bone Density (Densitometry) **21**

5.   Bone Scan (Skeletal Imaging) **27**

6.   Brain Scan/Death (Brain Flow) **34**

7.   Brain SPECT (Single Photon Emission Computed Tomography) **40**

8.   Breath Test for *H. Pylori:* Pytest® ^{14}C-Urea Breath Test (UBT) **46**

9.   Cardiac: Gated First-Pass Study **51**

10.   Cardiac: MUGA and MUGA-X (Stress MUGA) **56**

11.   Cardiac: Myocardial Infarction (MI) Scan **62**

12.   Cardiac: Resting Test (Perfusion) **67**

13.   Cardiac: Stress Test (Perfusion) **73**

14.   CEA-Scan® (Radioimmunoscinitigraphy [RIS]) **81**

15.   Cisternography **86**

16.   Cystography (Voiding Cystourethrogram): Direct and Indirect **91**

17.   DVT: AcuTect™ (Deep Venous Thrombosis) **96**

18.   DVT: Venography (Deep Venous Thrombosis) **102**

19.   Esophageal Transit Time **109**

20.   Gallium Scan **114**

21.   Gastric Empty (Solid and Liquid) **119**

22.   Gastroesophageal Reflux **125**

23 Gastrointestinal Bleed **129**

24 HIDA (Hepatobiliary or Gallbladder Scan) With Ejection Fraction **134**

25 LeVeen or Denver Shunt Patency **141**

26 Liver SPECT (Hepatic Hemangioma) **145**

27 Liver/Spleen Scan **149**

28 Lung Perfusion **154**

29 Lung Transmission **161**

30 Lung Ventilation: Gas and Aerosol **165**

31 Lymphoscintigraphy (Lymphangiogram) **171**

32 Meckel's Diverticulum **178**

33 NeoTect™ (Lung Mass) **183**

34 OctreoScan® **188**

35 OncoScint® (Radioimmunoscintigraphy [RIS]) **194**

36 Parathyroid Scan **199**

37 Positron Emission Tomography (PET) (Coincidence Imaging: An Overview) **205**

38 ProstaScint® Scan **212**

39 Renal: Cortical Imaging (^{99m}Tc-DMSA) **217**

40 Renal: Glomerular Filtration Rate (GFR:^{99m}Tc-DTPA) **222**

41 Renal: Tubular Function (MAG$_3$®, ^{131}I-OIH) **229**

42 Salivary Gland Imaging **236**

43 Schilling Test **240**

44 Scintimammography **246**

45 SPECT Imaging (Single Photon Emission Computed Tomography):
An Overview **252**

46 Testicular Scan **258**

47 Therapy: Bone Pain (Palliation) **262**

48 Therapy: Intra-articular (Joint); Synovectomy **268**

49 Therapy: Intracavitary (Serosal) **273**

50 Therapy: Polycythemia Vera **279**

51 Thyroid: Ablation **284**

52 Thyroid: Ectopic Tissue Scan (Substernal) **292**

53 Thyroid: Hyperthyroid Therapy (< 30 mCi) **298**

54 Thyroid Scan **304**

55 Thyroid Uptake **310**

56 Thyroid: Whole-Body ^{131}I Cancer Study and rTSH Augmentation **317**

57 Verluma™-Scan: Small Cell Lung Cancer **323**

58 White Blood Cell (^{111}In-oxime and ^{99m}Tc-Ceretec™) **329**

QUICK REFERENCE

A **CONVERSION TABLES** **339**

      lb/kg **340**
      in/cm **341**
      Target Heart Rates (Cardiac Studies) **342**
      mCi/MBq **343**

B **RADIOPHARMACEUTICALS** **344**

      Standard Adult Nuclear Medicine Dose Ranges **345**
      Routine Medical Radionuclides **347**
      Equations **348**
      Kit Preparations (Overview) **349**
      Pediatric Dosing in Nuclear Medicine **351**
      Radioactive Isotopes **356**

C **DECAY TABLES OF COMMON RADIONUCLIDES** **382**

      ^{137}Cs **383**
      ^{57}Co **384**
      ^{67}Ga **385**
      ^{111}In **386**
      ^{123}I **387**
      ^{131}I **388**
      ^{99}Mo **389**
      ^{99m}Tc **390**
      ^{201}Tl **391**
      ^{133}Xe **392**

D **STANDARD DRUG INTERVENTIONS** **393**

      Calculations, Preparations, and Administration **393**
      Infusion Rate Tables **397**
      Side Effects of Common Drugs **401**
      Drugs and Studies Affecting ^{123}I Uptake **403**

(E) LABORATORY TESTS **404**

    Normal Ranges **405**

    Enzymes and Hormones **409**

(F) LANGUAGE BARRIER BUSTER™/INTERPRETECH™ **415**

    Chinese-Mandarin **415**

    French **417**

    German **418**

    Italian **420**

    Japanese **421**

    Polish **423**

    Portuguese **424**

    Russian **426**

    Spanish **427**

(G) REGULATIONS **430**

    Misadministration **430**

    Radiation Safety **432**

(H) PATIENT INFORMATION FOR THYROID THERAPIES **435**

    Ablation (> 30 mCi) **436**

    Hyperthyroid (< 30 mCi) **437**

(I) PATIENT HISTORY SHEETS **438**

    Adrenal Scans, mIBG, and NP59 . . . . **439**

    Bone Scan **440**

    Brain Scan (SPECT) **441**

    Cardiac/MUGA **442**

    Gallium/Indium/Ceretec™ Scan **443**

    Gastric Empty Scan **444**

    GI Bleed/Meckel's **445**

    HIDA Scan **446**

    Lung Scan (Aerosol) **447**

    Lung Scan (Gas) **448**

    Liver/Spleen Scan **449**

    Miscellaneous Worksheet **450**

    Octreoscan® **451**

    OncoScint®/CEA-Scan®/Verluma™ **452**

    ProstaScint® **453**

    Renal/Renogram Scan **454**

    Renal/Renogram/Captopril Scan **455**

    Scintimammography **456**

    Thyroid Uptake and Scan **457**

(J) ABBREVIATIONS COMMONLY USED IN NUCLEAR MEDICINE **459**

REFERENCES **463**

ACKNOWLEDGMENT OF TRADEMARKS **464**

This manual is the property of_____

Name	Number	Name	Number

Quick reference for phones, beepers, and extensions

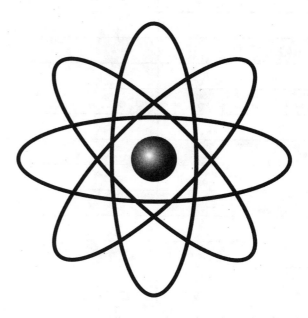

SECTION | ONE

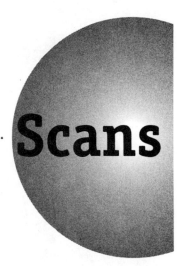

Scans

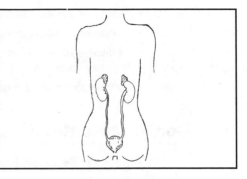

CHAPTER 1

Adrenocortical Scan

Radiopharmacy

Radionuclide

- ^{131}I $t_{1/2}$: 8.1 days

  Energies: 364 keV

  Type: β^-, γ, fission product

Radiopharmaceutical

- ^{131}I-6β Iodomethylnorcholesterol (NP-59). Available from the University of Michigan Nuclear Pharmacy under an Investigational New Drug (IND) application.

Localization

- Compartmental, blood flow, into the adrenal cortex, bound to plasma low-density lipoproteins.

Quality Control

- Done at factory, NP-59 > 90%. Dose calibrate for activity.

Adult Dose Range

- 2 mCi (74 MBq)

Method of Administration

- IV slow push over 2–3 minutes. Observe patient for 30 minutes after injection for reaction to injection. Injection may be required to be performed by physician as per institution protocol.

Indications

- Detection and localization of adrenal glands.
- Evaluation of documented primary hyperaldosteronism.

- Detection and localization of abnormal adrenal function in adrenocorticotropic hormone (ACTH)-independent Cushing's syndrome.
- Detection and localization of adrenal incidentalomas.
- Evaluation of adrenal lesions visualized on other imaging techniques.
- Evaluation of virilization or amenorrhea secondary to suspected adrenal hyperandrogenism.
- Differentiation of bilateral hyperplasia from adenoma in hyperaldosteronism.

Contraindications

- Allergy to iodine may be a consideration, although doses are small.
- Patient taking interfering medications.

Patient History *(or use complete patient history in reference section)*

The patient should answer the following questions.

Do you have a history of hypertension or hypotension?	Y	N
Do you have a history or family history of cancer?	Y	N
Have you had any recent weight gain?	Y	N
Have you experienced hirsutism (abnormal hair growth)?	Y	N
Have you had any chemotherapy or radiation therapy?	Y	N
Have you had any recent examinations such as CT, ultrasonography (US), MRI?	Y	N

If so, when and what facility?

What medications are you currently taking?

Have you had any recent blood or laboratory work done (of interest will be cholesterol

levels, ACTH, aldosterone, catecholamines and metabolites, plasma renin activity, blood sugar)?	Y	N

Female patients:

Are you pregnant or nursing?	Y	N

When was your last menstrual period?

Have you experienced amenorrhea (suppression of menstruation)?	Y	N

Other department-specific questions.

Patient Preparation

Before Day of Injection

- Physician instructs the patient to take SSKI (saturated solution potassium iodide) or Lugol's solution to block free iodine uptake in thyroid. This is administered 1 drop, t.i.d., beginning the day before radiotracer administration and continuing for 10 days after injection. If there is an allergy to iodine, perchlorate may be used.
- Physician instructs the patient to take bisacodyl (e.g., Dulcolax®) 10 mg PO, b.i.d. × 3 days before imaging, to reduce bowel activity. Patient may be required to take laxatives and/or enemas on afternoons before imaging days; check with radiologist.
- Physician instructs patients with atopic history (genetic disposition to hypersensitivity or allergy to medications such as iodine or steroids) to be treated with oral antihistamine (e.g., Benadryl® 50 mg) 1 hour before injection of radiotracer.

Day of Injection

- Identify the patient. Verify doctor's order. Explain the procedure.
- Obtain signed consent from patient and a prescription for the iodine.
- Ensure that the patient is not taking the following drugs: steroids, antihypertensives, reserpine, tricyclic antidepressants, sympathomimetics (adrenergic, stimulates release of epinephrine), diuretics as per physician's order.

Equipment

Camera

- Large field of view

Collimator

- Medium or high energy, parallel hole

Computer Set-up

Statics

- ^{131}I: 100,000 counts or up to 20 min/image

Single Photon Emission Computed Tomography (SPECT)

- 360°, 64 stops at 20 sec/stop

Procedure *(time: ~45 min/session)*

Single Isotope: NP-59

- Begin imaging 5 days (120 hours) after injection, followed by images on day 6 and 7 if required.

- Place patient in supine position, with camera posterior and kidneys centered (~12th rib).

- Collect statics to at least 100,000 counts or 5–20 minutes.

- Obtain lateral and posterior views with markers along spine on one of the imaging days to allow for determination of depth of each adrenal gland. (5 µCi ^{131}I capsule or store injection syringe for markers until imaging is done.)

- Record percent uptake using regions of interest (ROIs) for counts and correcting for depth differences. (Some processing systems have this software.)

- Determine whether SPECT images need to be taken.

Dual Isotope: NP-59 and ^{99m}Tc-DTPA

- Begin imaging 48 hours after injection and repeat at 2- to 3-day intervals until results are satisfactory.

- Place patient in supine position, with camera posterior and renal area centered.

- Collect ^{131}I images up to 20 minutes (1200 seconds).

- Change energy window; without moving patient, inject 5 mCi ^{99m}Tc-DTPA (diethylenetriaminepentaacetic acid) and collect 500,000–1,000,000 counts for subtraction image (computer protocol).

- Proceed with anterior views of chest and abdomen if adrenals are not visualized.

Procedure for Adrenocortical Scan With Suppression

- This scan differentiates bilateral hyperplasia from adenoma in hyperaldosteronism and hyperandrogenism. Unilateral visualization indicates adenoma. Bilateral visualization is indicative of hyperplasia. Dexamethasone suppresses pituitary ACTH secretion, thus embellishing NP-59 uptake into the ACTH-independent zona glomerulosa, while inhibiting NP-59 uptake into the ACTH-dependent zona fasciculata-reticularis.

- Patient preparation is the same. ADD: Give patient 2–4 mg dexamethasone b.i.d. beginning 2–7 days before injection of nuclide and continuing until completion of the study.

- Scan using same procedures through first 24–48 hours after injection.

Procedure for Adrenocortical Scan With ACTH Augmentation

- Patient preparation is the same. ADD: Give patient 50 IU of ACTH IV daily beginning 2 days before radiotracer injection.
- Scan using single isotope or dual isotope procedures.

Normal Results

- Both adrenal glands can be visualized, with the right slightly superior to the left.
- On posterior image, most normal patients present with the right adrenal gland showing greater intensity than the left because of the difference in depth and because the left adrenal gland is partially shielded by the kidney.
- Liver and gallbladder present brightly. If there is interference, laterals or SPECT can help localize. A fatty meal or cholecystokinin can also diminish the activity in the gallbladder.
- Dexamethasone will suppress about 50% of adrenal uptake of NP-59 that is ACTH-dependent. These studies will show only faint visualization or bilateral nonvisualization by day 5. Imaging may be discontinued after the 24- or 48-hour studies.

Abnormal Results

- In the nonsuppression study, faint visualization or nonvisualization (usually bilateral) indicates adrenal carcinoma.
- Asymmetric, bilateral, intense uptake suggests autonomous, ACTH-independent cortical nodular hyperplasia.
- Unilateral, intense uptake in the presence of known Cushing's syndrome is highly suggestive of adrenal cortical adenoma.
- No uptake in the presence of known Cushing's syndrome is suggestive of carcinoma.
- In primary aldosteronism, bilateral early visualization indicates bilateral adrenocortical hyperplasia, unilateral early visualization indicates aldosterone-secreting adenoma (Conn's tumor), and bilateral late visualization or nonvisualization is usually not diagnostic.
- Incidentally discovered (nonhyperfunctioning) adrenal mass lesion, with increased uptake on the same side, indicates benign nonhyperfunctioning adenoma; reduced uptake indicates a malignant lesion or infarction.
- In the suppression study, failure to suppress uptake with dexamethasone indicates adenoma if unilateral, hyperplasia if bilateral.
- In androgen excess, also with suppression, bilateral early visualization indicates bilateral adrenocortical hyperplasia and unilateral early visualization indicates adrenal adenoma. Oral contraceptives may give a false-positive result.

Artifacts

- Attenuating articles in clothing.
- Images not taken for enough counts.

- Focal areas of interest usually linger over time and grow in intensity. False-positive results can be limited by delayed images and lateral views.

Note

The adrenal cortex makes up about 90% of the adrenal gland. It contains three zones: (1) The zona glomerulosa, which is outermost, produces aldosterone, the principal mineralocorticoid hormone. (2) The zona fasciculata produces cortisol, the principal glucocorticoid hormone. (3) The zona reticularis produces androgenic steroids, principally androstenedione.

The adrenal medulla secretes the catecholamines epinephrine and norepinephrine.

Secretion from the adrenal cortex is controlled by ACTH from the anterior pituitary. The exception is aldosterone from the zona glomerulosa, which is controlled by angiotensin II, blood volume, and electrolyte concentrations. Cholesterol is stored in the cortex as the metabolic precursor for the synthesis of adrenocorticosteroids, e.g., aldosterone. NP-59 uses the similarity to cholesterol for uptake into the cortex. Increased ACTH increases the uptake, occurring gradually over a period of days.

SUGGESTED READINGS

Datz FL. Handbook of Nuclear Medicine. 2nd ed. St. Louis: Mosby, 1993.

Early PJ, Sodee DB. Principles and Practice of Nuclear Medicine. 2nd ed. St. Louis: Mosby, 1995.

Murray IPC, Ell PJ, eds. Nuclear Medicine in Clinical Diagnosis and Treatment. Vols. 1 and 2. New York: Churchill Livingstone, 1994.

Wilson, Michael A. Textbook of Nuclear Medicine. Philadelphia: Lippincott-Raven, 1998.

Benadryl® is a registered trademark of Parke-Davis, Morris Plains, NJ
Dulcolax® is a registered trademark of CIBA Consumer Pharmaceuticals, Edison, NJ

Notes

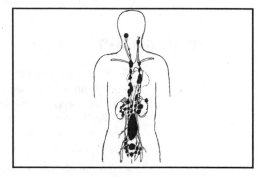

CHAPTER 2

Adrenal Medulla: Pheochromocytoma Scan (mIBG)

Radiopharmacy

Radionuclide

- ^{123}I $t_{\frac{1}{2}}$: 13.1 hours

  Energies: 159 keV

  Type: EC, γ, accelerator

- or: ^{131}I $t_{\frac{1}{2}}$: 8.1 days

  Energies: 364 keV

  Type: β⁻, γ, fission product

Radiopharmaceutical

- ^{123}I- or ^{131}I-mIBG (-*meta*-iodobenzylguanidine). Available from the University of Michigan Nuclear Pharmacy under an Investigational New Drug (IND) application.

Localization

- Blood flow, absorbed much the same as norepinephrine into adrenergic tissue and stored in adrenergic granules.

Quality Control

- ^{123}I- and ^{131}I-mIBG > 90%

Adult Dose Range

- ^{131}I: 500 μCi (18.5 MBq), 1 mCi (37 MBq) for suspected metastatic pheochromocytoma

- ^{123}I: 3–10 mCi (111–370 MBq)

Method of Administration
- IV slow push over 30 seconds

Indications

- Detection and localization of benign and malignant intra-adrenal and extra-adrenal pheochromocytomas (usually benign chromaffin cell tumors of the sympathoadrenal system that produce and secrete catecholamines, e.g., norepinephrine and epinephrine, producing hypertension and orthostatic [standing] hypotension). Occur within the adrenal medulla and are frequently associated with hereditary multiple endocrine neoplasia.
- Localization of site(s) of hormonal overproduction.
- Detection and localization of neuroectodermal (nerve tissue) tumors.
- Detection and localization of neuroblastomas (malignant hemorrhagic tumors of cells resembling neuroblasts of the sympathetic system, especially the adrenal medulla, and usually occurring in childhood).
- Detection and localization of other neuroendocrine tumors that share the property of amine precursor uptake in decarboxylation (APUD), such as:
    - carcinoid (argentaffin cells of the intestinal tract, bile ducts, pancreas, bronchus, or ovary that secrete serotonin) tumors
    - medullary thyroid tumors
    - paragangliomas (tumors of the adrenal medulla, chromaffin cells, and the paraganglia)
    - Merkel cell skin tumors
    - chemodectomas (tumors of the chemoreceptor system)
    - small cell lung carcinoma
    - schwannoma
- Evaluation of myocardial norepinephrine receptors.
- Distinguishing neuroendocrine tumors from nonneuroendocrine tumors.
- Detection and localization of metastatic deposits from previously diagnosed pheochromocytoma.

Contraindications

- Allergy to iodine may be a consideration although doses are small.
- Patient taking interfering medications.

Patient History *(or use complete patient history in reference section)*

The patient should answer the following questions.

Do you have a history or family history of cancer? Y   N

If so, what type and for how long?

Do you have a history of hypertension
   or hypotension?   Y   N
_____

Do you have palpitations?   Y   N
_____

Have you felt anxiety or apprehension?   Y   N
_____

Have you experienced excessive
   diaphoresis (sweating)?   Y   N
_____

Do you have headaches?   Y   N
_____

Have you experienced a flushed face?   Y   N
_____

Do you experience nausea or vomiting?   Y   N
_____

Have you experienced tingling of extremities?   Y   N
_____

Are you taking oral contraceptives?   Y   N
_____

Have you had any recent surgery?   Y   N

   If so, where and when?

_____

Have you had any chemotherapy or
   radiation therapy?   Y   N
_____

Are there any recent or planned CT,
   ultrasonography (US), MRI, or
   nuclear medicine (NM) scans?   Y   N
_____

What medications are you taking?
_____

Have you had any recent laboratory reports
   (with attention to adrenocorticotrophic
   hormone, aldosterone, catecholamines
   and metabolites, Na, K)?   Y   N
_____

Other department-specific questions.
_____

Patient Preparation

Before Day of Injection

- Physician instructs the patient to take SSKI (saturated solution potassium iodide) or Lugol's solution to block free iodine uptake in thyroid. This is administered 1 drop, t.i.d., beginning the day before radiotracer administration and continuing for 6 days after injection. If there is an allergy to iodine, perchlorate may be used.

- Physician instructs the patient to take bisacodyl (e.g., Dulcolax®) 10 mg PO, b.i.d. × 3 days before imaging, to reduce bowel activity. Patient may be required to take laxatives and/or enemas on afternoons before imaging days; check with radiologist.

- Physician instructs patients with atopic history (genetic disposition to hypersensitivity or allergy to medications such as iodine or steroids) to be treated with oral antihistamine (e.g., Benadryl® 50 mg) 1 hour before injection of radiotracer.

Day of Injection

- Identify the patient. Verify doctor's order. Explain the procedure.

- Obtain signed consent from patient and a prescription for the iodine.

- Ensure that the patient is not taking the following drugs: steroids, antihypertensives, reserpine, tricyclic antidepressants, sympathomimetics (adrenergic, stimulates release of epinephrine), diuretics as per physician's order. Ideally, no medications for 2-3 weeks before the examination (see Drugs to Withhold).

Equipment

Camera

- Large field of view

Collimator

- ^{131}I: medium energy, general purpose, or medium energy, high resolution
- ^{123}I: low energy, all purpose, or low energy, high resolution

Computer Set-up

Statics

- ^{131}I: 100,000 counts or up to 20 min/image
- ^{123}I: 500,000 counts or time

Whole Body

- 5-10 cm/min, cover at least head to pelvis

Single Photon Emission Computed Tomography (SPECT)

- 360°, 64 stops at 20 sec/stop

Procedure *(time: ~30-60 min/session)*

- Ensure patient is off medications and has taken thyroid blocker the night before.
- Instruct patient to empty bladder.
- Place patient in supine position.

^{131}I-mIBG: Images at 24, 48, and 72 Hours

- Acquire anterior/posterior images of head/neck, thorax, abdomen, and pelvis.

- Set whole body sweep slow (10 cm/min or less).

- Acquire static images of areas of interest if preferred or protocol. Statics should run at least 100,000 counts or 5–20 minutes.

- Acquire lateral views of abnormal uptake to aid in localization.

- Acquire marker images if protocol (on axillae, lower ribs, and iliac crests). Use 5 μCi ^{131}I capsule or perhaps store injection syringe for markers until imaging is done.

- Acquire SPECT images if protocol.

^{123}I-mIBG: Images at 3, 18, and 40 Hours (and possibly 72 hours)

- Same imaging procedures as above.

Normal Results

- Uptake occurs in the pituitary, salivary glands, thyroid, liver, and spleen.

- The gallbladder will be visualized in patients with renal failure.

- The heart is visualized in patients with normal catecholamine levels.

- The colon is visualized in some patients.

- The adrenal medulla is seldom visualized.

- The heart and adrenal medulla are visualized more clearly with ^{123}I-mIBG.

- Areas of normal uptake diminish in intensity over time.

Abnormal Results

- Focal areas of increased activity that increase more over time occur.

- Sporadic, unilateral tumors show focal intense uptake.

- Metastatic disease is visualized in the axial skeleton, heart, lung, mediastinum, lymph nodes, and liver.

- Neuroblastomas may arise in any location of sympathetic nervous system tissue but most often are visualized as an abdominal mass, metastasizing early to bone and bone marrow.

- Images at 72 hours will provide maximal contrast between foci of activity and background.

Artifacts

- Attenuating articles in clothing.

- Images not taken for enough counts.

- False-positive results may be caused by recent surgical sites, x-ray therapy to the lungs, and bleomycin-induced pulmonary changes.

- Focal areas of interest usually linger over time and grow in intensity. Limit false-positive results by delayed images (with obliques and laterals).

- Because of the nature of the disease and because they are off medications, patients may be agitated and not lie still.

Drugs to Withhold *(ideally, no medications 2–3 weeks before the examination)*

For Three Weeks (affect reuptake mechanism)

- Tricyclic antidepressants

For Two Weeks (affect depletion of storage vesicle)

- Amphetamines
- Bretylium tosylate
- Cocaine
- Guanethidine
- Haloperidol
- Phenothiazine
- Pseudoephedrine (nasal decongestants)
- Phenylpropanolamine (diet-control drugs)
- Phenylephrine (nasal decongestants)
- Reserpine
- Thiothixene

Alpha- and beta-adrenergic blocking drugs will not affect study with the exception of labetalol (affects both reuptake and storage depletion).

Note

mIBG is similar to the catecholamine norepinephrine. Epinephrine and norepinephrine are hormones that regulate smooth muscle tone, heart rate and force of contraction, and physiologic responses associated with stress. Pheochromocytomas produce excess amounts of these hormones resulting in hypertension and other symptoms associated with overabundance of catecholamines.

Renal and skeletal imaging with ^{99m}Tc agents can be used in conjunction with this test to aid in localization. Their injections can be timed for optimal scan times at the 24- or 48-hour images with two sets of images taken by changing the energy windows to suit the radiotracer.

SUGGESTED READINGS

Datz FL. Handbook of Nuclear Medicine. 2nd ed. St. Louis: Mosby, 1993.

Early PJ, Sodee DB. Principles and Practice of Nuclear Medicine. 2nd ed. St. Louis: Mosby, 1995.

Murray IPC, Ell PJ, eds. Nuclear Medicine in Clinical Diagnosis and Treatment. Vols. 1 and 2. New York: Churchill Livingstone, 1994.

Wilson MA. Textbook of Nuclear Medicine. Philadelphia: Lippincott-Raven, 1998.

Benadryl® is a registered trademark of Parke-Davis, Morris Plains, NJ
Dulcolax® is a registered trademark of CIBA Consumer Pharmaceuticals, Edison, NJ

Notes

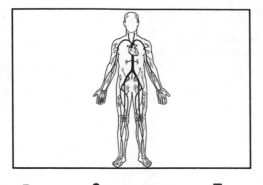

Angiography

Radiopharmacy

Radionuclide

- ^{99m}Tc $t_{1/2}$: 6 hours

  Energies: 140 keV

  Type: IT, γ, generator

Radiopharmaceutical

- Na^{99m}TcO$_4^-$ (pertechnetate). ^{99m}Tc-DTPA (diethylenetriaminepentaacetic acid). Tagged red blood cells by pyrophosphate or stannous chloride to ^{99m}TcO$_4^-$ by in vivo, in vitro, or kit, e.g., UltraTag®.

Localization

- Compartmental to blood supply

Quality Control

- ^{99m}TcO$_4^-$: Moly-Al breakthrough, chromatography.
- ^{99m}Tc-DTPA: chromatography. > 90%, use within 1 hour.

Adult Dose Range

- 8–25 mCi (296–925 MBq)

Method of Administration

- IV injection, good bolus for flow

Indications

- Evaluation of blood flow through major vessels as with arteriograms and venograms (more venous than arterial because contrast radiography is now largely used for arterial flow).
- Evaluation of regional perfusion in organs and extremities.

- Evaluation of penetrating wounds to thorax, abdomen, or extremities.
- Detection and localization of known or suspected hematoma or bleeding from large vessel.
- Detection and localization of vessel obstruction (e.g., deep venous thrombosis).
- Detection and evaluation of vessel abnormalities.
- Detection and evaluation of vascularized tumors.
- Evaluation of vessel location and/or anatomic position.

Contraindications

- None

Patient History

The patient should answer the following questions.

Do you have a history or family history of cancer?   Y   N

If so, what type and for how long?

Do you have any pain and if so, where and for how long?

Do you have a history of aneurysm, blood clots, peripheral vascular disease, or any vessel abnormalities?   Y   N

If so, explain.

Have you been diagnosed with any major organ disorders?   Y   N

If so, which one(s) and for how long?

Do you have any discolored skin?   Y   N

Do you have any tingling in the extremities?	Y	N
Do you have any blood in your stool or urine?	Y	N
Do you have any unusual lumps or swelling?	Y	N
Have you had any recent or planned related studies?	Y	N
Do you have the results of any recent laboratory tests?	Y	N
Other department-specific questions.		

Patient Preparation

- Identify the patient. Verify doctor's order. Explain the procedure.
- For $^{99m}TcO_4^-$: administer 200–400 mg perchlorate PO 30 minutes before imaging to block thyroid uptake if that area is within the region of interest (ROI). Lemon can be used to stimulate and reduce uptake in salivary glands.

Equipment

Camera

- Large field of view

Collimator

- Low energy, all purpose, or low energy, high resolution

Computer Set-up

Flow

- 1–5 sec/image for 30–60 seconds.
- Time for flow is according to size of vessels of interest. Choose shorter times for structures with large vessels and quick blood flows, longer times for structures with smaller vessels and less blood flow. Suggested times:
  - 1 sec/image for heart
  - 2 sec/image for brain
  - 3 sec/image for kidneys
  - 5 sec/image for extremities
- Length of flow: 30–60 seconds.

Statics

- 300,000–750,000 counts or set for time, e.g., 180 seconds.
- Acquire anterior or posterior images (according to ROI).
- Acquire added views (laterals, etc.) if needed for visualization.

Procedure *(time: ~20 minutes)*

- Position patient on table if torso is to be imaged, such that the entire area of interest (suspected side and normal side) is completely in camera view.
- Position extremities (left and right) in field of view if one or both is the area of interest.
- Position camera as close as possible to area or organ of interest.
- Consider a foot injection if the arterial or venous flow to arms is the area of interest.
- Inject patient and start camera at appropriate time to catch flow.
- Optional quantitative analysis can be done with computer software.
    - Acquire flow at 1 image/sec
    - Draw ROIs on desired structures
    - Generate time-activity curves with computer software
    - Calculate quantitative analysis of transit time, blood volume, and flow by this method
- Optional blood tagging:
    - In vitro method: extract ~2-2.5 mL of blood into heparinized syringe from patient and tag with UltraTag®
    - In vivo method: inject cold pyrophosphate, then 20 minutes later, inject radiotracer under camera for flow
    - Modified in vivo method: inject cold pyrophosphate and wait 20 minutes; then extract ~2-2.5 mL of blood into a heparinized, shielded syringe containing ~30 mCi ^{99m}Tc-O$_4$ and mix for 5-10 minutes
    - Inject patient (or reinject blood) under camera to image flow to ROI
    - Obtain static images of ROI at 5- to 10-minute intervals as per physician's request

Normal Results

- Depending on the position of the camera and the injection site, veins appear first, leading to the right heart, then out to the lungs, back to the left heart, then out the aorta to the body.
- Large vessels appear prominently and subsequently show branching. With extremities, approximate bilateral symmetry should be present.
- Organs present shortly after aorta, then vascularization of general body tissue.

Abnormal Results

- Punctures to a vessel will present with diffuse radiotracer collecting outside the vessel in that area.
- Obstruction presents as vessel to point of obstruction and no vessel appearing distal to the obstruction.
- Obstruction to organs presents as partial or complete lack of perfusion.
- Vascularized tumors and cysts will present as localized areas of increased uptake.
- Nonvascularized tumors and cysts will present as localized areas of decreased or no uptake.

Artifacts

- Attenuating articles obscuring ROI.
- Patient movement blurs image.

SUGGESTED READINGS

Alazraki NP, Mishkin FS, eds. Fundamentals of Nuclear Medicine. 2nd ed. New York: Society of Nuclear Medicine, 1988.

Datz FL. Handbook of Nuclear Medicine. 2nd ed. St. Louis: Mosby, 1993.

Early PJ, Sodee DB. Principles and Practice of Nuclear Medicine. 2nd ed. St. Louis: Mosby, 1995.

Klingensmith W, Eshima D, Goddard J. Nuclear Medicine Procedure Manual 1997–98. Englewood, CO: Wick, 1998.

Murray IPC, Ell PJ, eds. Nuclear Medicine in Clinical Diagnosis and Treatment. Vols. 1 and 2. New York: Churchill Livingstone, 1994.

Wilson MA. Textbook of Nuclear Medicine. Philadelphia: Lippincott-Raven, 1998.

UltraTag® is a registered trademark of Mallinckrodt Medical, Inc., St. Louis, MO

Notes

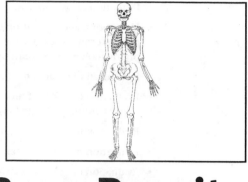

Bone Density

(Densitometry)

Radiopharmacy

Radionuclide

- Single radionuclide: ^{125}I $t_{\frac{1}{2}}$: 60.1 days

  Energies: 23–31 keV

  Type: EC, x, γ, accelerator

- or: ^{241}Am (americium) $t_{\frac{1}{2}}$: 432.7 years

  Energies: 60 keV

  Type: α, γ, spontaneous fission product.

- Dual radionuclide: ^{153}Gd (gadolinium) $t_{\frac{1}{2}}$: 241.6 days

  Energies: 44, 100 keV (γ); 35, 70 keV (x-ray)

  Type: x, γ, neutron irradiation of ^{152}Gd

Radiopharmaceutical

- N/A

Localization

- N/A

Quality Control

- N/A

Adult Dose Range

- N/A

Method of Administration

- Exposure to, not administration by injection

Indications

- Detection of osteoporosis.
- Monitoring and evaluation of treatment programs for osteoporosis (e.g., estrogen, progesterone, testosterone replacement, calcitonin therapy, exercise, or pharmacologic interventions with vitamins).
- Evaluation of osteopenia (diminished bone tissue).
- Evaluation of effect of menopause and premature spontaneous menopause on bone density (to help decide hormone therapy).
- Evaluation for premenopausal oophorectomy.
- Evaluation of effect of steroid therapy on bone density.
- Evaluation of effect of Cushing's syndrome on bone density (and other endocrinopathies, e.g., prolactinoma, hyperparathyroidism, hyperthyroidism, and male hypogonadism).
- Detection and evaluation of pathologic fractures.
- Evaluation of effect of chronic renal disease on bone density.
- Evaluation of effect of gastrointestinal syndromes on bone density.
- Evaluation of effect of postgastrectomy and other malabsorption diseases on bone density.
- Evaluation of effect of long-term immobilization on bone density.

Contraindications

- Dense vertebrae from degenerative disease, fracture, injury, or metastatic cancer should be excluded as area of interest.

Patient History

The patient should answer the following questions.

Do you have a history or family history of cancer?   Y   N

  If so, what type and for how long?

What is your age, height, and weight?

Do you have a history of bone disease?   Y   N

Is there a family history of osteoporosis or dowager's hump?   Y   N

Do you have any breaks or fractures?   Y   N

Have you had any recent surgery requiring
    metal or screws in back, hip, legs, or arms?   Y   N

Have you had any recent trauma to arms,
    hips, or legs?   Y   N

    If so, where and when?

Are you on steroid therapy?   Y   N

Are you taking calcium supplements?   Y   N

Are you taking didronel or alendronic
    sodium (Fosamax®)?   Y   N

    If so, for how long?

Do you have any prostheses?   Y   N

Have you had any recent barium studies?   Y   N

Have you had any of the following diseases:
    rheumatoid arthritis, lupus, hyperthyroidism,
    hypothyroidism, kidney disease, diabetes,
    Cushing's syndrome, Crohn's disease,
    colitis, gastrectomy?   Y   N

Are you physically inactive?   Y   N

Have you had any recent related studies or scans? Y   N

Female patients:

Are you pregnant?   Y   N

When was your last menstrual cycle?

Have you experienced a pregnancy?   **Y**   **N**

Have you experienced menopause?   **Y**   **N**

   If so, at what age?

Have you had your ovaries removed?   **Y**   **N**

**Are you on any female hormone
   replacement therapy?**   **Y**   **N**

Other department-specific questions.

Patient Preparation

- Identify the patient. Verify doctor's order. Explain the procedure.
- Remove metal objects from person and pockets.

Equipment

Camera
- Rectilinear-style scanner
- Bone densitometer—single or dual energy x-ray absorptiometry

Collimator
- Collimated x-ray pencil beam

Computer Set-up
- Factory settings

Procedure *(time: ~30–60 minutes)*

- SPA (single photon absorptiometry) is suggested in pediatric through adolescent patients because long bones are most metabolically active. It is useful in determining bone development in many childhood and pediatric diseases. There is also SEXA (single energy x-ray absorptiometry), which is more expensive but does not require replacement of the gamma source.
  - Position patient's region of interest (ROI) under the scanner. The denser the bone, the more absorption of photons.

- Image patient's nondominant arm unless there is a known fracture to that extremity.

- Because of the low energy of ^{125}I, it is used mainly on wrist or distal forearm studies (the junction of the middle and distal third of the radius is the preferred site). Most scanners have preprogrammed scan lengths and processing.

- Compare results with database table for that patient (usually contained in a software processing program).

- DPA (dual photon absorptiometry of gamma rays) or DEXA (dual energy x-ray absorptiometry) for other patients emphasizes lumbar spine and proximal femur at the hip.

  - Position patient supine on imaging table; elevate legs at knees to flatten pelvis and lumbar spine against scanning table.

  - Obtain scan of L1–L5, rectilinear fashion, with dual energy photon beam beneath table. Gamma or x-rays pass through patient and are picked up by detector on C-arm above the table.

  - Obtain scan of proximal femur.

  - Obtain scan of distal radius and/or wrist.

  - Compare values to those of a database established for patient's characteristics (e.g., age, sex, race, and weight).

Normal Results

- Values obtained from scan or scans fall within normal limits listed in established database table.

Abnormal Results

- Values $\geq$ 10% lower than published mean for patient's age are considered mildly osteoporotic.

- Clinically significant osteopenia.

- Patients with vertebral values between 0.8 and 0.99 g/cm^2 have about a 20% predictability of spontaneous fracture.

- Patients with vertebral values between 0.62 and 0.8 g/cm^2 are more likely to have a spontaneous fracture.

- Patients with vertebral values < 0.62 g/cm^2 will be found to have already had at least one spontaneous fracture 100% of the time.

Artifacts

- Overlying metal objects will cause falsely elevated results.

- A dense vertebrae from severe degenerative disease or fracture, injury, or metastatic cancer should not be used for analysis.

- Degenerative disease with severe facet sclerosis may result in artificially high values.

- A heavily calcified overlying aorta may result in artificially high values.

- Recent gastrointestinal barium studies may interfere because of attenuation of the photons by barium.

Note
· · · · · · ·

Usual analysis includes averaging anterior-posterior image values taken from the L2–L4 vertebrae. Studies include bone density (of trabecular and cortical bone), bone mineral content, percent fat, and lean body mass. The lifetime risk to women for hip fracture is 15%, compared with men, 5%. Vertebral fractures usually occur earlier and carry with them pain, decreased physical activity, and change in physical appearance, e.g., reduced height and "dowager's hump" or senile dorsal kyphosis. With the treatment available, the earlier the diagnosis of osteopenia or osteoporosis, the more likely the better outcome.

SPA and SEXA work extremely well for pediatric patients in determining bone density and mineral content of the radius by comparing values with published normal tables.

DEXA delivers improved precision (< 1%) because of increased photon flux of x-rays (35 and 70 keV), greater stability, and constancy of the photon source and hence at present is considered the superior system for measuring bone density. Scan time is ~4 minutes for lumbar spine with whole-body bone mineral content studies in 10-20 minutes (multiple detectors). These systems can also perform ROI studies on any bone in the body, opening application possibilities to a wide variety of orthopedic and metabolic studies not easily accommodated by other modalities.

DPA may soon surpass 1% precision as well because of refinements in equipment. Both deliver clinically useful data and both deliver low radiation exposure (1-2 mrem to the skin surface). If ^{153}Gd is used as the gamma source (44 and 100 keV), although the useful life might be up to 18 months, it is recommended that it be changed once a year.

CT can also be used for single or dual photon technique. The scanner can be programmed or modified to accommodate either. The radiation exposure, however, is 250-1000 mrem per study. Some of the positions required are awkward to achieve.

SUGGESTED READINGS

Early PJ, Sodee DB. Principles and Practice of Nuclear Medicine. 2nd ed. St. Louis: Mosby, 1995.

Wilson, MA. Textbook of Nuclear Medicine. Philadelphia: Lippincott-Raven, 1998.

Fosamax® is a registered trademark of Merke and Co., Inc., Fort Washington, PA.

Notes
· · · · · · ·

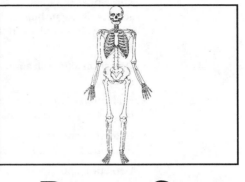

Bone Scan

(Skeletal Imaging)

Radiopharmacy

Radionuclide

- ^{99m}Tc $t_{1/2}$: 6 hours

  Energies: 140 keV

  Type: IT, γ, generator

Radiopharmaceutical

- MDP (methylene diphosphonate) or HDP (hydroxyethylene diphosphonate)

Localization

- Chemisorption; chemically bonds on surface of hydroxyapatite crystals. These hydrolyze and bind normally to bone as tin oxide and/or TcO_2, and present as prominent focal areas during the process of osteoblastic activity of bone repair.

Quality Control

- No O_2 in kit. Chromatography, 90–95% tagging. Use within 4 hours.

Adult Dose Range

- 20–30 mCi (740–1110 MBq), pediatrics by weight.

Method of Administration

- IV, straight stick or existing IV with saline flush. Flow requires good bolus injection.

Indications

- Detection of primary and staging metastatic disease. (Types known to frequently metastasize to bone are breast, lung, prostate, and kidney.)

- Differentiation between osteomyelitis (inflammation of bone and bone marrow) and cellulitis (inflammation of cellular or connective tissues). A flow study is indicated. Three-phase examines vascular, immediate blood pool, then osseous (osteoblastic) activity distinguishing cellulitis (activity in flow and immediate phases) from osteomyelitis (activity in third or all three phases). A fourth phase includes a 24-hour delay.
- Detection and evaluation of suspected infections, avascular necrosis, and prosthesis pain.
- Evaluation of bone pain, trauma, occult fractures, metabolic bone disease, osteoporosis, and osteomalacia (vitamin D deficiency) and other osteopathies.
- Detection and evaluation of Paget disease of the bone (bone inflammation and resorption replaced by soft bone).
- Detection and evaluation of arthritis and joint disease.
- Evaluation of bone graft viability, bone viability when blood supply is in question (infarct), and reflex sympathetic dystrophy.
- Evaluation of abnormal laboratory results (e.g., elevated prostate-specific antigen [PSA], alkaline phosphatase) or x-ray images.
- Evaluation of neoplasm or known lesion(s).
- Evaluation of response to chemotherapy, radiation therapy, antibiotic therapy, and other treatment.
- Differentiation of monostotic (single bone) from polyostotic primary bone tumors.
- Localization of sites for biopsy.

Contraindications

- Patient who has recently ingested contrast medium for a different study or has one scheduled between injection and imaging.
- Patient who has recently (24–48 hours) had a technetium-based nuclear medicine scan performed.
- Some institutions require approval from case management for inpatients before a scan can be performed.

Patient History *(or use complete patient history in reference section)*

The patient should answer the following questions.

Do you have history or family history of cancer?   Y   N

If so, what type and when was it diagnosed?

Have you had any chemotherapy or radiation therapy?   Y   N

Do you have any bone pain?	Y	N

If so, where? Since when?

Have you had any recent falls, fractures, breaks, or trauma?	Y	N
Do you have any old sports injuries?	Y	N
Have you had any recent surgery?	Y	N
Do you have any pumps, a pacemaker, or prostheses?	Y	N
Do you have a history of any bone or kidney disease?	Y	N
Have you had any recent dental work?	Y	N
Have you had recent abnormal blood tests?	Y	N
Have you had any previous scans or x-rays or have any scheduled diagnostic tests (e.g., CT with contrast)?	Y	N

If so, what type, when, and where?

Other department-specific questions.

Patient Preparation

- Identify the patient. Verify doctor's order. Explain the procedure.
- For flow; remove any attenuating material from region of interest (ROI).
- Instruct patient to drink lots of fluids (hydrate well) and urinate often before imaging.
- Instruct patient to return in 2–4 hours (usually 3 hours) after injection for delayed statics or whole body imaging.

Equipment

Camera

- Large field of view

Collimator

- Low energy, high resolution, or low energy, all purpose

Computer Set-up

Flow

- Dynamic, 2-4 seconds for 60 seconds with immediate blood pool image ~500,000 counts

Static Imaging

- Extremities 200,000-300,000 counts; torso 500,000-800,000 counts

Whole Body Sweep

- Check length of patient, usually 10-14 cm/min, patient orientation

Single Photon Emission Computed Tomography (SPECT)

- Circular or noncircular, 360°, 64 stops, 20-25 sec/stop; ROI centered

Procedure *(time: immediate flows, ~10 minutes; scans, acquired 2-4 hours [usually 3 hours] after injection; images take 20-60 minutes)*

- Instruct patient to empty bladder, empty pockets, remove jewelry and necklaces, check pants and shirts for buttons, etc., anything that can cause artifacts and attenuation.
- Remove cardiac monitors from field of view (FOV).
- Note location of pacemaker, pumps, colostomy bags, etc.
- For whole body scan, position patient supine (although prone, sitting, or standing is not uncommon), arms at side, with knee pillow and foot band (if protocol).
- For SPECT, position ROI in center FOV. Some require SPECT for all pars interarticularis spinal stress fractures or defects.

Images

- Obtain flow and immediate blood pool. Position ROI in camera view.
  - Inject radiotracer; start pictures after slight delay to capture the flow into ROI (watch for first sign of "blush" in persistence scope. It takes a little longer for feet or elderly patients).
  - Obtain immediate blood pool image after flow (~200,000-500,000 counts).
  - For extremities, obtain at least immediate blood pool image of ROI; also may take images including nearest joint and laterals/medials.
  - For reflex dystrophy syndrome (RDS), obtain flow to wrists, then bilateral statics for hands to shoulders. If hands or wrists need to be flowed, consider a foot vein injection.

- Obtain statics: 2–4 hours after injection, 24-hour delays (fourth phase) uncommon but can be requested.
  - Limited: ROI same as immediate blood pool.
  - Axial: acquire anterior/posterior, laterals, obliques.
  - Extremities: anterior/posterior, proximal and distal joints, legs—add laterals and medials. If knees are ROI, take laterals and medial with knees at 90° angle.
  - With flow: Obtain images the same as acquired with flow. Be sure to include ROI, images to closest proximal joint, and laterals/medials (especially with lower extremities).
  - For reflex sympathetic dystrophy, obtain images up to shoulder.
  - For carpal tunnel syndrome and all hand and wrist flows, obtain images up to elbow. Include shoulders if pain radiates there.
  - Other common static images: right and left posterior obliques, right and left anterior obliques, tail on detector (TOD), tail in air (TIA), laterals/medials, frog leg, plantar, palmar, vertex, etc.
- Whole body statics: 2–4 hours after injection. Overlapping images.
  - Anterior: pelvis, femur, knees, tibia/fibula, feet, abdomen, thorax, right shoulder, left shoulder, head.
  - Posterior: pelvis, abdomen, thorax arms down/arms up to move scapula, head. No extremities unless there is an area of interest that needs defining.
- Whole body sweep, single and dual head cameras: 2–4 hours after injection. Low energy, high resolution collimator(s). Matrix set for $256 \times 1025 \times 16$ or greater, time set for 20–30 minutes (10–20 cm/min), 24-hour delays if ordered.
  - If anything is visualized that cannot be easily identified or the position assessed, add static oblique and lateral views, particularly with an outpatient.
- SPECT: Position patient ROI in camera view. 360° rotation (dual head; 180° per head) at 60–64 steps/head, 20–40 sec/stop. Process as per protocol: transverse, coronal, and sagittal slices.

Normal Results

- Symmetric, uniform uptake with increased activity in joints, junctions, and scapulas.
- Kidneys show lightly, bladder shows brightly.
- Epiphysial plates and cranial sutures show brightly in growing children.
- It usually takes 3–5 days for new fractures to present positive but may present as early as 24 hours because of bone healing process.

Abnormal Results

- Asymmetric, focal areas of increased or decreased activity.
- "Super Scan" with bone uptake showing brightly, no kidney, bladder, distal extremities, facial bones, or soft tissue uptake apparent on film at normal intensities; caused by intense and widespread metastatic involvement. Tumors causing this type of osseous metastasis are prostate, breast, lung, renal, bladder, or lymphoma.
- Nontumor causes are hyperparathyroidism, osteomalacia, Paget disease of the bone (elevated alkaline phosphatase levels), or fibrous dysplasia.

- Metabolic diseases involve the calvarium (cranium) and long bones whereas metastases tend to spare them. Paget disease may present with "Halloween mask" skull and uptake in sacrum, pelvis, and long bones.

- Diminished activity or none is indicative of osteonecrosis, osteoporosis, osteomalacia, multiple myeloma (normal or lowered), radiation or steroid therapy, or end-stage cancer patients with diminished metabolism.

- Increased uptake in flow, blood pool, and delays indicates osteomyelitis.

- Increased uptake in flow and blood pool with mild or no uptake in delays indicates cellulitis.

- Increased vascular flow, blood pool, and delays focally indicate primary malignant tumors (osteogenic and chondrosarcomas).

- Increased blood pool and delays, focally intense, indicate benign primary tumors (osteoid osteoma). May have double intensity sign of hot area surrounded by less but increased intensity. Other types of benign lesions may show increased uptake.

- Arthritis presents as increased activity in and around joints in flow, blood pool, and delays.

Artifacts

- Belt buckles, medallions, buttons, glasses, zippers, prostheses, dental work, metal articles implanted with surgery, guns, knives, and other articles (money, keys, wallets, asthma sprays, etc.) in pockets cause cold spots.

- Bladder may need lead shield.

- Pubic lesions may be obscured by bladder activity.

- Catheters or urine seepage, IV infiltration, and contaminated clothing or linen cause hot spots.

- Patient movement or rotation may distort view.

- Radiotracer tag may break down, localizing in thyroid, gastrointestinal tract, or other systems.

- Imaging begun too soon or with patient not hydrating adequately before imaging may show excessive activity in soft tissue.

- Degenerative joint disease, surgery, and old trauma may give false-positives.

- Scan ordered too early for fractures. Although a nuclear scan can detect a hairline fracture before a radiograph, it usually takes 3–5 days for new fractures to present as positive. If looking for pseudoarthrosis or stress fracture, take 3-hour postinjection images.

- Take laterals, obliques, and/or any other helpful positions if there is any question about a visualization (better too many than too few, or needing the patient to return at radiologist's request).

Note

It takes 15% loss of calcium mineral to be detected by nuclear medicine procedure, 30–50% loss of calcium mineral to be detected by x-ray procedure.

SUGGESTED READINGS

Datz FL. Handbook of Nuclear Medicine. 2nd ed. St. Louis: Mosby, 1993.

Early PJ, Sodee DB. Principles and Practice of Nuclear Medicine. 2nd ed. St. Louis: Mosby, 1995.

Murray IPC, Ell PJ, eds. Nuclear Medicine in Clinical Diagnosis and Treatment. Vols. 1 and 2. New York: Churchill Livingstone, 1994.

Wilson, MA. Textbook of Nuclear Medicine. Philadelphia: Lippincott-Raven, 1998.

Notes
· · · · · · · ·

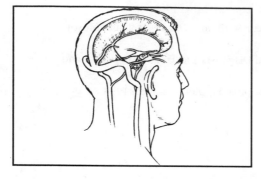

CHAPTER 6

Brain Scan/Death

(Brain Flow)

Radiopharmacy

Radionuclide

- ^{99m}Tc $t_{1/2}$: 6 hours

  Energies: 140 keV

  Type: IT, γ, generator

Radiopharmaceutical

- Non–blood–brain barrier (BBB)-penetrating: Na ^{99m}TcO$_4^-$ (pertechnetate), ^{99m}Tc-GH (Glucoheptonate), ^{99m}Tc-DTPA (diethylenetriaminepentaacetic acid)
- BBB-penetrating: ^{99m}Tc-HMPAO (*d,l*-hexamethylpropyleneamine oxime or Ceretec™) and others (see list at end)

Localization

- Compartmental to blood supply

Quality Control

- Moly-Al breakthrough, chromatography. > 90% tag.

Adult Dose Range

- 15–30 mCi (555–1110 MBq)

Method of Administration

- Bolus IV

Indications

- Determination of brain death. This is the most common usage of brain flow because other types of studies and modalities are as good or better for other indications.
- Evaluation of blood flow.

- Evaluation and localization of primary and metastatic tumors, abscesses, subdural hematomas, and lesions.
- Detection of vascular malformations, inflammatory or infectious diseases, cerebrovascular accidents (CVAs), and transient ischemic attacks (TIAs).
- Differentiation between contusions from simple concussions or brain tumors from vascular accidents.
- Evaluation of suspected arteriovenous malformations (AVMs).
- Evaluation of surgical procedure, radiation therapy, or chemotherapy.
- Evaluation of intracerebral inflammatory or degenerative diseases, e.g., acquired immune deficiency syndrome (AIDS), multiple sclerosis, collagen diseases.
- Evaluation of unexplained neurologic symptoms.

Contraindications

- Patient too agitated or uncooperative to remain still for acquisition.

Patient History

The patient should answer the following questions. Ask relative or care taker if patient's alertness is in question.

For brain death		
Any known head/neck trauma?	Y	N
Any known plates? (Check chart)	Y	N

Brain flow		
Do you have a history or family history of cancer?	Y	N
Do you have a history of recent or old trauma?	Y	N
Do you have any head pain?	Y	N
Are you suffering from headaches, speech problems, equilibrium or vision problems, unusual motor functions, unusual body function, mood changes, or seizures?	Y	N

If so, which and since when?

Have you had any recent surgery?	Y	N
Do you have a shunt or metal plates?	Y	N
Other department-specific questions.		

Patient Preparation

- Brain Death: None.
- Other: Identify the patient. Verify doctor's order. Explain the procedure.
- Instruct patient to remain motionless during imaging.

Equipment

Camera

- Large field of view

Collimator

Flow and blood pool

- Low energy, all purpose, or low energy, high sensitivity

Delays

- Low energy, all purpose, or low energy, high resolution

Computer Set-up

Flow

- 2 sec/frame, 60 seconds

Blood pool statics and delays

- 200,000–800,000 counts

Procedure *(time: initial flow and blood pool ~30 minutes; delays ~45 minutes)*

Flow: can be anterior (usually for adults) or posterior (usually for children) (for dual head, get both, position head straight up).

- Position patient supine, camera anterior, as close as possible, entire cranium in field of view (FOV), head flexed back facing straight up (head is held or strapped in place). Or
- Position patient supine, camera posterior, as close as possible, entire cranium in FOV, chin tucked down to expose posterior fossa and for better evaluation of transverse sinus, head straight up (head is held or strapped in place).

- Place a tourniquet or ace bandage around head to limit amount of scalp circulation.
- Inject good bolus, start camera immediately. Better too early than too late. The flow is extremely important to the diagnosis.
- Obtain at least one blood-pool image in same position at end of flow.
- Optional views include anterior, posterior, right and left laterals, and vertex (right side markers sometimes help in orientation, and if possible, use lead apron around patient's shoulders to shield body counts on vertex view) views at this time, 200,000–800,000 counts/image.

Delays

- Patient is returned after 1–2 hours (usually 2 hours) for delayed images.
- Anterior, posterior, right and left laterals, and vertex views are repeated (right side markers sometimes help in orientation). Radiologists may want them repeated again at 4 or more hours.
- With ^{99m}Tc-HMPAO, images acquired at 15 minutes after injection. Single photon emission computed tomography (SPECT) acquisition may also be performed if required.

Normal Results

- Flow: three phases

    Arterial phase: subclavian, carotid, cerebral arteries visualize symmetrically

    Capillary phase: symmetric diffuse activity in both cerebral hemispheres

    Venous phase: sagittal sinus and jugulars visualized

- Blood pool: soft tissue and venous sinus activity
- Delays: (depending on view)

    Superior rim, sagittal sinus, transverse sinus (small or absent left sinus not unusual), occipital sinus, facial vascularity, and salivary glands increased activity

    Cerebral cortex normally devoid of activity

Abnormal Results

- Brain death criteria

    Flow: no intracranial blood flow (arterial, capillary, or venous) from base of skull up. No perfusion with BBB-penetrators.

    Blood pool: no visualization of sagittal sinus on immediate postinjection images.

    Delays: no visualization of dural sinus. Occasionally, sagittal or transverse sinus seen faintly over time because of scalp circulation or drainage through basilar system. In pediatric patients, sutures may visualize because of diminished background.

- Other: (look for areas of increased uptake, "doughnut" sign, lack of uptake, or diminished flow)

    Flow: focal area(s) of increased or decreased uptake other than normal vascularity and/or abnormal appearance to vascularity. Asymmetric flow. "Flip-flop" sign, one side visualizing then the other. Unmatched activity in any phase.

    Blood pool: focal area(s) of increased or decreased uptake persist and/or abnormal appearance to vascularity.

Delays: focal area(s) of increased or decreased uptake persist. Perhaps visualization of new areas not present on initial dynamic study.

Artifacts

- The flow is all important. "Don't blow the flow!" If necessary, set for 120 seconds and start as soon as or just before the injection is in.

- Patient movement.

- Metal plates and respirator or life-support equipment attenuation.

Note

This procedure is nonspecific. It delineates areas of increased vascular permeability secondary to a variety of disease processes. Early strokes, abscesses, tumors of the pituitary, and grade I and II astrocytomas often visualize poorly. The latter two problems account for more than half of the false-negative results.

Non-BBB Penetrating Radiopharmaceuticals

	Delays
$^{99m}TcO_4^-$ (pertechnetate)	2–4 hours
^{99m}Tc-DTPA (diethylenetriaminepentaacetic acid)	0.5–1 hour
^{99m}Tc-GH (glucoheptonate)	1–4 hours
^{99m}Tc-RBCs (tagged red blood cells)	0.5–1 hour
^{99m}Tc-MDP (methylene diphosphonate)	2–4 hours
^{99m}Tc-HDP (hydroxymethylene diphosphonate)	2–4 hours
^{67}Ga-citrate	24–72 hours
^{201}Tl-chloride	None

BBB Penetrators

	Delays
^{133}Xe-gas	None
^{123}I-Iodoamphetamine	0.5–1 hour
^{99m}Tc-HMPAO (*d,l*-hexamethylpropyleneamine oxime or Ceretec™)	0.25–3 hours
^{99m}Tc-ECD (ethyl cysteinate dimer, bicisate, or Neurolite™)	2–3 hours

SUGGESTED READINGS

Datz FL. Handbook of Nuclear Medicine. 2nd ed. St. Louis: Mosby, 1993.

Early PJ, Sodee DB. Principles and Practice of Nuclear Medicine. 2nd ed. St. Louis: Mosby, 1995.

Murray IPC, Ell PJ, eds. Nuclear Medicine in Clinical Diagnosis and Treatment. Vols. 1 and 2. New York: Churchill Livingstone, 1994.

Wilson, MA. Textbook of Nuclear Medicine. Philadelphia: Lippincott-Raven, 1998.

Ceretec™ is a trademark of Amersham International Plc, Amersham, UK.
Neurolite™ is a trademark of DuPont Merck, Wilmington, DE.

Notes

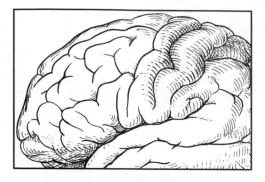

Brain SPECT

(Single Photon Emission Computed Tomography)

Radiopharmacy

Radionuclide

- ^{99m}Tc $t_{1/2}$: 6 hours

  Energies: 140 keV

  Type: IT, γ, generator

Radiopharmaceutical

- ^{99m}Tc-HMPAO (*d,l*-hexamethylpropyleneamine oxime or Ceretec™)
- ^{99m}Tc-ECD (ethyl cysteinate dimer, bicisate, or Neurolite™)

Localization

- Compartmental, blood flow, blood–brain barrier (BBB)-penetrating

Quality Control

- Chromatography, > 95% radiochemical purity

Adult Dose Range

- 20–30 mCi (740–1110 MBq)

Method of Administration

- Usually through catheter or butterfly, IV slow push with 10 mL flush

Indications

- Evaluation of cerebrovascular diseases (CVAs), e.g., infarction, hemorrhage, transient ischemic attacks (TIAs).
- Evaluation of neuropsychiatric disorders, e.g., Alzheimer's, memory loss, behavioral changes, schizophrenia, manic depression, and dementias.

- Evaluation of head trauma (acute or chronic).
- Evaluation and localization of cerebral ischemia and brain perfusion.
- Evaluation of brain death.
- Evaluation of convulsive disorders (grand mal and petit mal).
- Assessment of cognitive functions.
- Detection and localization of recurring brain tumors, especially using dual-isotope method with ^{99m}Tc-HMPAO and ^{201}Tl-thallous chloride for tumor viability study.
- Assessment of brain tissue viability using ^{123}I-Imp (N-isopropyl-P-[^{123}I] iodoamphetamine) imaging 3–4 hours after injection for redistribution and possible viability.

Contraindications

- Patient too agitated or uncooperative to hold head still.

Patient History *(or use complete patient history in reference section)*

The patient should answer the following questions. Ask relative or care taker if patient's alertness is in question.

Is there a history or family history of cancer?   Y   N

   If so, what type and when was it diagnosed?

Has there been any recent memory loss?   Y   N

   If so, is it long or short memory?

Is there a history of any brain disorders?   Y   N

Have there been any recent behavioral changes?   Y   N

**Has there been any recent head trauma or
   headaches?**   Y   N

Has there been any recent infection?   Y   N

**Have there been any recent seizures or
balance problems?**   Y   N

Have there been any surgeries?	Y	N

Does the patient have a shunt or metal plate?	Y	N

Are there any recent CT or MRI scans?	Y	N

If so, what type and at what institution?

What is the patient taking for medications?

Other department-specific questions.

Patient Preparation

- Identify the patient. Verify doctor's order. Explain the procedure.
- Instruct patient to remain motionless during imaging.
- Place patient in a quiet environment before injection and examination if protocol.

Equipment

Camera
- Rotating large field of view camera, single- or multihead

Collimator
- Low energy, high resolution

Computer Set-up
- Single photon emission computed tomography (SPECT) acquisition, e.g., 360° rotation, 64 projections per rotation, 20 sec/stop (200,000 counts), 128 × 128 or 64 × 64 matrix, magnified.

Procedure *(time: ~45 minutes)*

- Inject patient with radiotracer via butterfly and flush.
- Obtain images beginning 15 minutes to 3 hours after injection.
- Position patient supine on table, head in toward camera(s).
- Place an ace bandage around patient's head and table to hold in place.
- Position head into camera view so that cerebrum and cerebellum are visualized.
- Remind patient of absolutely no movement during acquisition.
- Camera(s) mapped around head and SPECT acquisition taken as per protocol. Acquisition should begin anterior or lateral, 360°.
- Use subdued lighting and noise if possible to limit extraneous brain activity.

Normal Results

- Symmetric uptake, especially of gray matter of brain.

Abnormal Results

- Asymmetric areas of increased or decreased activity.
- Alzheimer's usually follows a pattern of decreased activity in the parietal, then temporal, then frontal lobes, but not always.

Brain SPECT With Diamox® (acetazolamide)

- This drug is a diuretic, anticonvulsant, glaucoma pressure reducer, ventilation stimulant, and a potent cerebral vasodilator.

Indications

- Evaluation of cerebrovascular ischemia and regional cerebral blood flow (rCBF).
- Evaluation of possible neurovascular shunt surgery.

Contraindications

- Sulfonamide allergy

Procedure

- Two-part test, first with chemical, second (baseline) without chemical 1 or 2 days later.
- Start IV on patient.
- Inject patient with 1 g Diamox® slowly over 2 minutes (or oral caplet).
- Monitor for reaction for 25 minutes (visually, take blood pressure).
- Inject radiotracer slowly, flush with 10 mL saline.
- Wait 20 minutcs.
- Image using SPECT procedure as above.
- Repeat procedure without chemical after 24–48 hours.

Possible Reactions to Drug Intervention (usually short acting, ~15 minutes)

- Numbness in extremities or around mouth.
- Feeling flushed or lightheaded, or having blurred vision.

Artifacts

- Movement blurs or disallows acquisition.
- TIAs can fill back in between attacks.
- May clip bottom of cerebellum.
- Because the patient population that generally needs this scan may be confused, uncooperative, incoherent, or encumbered with involuntary movement, patience is

needed with these patients. Get a history from whomever might be accompanying the patient.

Processing

• SPECT, some use ramp and Butterworth filters. Include transverse, coronal, and sagittal slices for presentation.

Medications Held on Physician's Orders for Brain SPECT (benzodiazepines)

Alprazolam (Xanax®)

Chlordiazepoxide HCl (Librium®)

Clonazepam (Klonopin®)

Diazepam (Valium®)

Flurazepam (Dalmane®)

Halazepam (Paxipam®)

Lorazepam (Ativan®)

Oxazepam (Serax®)

Prazepam (Centrax®)

Quazepam (Doral®)

Temazepam (Restoril®)

Triazolam (Halcyon®)

SUGGESTED READINGS

Datz FL. Handbook of Nuclear Medicine. 2nd ed. St. Louis: Mosby, 1993.

Early PJ, Sodee DB. Principles and Practice of Nuclear Medicine. 2nd ed. St. Louis: Mosby, 1995.

Murray IPC, Ell PJ, eds. Nuclear Medicine in Clinical Diagnosis and Treatment. Vols. 1 and 2. New York: Churchill Livingstone, 1994.

Wilson, MA. Textbook of Nuclear Medicine. Philadelphia: Lippincott-Raven, 1998.

Ativan® is a registered trademark of Wyeth-Ayerst Laboratories, Philadelphia, PA.
Centrax® is a registered trademark of Parke-Davis, Morris Plains, NJ.
Ceretec™ is a trademark of Amersham International Plc, Amersham, UK.
Dalmane® is a registered trademark of Roche Laboratories, Nutley, NJ.
Diamox® is a registered trademark of Lederle Laboratories, Wayne, NJ.
Doral® is a registered trademark of Wallace Laboratories, Cranbury, NJ.
Halcyon® is a registered trademark of The Upjohn Company, Kalamazoo, MI.
Klonopin® is a registered trademark of Roche Laboratories, Nutley, NJ.
Librium® is a registered trademark of Roche Laboratories, Nutley, NJ.
Neurolite™ is a trademark of DuPont Merck, Wilmington, DE.

Paxipam® is a registered trademark of Schering Corporation, Kenilworth, NJ.
Restoril® is a registered trademark of Sandoz Pharmaceuticals, East Hanover, NJ.
Serax® is a registered trademark of Wyeth-Ayerst Laboratories, Philadelphia, PA.
Valium® is a registered trademark of Roche Laboratories, Nutley, NJ.
Xanax® is a registered trademark of The Upjohn Company, Kalamazoo, MI.

Notes

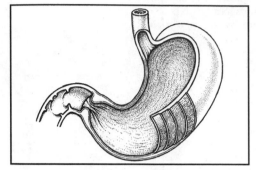

Breath Test for *H. Pylori:* PYtest® C-14 Urea Breath Test (UBT)

Radiopharmacy

Radionuclide

- ^{14}C $t_{1/2}$: 5,730 years

  Energies: 156 keV(max), 49 keV(mean)

  Type: β^-, fission byproduct

Radiopharmaceutical

- Urea (NH_2 $^{14}CONH_2$)

Localization

- Gastric urease from *Helicobacter pylori* splits urea molecule to form CO_2 and NH_3 at the interface between gastric epithelium and lumen. The $^{14}CO_2$ is absorbed into the blood and exhaled in the breath, $T_b = \sim15$ minutes. Urea that is not hydrolyzed by *H. pylori* is excreted in urine, $T_b = \sim12$ hours, with the last 10% $T_b = \sim40$ days.

Quality Control

- Capsule is precalibrated at factory.

Adult Dose Range

- 1 µCi (0.037MBq)

Method of Administration

- PO by capsule taken from cup. Patient or technologist should have no other contact with capsule.

Indications

- Detection of gastric urease as an aid in the diagnosis of *H. pylori* infection in the human stomach.

Contraindications: The following may give false-negative results.

- Antibiotics within the last 30 days.
- Bismuth: Pepto-Bismol® within the last 30 days.
- Sucralfate within the last 14 days.
- Nonfasting: Patient should be NPO for 6 hours before test.
- Proton pump inhibitors within the last 14 days.

Patient History

The patient should answer the following questions.

Do you have a history or family history
  of cancer?   Y   N

If so, what type and for how long?

Do you have a history of any type of
  gastric disease?   Y   N

Do you have gastric or abdominal pain?   Y   N

If so, exactly where and for how long?

When does it occur, after meals, what type of meals?

When did you last have a meal?

Do you have a history of ulcers?   Y   N

Do you have a history of gastritis?   Y   N

Have you had any gastric surgery?	Y	N
Do you have a history of pernicious anemia?	Y	N
Do you have a history of adrenal insufficiencies?	Y	N
Are you a diabetic?	Y	N
Are you taking any medications?	Y	N
Are you taking any bismuth products like Pepto-Bismol®?	Y	N
Are you on antibiotic therapy?	Y	N
Are there any prior or pending related tests (endoscopy, biopsy, blood samples, CLOtest® [urease test], NM-gastric empty Schilling)?	Y	N
Other department-specific questions.		

Patient Preparation

- Identify the patient. Verify doctor's order. Explain the procedure.
- Instruct patient to be NPO for 6 hours minimum before test.
- Physician to instruct patient to be off antibiotics and bismuth (e.g., Pepto-Bismol®) for 1 month.
- Physician to instruct patient to be off proton pump inhibitors and sucralfate for 2 weeks.
- Instruct patient to bring list of pending related exams and results from past related exams.

Equipment

Camera
- Liquid scintillation counter (LSC). Single-sample (Tri-Med) or multi-sample versions available.

Collimator
- N/A

Computer Set-up
- 300-second counting statistics are needed for sample and background.

Procedure: Supplied by kit. Have stopwatch available. *(time: ~20 minutes)*

- Order kit from radiopharmacy or directly from Tri-Med.
- Label balloon provided, check all materials.
- Place capsule into cup provided, fill second cup provided with 20 mL of water.
- Administer capsule to patient. Ensure no other contact with capsule. Administer 20 mL of water to patient. Time for 3 minutes.
- At 3 minutes, administer 20 mL more water to patient. Time for 10–15 minutes.
- Place straw into neck of balloon provided.
- Instruct patient to hold breath for 5–10 seconds, then blow into balloon (the balloon should be filled completely to comply with manufacturer's protocol). If the patient fails to fill the balloon with the first breath, pinch off the straw, instruct patient to hold breath for 10 more seconds, then blow second (or more) breath into balloon until it is full. In the event of a leak, locate leak and tape it, or use any 2-L Mylar balloon as backup.
- Tie neck of balloon into tight knot.
- Prepare sample as to manufacturer's protocol. Balloon is sent back to radiopharmacy or can be sent directly to Tri-Med by means provided. Results are faxed within 24 hours of when Tri-Med receives the package or counted in-house with proper equipment.
- For counting in-house: sample is counted in LSC for 5 minutes (300 seconds) Tri-Med supplies a detailed description as to measurements, background, and efficiency ratings to use for analysis.
- If the count is between 50 and 300 disintegrations per minute (DPM), wait for 30 minutes, up to several hours, or the next day, then count again because chemical activity called chemiluminescence can temporarily produce false counts on the order of 100 DPM. Samples outside this range need not be recounted.

Normal Results

- < 50 DPM, background subtracted, is negative.

Abnormal Results

- 50–199 DPM, background subtracted, is indeterminate.
- ≥ 200 DPM, background subtracted, is positive for urease and *H. pylori*. The numbers could range into the thousands.

Artifacts

- Negative results do not completely rule out the presence of *H. pylori*. Other diagnostic tests should be performed.
- False-positive results could occur in patients with achlorhydria (absence of free hydrochloric acid in stomach), antacid use, H_2-receptor antagonist use, and uremia.

These will allow the gastric pH to rise, allowing colonization of urease-producing flora.

- False-positive results could occur in patients having urease associated with *Helicobacter* organisms other than *H. pylori* (e.g., *H. heilmanni*).

- There is a risk for false-negative results if the patient is not off of antibiotics, bismuth, sucralfate, or omeprazole (7 days), has rapid gastric emptying, e.g., dumping syndrome or surgery, or is nonfasting (6 hours).

- Test may not work well with the physiology of the elderly or in patients who have no systemic antibody response to *H. pylori*.

- Proton pump inhibitors

  Omeprazole (Prilosec®)

  Lansoparazole (Prevacid®)

- H_2 blockers (e.g., cimetidine [Tagamet®], ranitidine [Zantac®], nizatidine [Axid®], famotidine [Pepcid®]) and antacids (e.g., Maalox®, Rolaids®, Tums®, Mylanta®, Gelusil®) are not contraindicated.

Note

Urease enzyme is not normally present in mammalian cells. If found to be present, it is evidence of the presence of bacteria.

SUGGESTED READINGS

Manufacturer's pamphlet, insert, and User's Guide. Tri-Med Specialties, Inc., Lenexa, KS.

Axid® is a registered trademark of Whitehall-Robins Laboratories, New York, NY.
CLOtest® is a registered trademark of Tri-Med Specialties, Lenexa, KS.
Gelusil® is a registered trademark of Warner-Lambert, Morris Plains, NJ.
Maalox® is a registered trademark of CIBA Consumer Pharmaceuticals, Edison, NJ.
Mylanta® is a registered trademark of Merck & Co., Fort Washington, PA.
Pepcid® is a registered trademark of Merck & Co., Fort Washington, PA.
Pepto-Bismol® is a registered trademark of Proctor & Gamble, Cincinnati, OH.
Prevacid® is a registered trademark of TAP, Deerfield, IL.
Prilosec® is a registered trademark of Astra Merck, Wayne, PA.
Pytest® is a registered trademark of Tri-Med Specialties, Lenexa, KS.
Rolaids® is a registered trademark of Warner-Lambert, Morris Plains, NJ.
Tagamet® is a registered trademark of SmithKline Beecham Pharmaceuticals, Pittsburgh, PA.
Tums® is a registered trademark of SmithKline Beecham Pharmaceuticals, Pittsburgh, PA.
Zantac® is a registered trademark of Glaxo Wellcome, Morris Plains, NJ.

Notes

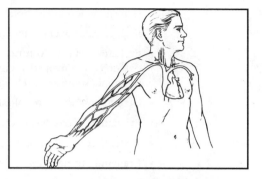

CHAPTER 9

Cardiac: Gated First-Pass Study

Radiopharmacy

Radionuclide

- ^{99m}Tc $t_{1/2}$: 6 hours

  Energies: 140 keV

  Type: IT, γ, generator

Radiopharmaceutical

- ^{99m}Tc-pertechnatate, ^{99m}Tc-sestamibi (hexakis[2-methoxyisobutylisonitril]), ^{99m}Tc-1,2-bis (bis[2-ethoxyethyl]phosphino) ethane

Localization

- Compartmental to blood flow

Quality Control

- ^{99m}Tc-sestamibi, ^{99m}Tc-tetrofosmin, chromatography > 90%

Adult Dose Range

- 8–30 mCi (296–1110 MBq). Small volume, < 1 mL; 6-inch or greater extension tubing attached to IV catheter and three-way stopcock for radiotracer and 10–20 mL or greater of saline flush. Use large-bore (18–22 gauge) IV catheter.

Method of Administration

- IV catheter, butterfly, or straight stick. Small volume, good bolus shot. Example of preparation listed below.

(done separately, in conjunction with gated or nongated resting study at injection, or at injection with some types of stress studies)

Indications

- Determination of ejection fraction of right or left ventricle.
- Evaluation of overall function of heart for congenital heart disease or defects.
- Evaluation of right ventricular dysfunction, e.g., infarct, atrial or ventricular septal defect, cardiomyopathy, chronic lung disease, primary pulmonary hypertension, pulmonic stenosis, and lung transplantation.
- Detection of aortic or mitral valve insufficiency.
- Evaluation of baseline study for surgery candidates.
- Evaluation of follow-up study for posttherapy or postsurgical patients.
- Evaluation of right and/or left ventricular wall motion.
- Detection of prolapse or shunts.
- Evaluation of chamber-to-chamber transit times.

Contraindications

- None.

Patient History *(or use complete patient history in reference section)*

The patient should answer the following questions.

Do you have a history of or family history of heart disease?	Y	N
Do you have a history of heart attacks?	Y	N
Have you had any chest pain?	Y	N
If so, when, and are you having chest pain now?		
Have you been short of breath or had trouble breathing, or do you have asthma?	Y	N
Do you or did you smoke? How much? When did you quit?	Y	N
Do you have a pacemaker?	Y	N
Have you had any recent surgery?	Y	N

Have you had any recent chemotherapy?	Y	N
Do you have high blood pressure or diabetes?	Y	N
Are you allergic to any medications?	Y	N
What medications are you presently taking?		
Have you had any prior ECG tests or related tests (e.g., echocardiography, stress tests, etc.)?	Y	N
Other department-specific questions.		

Patient Preparation

- Identify the patient. Verify doctor's order. Explain the procedure.
- Instruct patient to be NPO for 4–12 hours (no sugar, caffeine, or dairy products).
- Place five- or three-lead ECG setup on patient.
- Position patient supine on table; if possible have right antecubital basilic vein accessible for injection site. Some prefer jugular vein.

Equipment

Camera

- Large field of view gamma camera or multicrystal

Collimator

- Low energy, all purpose, or low energy, high resolution

Computer Set-up

- Most have a preprogrammed study. List mode, 16 frames/cycle or frame mode, 20–35 frames/sec, 64×64 matrix or can use 32×32 matrix for a 20-cm field of view (FOV). Study is usually about 20–120 seconds or 800–1200 frames.

Procedure *(time: 15 minutes, usually in conjunction with another test)*

- Position patient supine on bed.
- Connect three-lead ECG for gate.
- Position camera anterior (though RAO or LAO can be used depending on intent) with right arm (or IV arm) and heart in camera view.
- Start IV or butterfly, preferably in basilic vein of right arm (left will do if need be; some use right external jugular vein).
- Start camera and inject quickly to catch bolus.
- When program is done, IV or butterfly is removed if not required for second study to follow, e.g., patient may be scheduled for a 1-day perfusion protocol.

- Options: Position patient and camera for single photon emission computed tomography (SPECT) perfusion study, ask to return at specified time for resting SPECT, image for a multi-gated acquisition (MUGA) study if patient was administered pyrophosphate-labeled red blood cells, ask to return for myocardial infarction scan if ^{99m}Tc-stannous pyrophosphate was used, or dismiss if patient is finished with procedure.

Normal Results

- Left ventricular ejection fraction: 50–80%.

- Right ventricular ejection fraction: 40–60%.

- Bolus travels through right atrium and ventricle to lungs and back through left atrium and ventricles with no obvious obstruction or alteration in path.

- No deviations in full contraction of heart; all walls working and pushing in a coordinated manner.

Abnormal Results

- Cine showing one or more walls with abnormal movement (dyskinesis–paradoxic passive expansion, rather than contraction, of a myocardial segment during systole, e.g., a left ventricular aneurysm is characterized by localized dyskinesis), decreased wall motion (hypokinesis), or no movement (akinesis).

- Low ejection fraction, i.e., 35–45%, or less. Severe impairment is present below 30%.

- Regional wall abnormalities indicate coronary artery disease.

Example of a Set-up (others are not so elaborate)

- Fill a 35-mL syringe with saline.

- Attach a three-way stopcock to syringe, attach 20-inch extension tubing to three-way stopcock, prime tubing with saline from the 35-mL syringe.

- Using a 3-mL syringe, pull plunger back to draw in 0.5 mL air. Attach 3-mL syringe to stopcock. With stopcock turned off toward the 35-mL syringe, add the 0.5 mL air into the tubing. Close off the stopcock.

- Using the dose syringe (provided by the radiopharmacy), carefully pull back plunger and draw in 0.5 mL air. Carefully invert syringe upside down and ensure all the air moves upward toward the plunger.

- Carefully remove needle on dose syringe, add dose with 0.5 mL air to extension through three-way stopcock (turned off toward 35-mL syringe), close off three-way stopcock. The 20-inch extension tubing should have an 18-gauge needle on the end.

- Place lead cylinder over dose in extension tube or keep covered with lead.

- To a 3-mL syringe, add 0.5 mL of heparin; fill with saline.

- Add 5-inch extension tube (must have pinch-off plastic) with "T" attachment to 3-mL syringe; prime.

- These two setups are brought out to the patient, who is attached to the ECG and under the camera.

- On a portable table beside the patient, start the IV catheter.

- Attach "T" with 5-inch tubing and syringe; draw to test patency, tape well, and test again.

- Pinch off the 5-inch tubing. This is important, otherwise it blows technetium everywhere when bolus is pushed!
- Insert 18-ga needle on 20-inch extension into "T"; tape to make sure it is secure, and open three-way stopcock for 35-mL syringe push.
- Optional, cover site with towel in the event of a blowout.
- Start camera; when it begins to acquire, push hard, fast, and steady for good bolus. Should only run for a minute or two.
- Remove apparatus and proceed.

Artifacts

- Because initial push must be fairly hard for good bolus, IV might blow when injecting. Make sure everything is secure and covered with a towel in the event of a mishap.
- Arrhythmia may hamper acquisition. Run ECG to verify status of rhythm.
- May not get good bolus. Bolus should be tight and together; a mean transit time of 1–3 seconds is considered adequate for the study.

SUGGESTED READINGS

Early PJ, Sodee DB. Principles and Practice of Nuclear Medicine. 2nd ed. St. Louis: Mosby, 1995.

Murray IPC, Ell PJ, eds. Nuclear Medicine in Clinical Diagnosis and Treatment. Vols. 1 and 2. New York: Churchill Livingstone, 1994.

Wilson, MA. Textbook of Nuclear Medicine. Philadelphia: Lippincott-Raven, 1998.

Notes

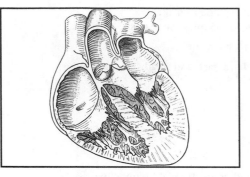

CHAPTER 10

Cardiac: MUGA and MUGA-X (Stress MUGA)

Radiopharmacy

Radionuclide
- ^{99m}Tc $t_{1/2}$: 6 hours

  Energies: 140 keV

  Type: IT, γ, generator

Radiopharmaceutical
- Tagged red blood cells (RBC) by pyrophosphate (pyp) or stannous chloride kit e.g., UltraTag® RBC in combination with ^{99m}TcO$_4^-$.

Localization
- Compartmental, tagged to and circulating with blood

Quality Control
- ^{99m}TcO$_4^-$, chromatography. Tagging, 90% in vivo; 95% in vitro.

Adult Dose Range
- 20–50 mCi (740–1850 MBq)

Method of Administration
- Two IV straight sticks into opposite arms (pyp, then after 20–30 minutes, ^{99m}TcO$_4^-$).
- Two IV straight sticks, blood draw (~3 mL into heparinized hot pyp), then reinject tagged RBCs after ~30 minutes.
- IV setup (IV catheter or butterfly, large bore). Use modified in vivo or UltraTag® preparation.

(Multi-Gated Acquisition/Equilibrium Gated Ventriculography/Gated Blood Pool Study/Ventricular Wall Motion Study)

Indications

MUGA

- Evaluation of left and sometimes right (for congestive heart failure) wall motion.
- Calculation of ejection fraction.
- Evaluation of patient's heart condition for pending surgery, chemotherapy, or radiation therapy.
- Evaluation of cause of dyspnea: cardiac or pulmonary.
- Evaluation of physical indicators: myocardial infarction, chest pain, shortness of breath, or history of heart disease.
- Evaluation of laboratory indicators: elevated levels of creatine phosphokinase, lactate dehydrogenase, and the newer tests for troponin and myoglobin (specific indicators for heart damage).

MUGA-X (all of the above, with emphasis on the following)

- Diagnosis and prognostication of coronary artery disease (CAD).
- Detection and evaluation of valvular dysfunction.
- Evaluation of cardiomyopathy.
- Evaluation of precardiac and postcardiac transplantation.

Contraindications

- Patient experiencing chest pain.
- Patient in an unstable medical condition.
- Patient with known severe arrhythmia.
- Patient known to be allergic to pyrophosphate or phosphates.

Patient History *(or use complete patient history in reference section)*

The patient should answer the following questions.

Do you have a history of or family history of heart disease?	Y	N
Do you have a history of heart attacks?	Y	N
Have you had any chest pain?	Y	N

If so, when, and are you having chest pain now?

Have you been short of breath, had trouble breathing, or do you have asthma?	Y	N
Do you or did you smoke? How much? When did you quit?	Y	N
Do you have a pacemaker?	Y	N
Have you had any recent surgery?	Y	N
Have you had any recent chemotherapy?	Y	N
Do you have high blood pressure or diabetes?	Y	N
Are you allergic to any medications?	Y	N
What medications are you presently taking?		
Have you had any prior ECG tests or related tests (e.g., echocardiography, stress tests, radiographs, etc.)?	Y	N
Other department-specific questions.		

Patient Preparation

- Identify the patient. Verify doctor's order. Explain the procedure.
- Instruct patient to be NPO 4–8 hours before the study.
- Physician is to discontinue patient's cardiac medications and caffeine ~4 hours before.
- Start IV setup (except for in vivo method).
- Prepare patient with three-lead or five-lead ECG.
- Remove articles from chest area that may attenuate images, e.g., buttons, medallions, or breast prostheses.

Equipment

Camera

- Large field of view

Collimator

- 30° slant hole, low energy, high resolution or low energy, all purpose

Computer Set-up

- Typically, 16 frames/sec, 20–50 ms/frame, matrix 64 × 64, reject ±20%, 600 sec/view, or 3 million counts.

Procedure *(time: ~1 hour)*

Blood Preparation (tagging the RBCs)
Procedure one (in vivo)

- Make up cold pyp kit; 2–3 mL normal saline into pyp vial. Mix. Let sit for 5 minutes.
- Inject 1–3 mL pyp. Wait ~20 minutes.
- Inject 20–30 mCi $^{99m}TcO_4^-$ into opposite arm.
- Follow acquisition steps below.

Procedure two (modified in vivo)

- Make up cold pyp kit; 2–3 mL normal saline into pyp vial. Mix. Let sit for 5 minutes.
- Inject patient with pyp, straight stick whenever possible; 1.5 mL for small patient or patient not on blood thinners; 3 mL for large patients or those on blood thinners.
- Wait 20 minutes; meanwhile start butterfly IV, hook up three- or five-lead ECG and run a test strip for baseline (and to make sure there is a good heart rhythm for gate).
- At 20 minutes, carefully draw 3–5 mL of blood into a 5- to 10-mL syringe containing 1 mL heparin and ~25 mCi (925 MBq), $^{99m}TcO_4^-$.
- Mix for 5–10 minutes, then reinject.
- Follow acquisition steps below.

Procedure three (in vitro commercial kits, e.g., UltraTag® RBC)

- Start catheter, large bore. (Straight stick with large-bore needle is an option.)
- Draw 1.5–3 mL blood slowly into 5- to 10-mL syringe containing 0.3–0.5 mL of heparin (or ADC). Inject into reaction vial. Swirl for 5 minutes.
- Add contents of syringe I, swirl; then add contents of syringe II, swirl; then add ~50 mCi $^{99m}TcO_4^-$.
- Wait 20 minutes, swirling occasionally; reinject slowly through catheter (or straight stick).
- Follow acquisition steps below.

MUGA Imaging

- Position patient supine on bed.
- Hook up three- or five-lead ECG. Check R-R wave, adjust acquisition parameters accordingly. Run a 15-second test ECG sheet if protocol.
- Position camera anteriorly, typically, ANT, LAO (two positions, ~35–60° looking for best septal wall separation for ejection fraction (EF) calculation and processing, slight caudal tilt, 5–10%, to camera can help), LLAT, and sometimes RLAT or RAO (looking for "shoe" picture), displaying anterior and inferior wall motion and apex.
- Collect 300–600 beats/image or go by preset time (~5–10 min/image).
- Process for EF. Use auto, then manual. If skeptical about results, have another technologist try the EF or try different color schemes.

MUGA-X Imaging

- Prepare patient as above. Position patient in exercise device, e.g., a bicycle ergometer.

- Position patient supine, feet in pedals, connect ECG leads, and position camera for test as per protocol.

- If resting images are first, obtain ANT, best LAT, then best LAO for septal separation as above or as per protocol.

- Physician is to determine stress settings, e.g., 25 W or 50 W, etc. Ensure patient's feet are secure in pedals. Ensure camera has best septal separation.

- Start camera, start stress, collect for up to 3 million counts if possible.

- Obtain blood pressures and record ECGs at each level if protocol (some institutions have nurses and specialized technicians available for these functions).

Processing

- Draw regions of interest manually and/or automatically on computer.

- Calculate $EF = (ED - ES) / ED \times 100$

  where ED is end-diastolic volume and ES is end-systolic volume.

- Calculate SV (stroke volume) $= ED - ES$.

- Calculate CO (cardiac output in mL) $= SV \times HR$ (heart rate).

Normal Results

- Should get good tag with blood. Circulation and heart should present clearly.

- Septal image should show easily definable separation between right and left ventricles.

- Cine should show fair amount of motion in all (septal, anterior, lateral, inferior, and apex) walls (no defects).

- $EF = 50-70\%$ or better left ventricle, 40–60% right ventricle.

Abnormal Results

- Cine showing one or more walls with abnormal movement (dyskinesis–paradoxic passive expansion, rather than contraction, of a myocardial segment during systole, e.g., a left ventricular aneurysm is characterized by localized dyskinesis), decreased wall motion (hypokinesis), or no movement (akinesis).

- Low EF, i.e., 35–45%, or less. Severe impairment is present below 30%.

- Regional wall abnormalities indicate CAD.

Artifacts

- Arrhythmias may make the study impossible to gate.

- Cold pyp may oxidize if not used soon after mixing.

- If reseals or IV lines are used, heparin or other pharmaceuticals may interact. Flush extremely well. Patient may be taking chemicals or drugs that interfere. All may cause a poor tag.

- Do not use chest ports as they will show in pictures and distort count information.

- If patient is obese, heart may be oriented more laterally; if thin, more anteriorly.

- Test should be performed before any contrast material type examination.

- Check clothing for articles in pockets, big buttons on shirts, ECG electrodes in way, medallions, or pacemakers (at least there should be a good R–R).

- Get good separation of right and left ventricles and good regions of interest for EF. It is not unusual to do automatic and manual EFs to compare results, or to have other technologists try their luck for comparison if time allows.

SUGGESTED READINGS

Datz FL. Handbook of Nuclear Medicine. 2nd ed. St. Louis: Mosby, 1993.

Early PJ, Sodee DB. Principles and Practice of Nuclear Medicine. 2nd ed. St. Louis: Mosby, 1995.

Murray IPC, Ell PJ, eds. Nuclear Medicine in Clinical Diagnosis and Treatment. Vols. 1 and 2. New York: Churchill Livingstone, 1994.

Wilson, MA. Textbook of Nuclear Medicine. Philadelphia: Lippincott-Raven, 1998.

UltraTag® is a registered trademark of Mallinckrodt Medical, Inc., St. Louis, MO.

Notes
. . . .

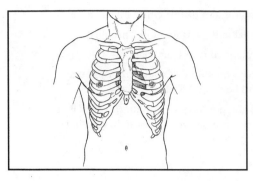

CHAPTER 11

Cardiac: Myocardial Infarction (MI) Scan

Radiopharmacy

Radionuclide

- ^{99m}Tc $t_{1/2}$: 6 hours

  Energies: 140 keV

  Type: IT, γ, generator

Radiopharmaceutical

- ^{99m}Tc-stannous pyrophosphate ("hot pyp")

Localization

- Flows with blood stream, pyrophosphate deposition accumulates with calcium in the mitochondria and within the cytoplasm of necrotic myocardial tissue. Maximum concentration occurs when myocardial blood flow decreases to 30–40% of normal. Maximum pyrophosphate deposition occurs usually 48–72 hours after infarction.

Quality Control

- ^{99m}TcO$_4^-$; chromatography. Tagging, 90% in vivo; 95% in vitro.

Adult Dose Range

- 15–30 mCi (555–1110 MBq)

Method of Administration

- IV, good bolus if flow is required.

Indications

- Evaluation of myocardial infarction (MI) several days after acute event.
- Evaluation of patients having chest pain at least 48 hours before. The imaging window considered by some is from 24 to 72 hours.
- Evaluation of equivocal ECG or elevated cardiac laboratories indicating an event.
- Evaluation of bundle branch block ECGs difficult to interpret.
- Evaluation of right ventricular infarction.
- Evaluation of infarctions after coronary artery surgery.

Contraindications

- Patient presently has severe angina.
- Too soon after the event.
- Too late after the event.

Patient History *(or use complete patient history in reference section)*

The patient should answer the following questions.

Do you have a history of or family history of heart disease?	Y	N
Do you have a history of heart attacks?	Y	N
Have you had any chest pain?	Y	N
If so, when, and are you having chest pain now?		
Have you been short of breath, had trouble breathing, or do you have asthma?	Y	N
Do you or did you smoke? How much? When did you quit?	Y	N
Do you have a pacemaker?	Y	N
Have you had any recent surgery?	Y	N
Have you had any recent chemotherapy?	Y	N

Do you have high blood pressure or diabetes?	Y	N
Are you allergic to any medications?	Y	N
What medications are you presently taking?		
Have you had any prior ECG tests or related tests (e.g., echocardiography, stress tests, etc.)?	Y	N
Other department-specific questions.		

Patient Preparation

- Identify the patient. Verify doctor's order. Explain the procedure.
- No preparation for injection.
- Instruct the patient to hydrate well and urinate often after the injection.

Equipment

Camera

- Large field of view

Collimator

- Low energy, all purpose, or low energy, high resolution

Computer Set-up

Statics

- 500,000–1,000,000 counts, 20% window, ^{99m}Tc

Flow

- List mode for first-pass or 1 sec/frame for 30 seconds

Single Photon Emission Computed Tomography (SPECT)

- 360°, 64 steps at 25 sec/step

Procedure *(time: ~ 30 min/session)*

- Position patient supine on table.
- Obtain flow if protocol; inject good bolus under anterior camera for a first-pass type study (list mode, ANT or RAO for right and left ventricular ejection fractions), followed by some or all of the static images for immediate blood pool.
- Obtain only the immediate blood pool images if protocol. Check with radiologist.
- Obtain the following static images at 2–3 hours after the injection: ANT, LAO, LLAT, and RAO, adjusting views to separate and/or discern any cardiac visualization from sternum and rib cage. Check with radiologist if unsure as to other images.

- Obtain SPECT images, usually performed at 3 hours with thorax in region of interest, if protocol.
- Obtain extra-delayed images at 6 hours or longer if requested.

Normal Results

- ^{99m}Tc-pyp is a skeletal imaging agent.
- Sternum and ribs should show evenly along with vertebrae and other bones in field of view.
- There should be no cardiac muscle visible in any of the thorax views.

Abnormal Results

- Part or all of the myocardium will present to varying degrees within the rib cage and sternum.
- Image interpretation (level of activity in the region of the heart) may be reported as follows:

  0 = no increase above background, no cardiac uptake.

  1+ = faint, diffuse definite increase but less than rib cage levels.

  2+ = definite activity increase equal to rib levels but less than sternum.

  3+ = activity level equal to that of sternum levels.

  4+ = activity level greater than that of sternum levels.

- A positive study will usually return to normal within a week to a month after the acute event. Repeating the scan in 7–10 days may help the assessment of sustained abnormal uptake. Persistent abnormal uptakes indicate a poor prognosis.
- 2+ indicates subendocardial infarction and/or unstable angina. Patients with unstable angina have focal areas of myocardial necrosis even though there are no corroborating laboratory results for myocardial damage.
- 3+ and 4+ indicate acute transmural myocardial damage.

Artifacts

- Attenuating objects on necklaces, shirt pockets, etc.
- Unexpected bone metastasis in thorax region may obscure cardiac visualization.
- Background from inadequate hydration may hinder visualization.
- Pyrophosphate has been shown to localize in regions of old myocardial infarcts several months after the acute episode, yielding a possible false-positive result.
- Recent thoracic injury or surgery involving skeletal muscle would have to be localized by various oblique views.

Note

Trials were performed with a cardiac drug called cariporide, which may prevent damage to cardiac tissue during and immediately after an MI. Normally, calcium is needed in muscle cell contraction by interacting with myosin and actin, causing them to attach and move against each other, and thus causing the contraction. The calcium then displaces, the cell relaxes, and the process is repeated. During an attack, blood flow is restricted, the affected cells become too acidic, sodium is pumped in to replace the acid, and calcium is then exchanged for the sodium. The excess calcium causes a sustained contraction until the cell dies. By blocking the initial acid/sodium exchange, Cariporide interferes with these reactions, leaving the cell acidic but still alive.

SUGGESTED READINGS

Datz FL. Handbook of Nuclear Medicine. 2nd ed. St. Louis: Mosby, 1993.

Early PJ, Sodee DB. Principles and Practice of Nuclear Medicine. 2nd ed. St. Louis: Mosby, 1995.

Murray IPC, Ell PJ, eds. Nuclear Medicine in Clinical Diagnosis and Treatment. Vols. 1 and 2. New York: Churchill Livingstone, 1994.

Wilson, MA. Textbook of Nuclear Medicine. Philadelphia: Lippincott-Raven, 1998.

Notes

CHAPTER 12

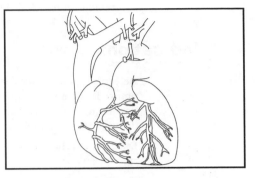

Cardiac: Resting Test

(Perfusion)

Radiopharmacy

Radionuclide

- ^{99m}Tc $t_{\frac{1}{2}}$: 6 hours

  Energies: 140 keV

  Type: IT, γ, generator; or

- ^{201}Tl $t_{\frac{1}{2}}$: 73 hours

  Energies: 68–80 keV k x-ray, 135, 167 keV

  Type: EC, γ, accelerator

Radiopharmaceutical

- ^{99m}Tc-sestamibi (hexakis[2-methoxyisobutylisonitril]), ^{99m}Tc-1,2-bis (bis[2-ethoxyethyl]phosphino) ethane, ^{201}Tl-thallous chloride

Localization

- ^{99m}Tc-sestamibi; passive transport into myocardial mitochondria in proportion to blood flow. ^{99m}Tc-tetrofosmin; same, binds to myocytes. ^{201}Tl-thallous chloride; similar to potassium, distributes with Na/K pump within 20 minutes of injection, then seeps out of myocardium and redistributes.

Quality Control

- ^{99m}Tc-sestamibi, ^{99m}Tc-tetrofosmin, chromatography > 90%; ^{201}TlCl, chromatography > 95%, use within 7 days.

Adult Dose Range

- ^{99m}Tc-sestamibi, ^{99m}Tc-tetrofosmin; 8–30 mCi (296–1110 MBq), ^{201}TlCl; 2–5 mCi (74–185 MBq)

Method of Administration

- Tetrofosmin, sestamibi, or thallium: IV

- Thallium redistribution (3–4 hours after injection): no injection for redistribution needed unless it is a rest-only study. Some stress or redistribution protocols call for a second injection (~1 mCi IV). Separate day: IV

Indications

- Detection and evaluation of coronary artery disease. For both sestamibi and thallium, uptake in the myocardium is proportional to flow. At rest there are no increased flow requirements. Diminished or restricted flow will be detected in areas served by diseased vessels. Results are usually compared with the cardiac stress test.
- Evaluation of those patients who may be candidates for coronary bypass surgery or angioplasty.
- Detection and evaluation for viable or hibernating myocardial tissue (particularly with thallium).
- Evaluation of physical indicators: myocardial infarction, chest pain, shortness of breath, history or family history of heart disease.
- Evaluation of laboratory indicators: elevated levels of creatine phosphokinase, lactate dehydrogenase, and the newer tests for troponin and myoglobin (specific indicators for heart damage).

Contraindications

- Patient should not be taking chemical stressors, e.g., caffeine, dipyridamole, nitroglycerin drips and patches, etc. Most prefer to discontinue heart medications until after test.
- Patient should be NPO for 4–12 hours.

Patient History *(or use complete patient history in reference section)*

The patient should answer the following questions.

Do you have a history of or family history of heart disease?	Y	N
Do you have a history of heart attacks?	Y	N
Have you had any chest pain?	Y	N
If so, when, and are you having chest pain now?		
Have you been short of breath, had trouble breathing, or do you have asthma?	Y	N

Do you or did you smoke? How much? When did you quit?	Y	N
Do you have a pacemaker?	Y	N
Have you had any recent surgery?	Y	N
Have you had any recent chemotherapy?	Y	N
Do you have high blood pressure or diabetes?	Y	N
Are you allergic to any medications?	Y	N
What medications are you presently taking?		
Have you had any prior ECG tests or related tests (e.g., echocardiography, stress tests, etc.)?	Y	N
Other department-specific questions.		

Patient Preparation

- Identify the patient. Verify doctor's order. Explain the procedure.
- Instruct patient to be NPO for 4–12 hours (no sugar, caffeine, or dairy products).
- Remove 10 ECG leads and electrodes if necessary or use three-lead ECG if it is a gated test.
- Position patient sitting upright for 15 minutes before injection to reduce pulmonary and splanchnic blood flow.

Equipment

Camera
- Large field of view

Collimator
- Low energy, all purpose, or low energy, high resolution

Computer Set-up
- ^{99m}Tc window at 140 keV, ^{201}Tl windows at (minimum) Hg k x-rays (68–80 keV) and 167 keV at 20%

Static
- Timed for 300 seconds

Single Photon Emission Computed Tomography (SPECT)

- 180°, 32 or 64 projections at 20 sec/frame, 8 frames/cycle if gated, matrix at 64 × 64, runs ~25 minutes.

Procedure *(many protocols; time: ~15-30 minutes)*

- Thallium: rest only; patient waits 5-20 minutes after injection before imaging.

- Sestamibi: patient waits 45-60 minutes after injection before imaging. Give patient a glass of cold water before imaging to clear thyroid, liver, and bowel.

- Tetrofosmin: patient waits 5-30 minutes after injection before imaging (give water).

- Position patient supine with heart in center field of view and left arm up over head if possible. If arm is down at side because of problems with shoulder joint or recent surgery, both the rest and stress images should be taken the same way.

- Images may include a static anterior picture first (300 seconds).

- Start SPECT images at appropriate time with camera right anterior oblique to left posterior oblique (except for patients with dextrocardia).

- Processing: computer analysis of left ventricle showing the vertical long axis, horizontal long axis, and short axis. Usually done at the same time as stress images; the results of the two are compared. Can be processed separately.

Normal Results

- Heterogeneous uptake of the left ventricular myocardium.

Abnormal Results

- Area(s) of little or no uptake exhibiting a cold spot. If the lack of uptake matches the stress results in the same area, it may be infarcted myocardium or severe ischemic tissue.

- Left ventricular walls of interest and their supply arteries

    Apical: left anterior descending, distal end, and/or right coronary artery, posterior descending

    Septal: left anterior descending

    Anterior: left anterior descending

    Lateral: left circumflex

    Inferior: right coronary artery

Artifacts

- Patient may not be NPO for 4 plus hours.

- Articles in pockets, medallions, necklaces, heart monitors, pacemakers, or metal buttons may cause artifacts.

- If patient has left arm down to side, it may cause unwanted attenuation.

- With sestamibi, possibly shield gall bladder because of uptake.

Protocols *(there are several stress-rest protocols being followed at present)*

- Thallium (only): The stress is done first, imaged as soon as possible (some perform an anterior view first for heart:lung ratio), then imaged again 3–4 hours later (sometimes with a small reinjection of ~1 mCi). The rest study is completed using its ability to redistribute. Some perform a 24-hour delay rest study with a 1 mCi reinjection (wait 5–20 minutes to image), looking for hibernating tissue.

- Thallium-Thallium: Both tests are done with thallium but on different days.

- Thallium-Sestamibi (dual energy-dual isotope): The thallium rest study (3 mCi) is done first (inject, wait ~20 minutes, image), followed fairly quickly (within the hour) by the stress test using sestamibi. Some add 24-hour resting thallium for viability.

- Sestamibi-Sestamibi: Both tests are done with sestamibi but on different days. The stress test can be done first. If no defects are observed, some choose not to do the rest study.

- Sestamibi-Sestamibi: Both tests are done on the same day. Either rest or stress can be done first; however, most prefer to do resting pictures first, then stress. The first study is done with a low dose, ~8 mCi, and the second (an hour or more later) with a high dose, ~25–30 mCi. Gated images are usually taken with whichever study used the higher dose.

Note

Many departments are now substituting tetrofosmin (Myoview®) for sestamibi (Cardio-lite®). Some facilities may be performing cardiac SPECT using these radiotracers on emergency room patients with chest pain if their initial ECG is suspicious.

PDR®: Cardiovascular Preparations (has full list of drugs).

Beta Blockers:	Calcium-Channel Blockers:
Blocadren®	Adalat®
Brevibloc®	Calan®
Cartrol®	Cardene®
Corgard®	Cardizem®
Inderal®	DynaCirc®
Inderide®	Isoptin®
Kerlone®	Nimotop®
Levatol®	Plendil®
Lopressor®	Procardia®
Normozide®	Vascor®
Sectral®	
Tenoretic Tablets®	
Tenormin®	
Timolide Tablets®	
Visken®	

SUGGESTED READINGS

Datz FL. Handbook of Nuclear Medicine. 2nd ed. St. Louis: Mosby, 1993.

Early PJ, Sodee DB. Principles and Practice of Nuclear Medicine. 2nd ed. St. Louis: Mosby, 1995.

Murray IPC, Ell PJ, eds. Nuclear Medicine in Clinical Diagnosis and Treatment. Vols. 1 and 2. New York: Churchill Livingstone, 1994.

Wilson, MA. Textbook of Nuclear Medicine. Philadelphia: Lippincott-Raven, 1998.

Notes

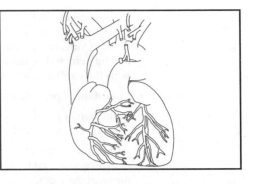

CHAPTER 13

Cardiac: Stress Test

(Perfusion, Usually With Cardiac Rest Test)

Radiopharmacy

Radionuclide

- ^{99m}Tc $t_{1/2}$: 6 hours

  Energies: 140 keV

  Type: IT, γ, generator; or

- ^{201}Tl $t_{1/2}$: 73 hours

  Energies: 68–80 keV k x-ray, 135, 167 keV

  Type: EC, γ, accelerator

Radiopharmaceutical

- ^{99m}Tc-sestamibi (hexakis[2-methoxyisobutylisonitril]), ^{99m}Tc-1,2-bis
  (bis[2-ethoxyethyl]phosphino) ethane, ^{201}Tl-thallous chloride

Localization

- ^{99m}Tc-sestamibi; passive transport into myocardial mitochondria in proportion to
  blood flow. ^{99m}Tc-tetrofosmin; same, binds to myocytes. ^{201}Tl-thallous chloride;
  similar to potassium, distributes with Na/K pump within 20 minutes of injection,
  then seeps out of myocardium and redistributes.

Quality Control

- ^{99m}Tc-sestamibi, ^{99m}Tc-tetrofosmin, chromatography > 90%; ^{201}TlCl,
  chromatography > 95%, use within 7 days (T_b = 56 hours)

Adult Dose Range

- ^{99m}Tc-sestamibi, ^{99m}Tc-tetrofosmin; 20–30 mCi (740–1110 MBq), ^{201}TlCl; 3–5 mCi
  (111–185 MBq)

Method of Administration

- IV catheter or butterfly setup, which can include a three-way stopcock, 10-mL
  syringe filled with normal saline, and an injection port.

Indications

- Detection and evaluation of coronary artery disease. For sestamibi, tetrofosmin, and thallium, uptake in the myocardium is proportional to blood flow. With stress, there are increased flow requirements. Diminished or restricted flow will occur and be detected in areas served by diseased vessels. Results are usually compared with the cardiac rest test (though some order no rest test if stress is normal).

- Evaluation of possible candidates for coronary bypass surgery or angioplasty.

- Evaluation of physical indicators: myocardial infarction, chest pain, shortness of breath, history or family history of heart disease.

- Evaluation of laboratory indicators: elevated levels of creatine phosphokinase, lactate dehydrogenase, and the newer tests for troponin and myoglobin (specific indicators for heart damage).

Contraindications

- Patient experiencing chest pain.

- Patient should discontinue chemical stressors, e.g., caffeine, Persantine®, theophylline.

- Patient with extremely high blood pressure.

- Patient who is not comfortably weaned from nitroglycerin drip or is medically unstable.

- Patient may have allergies to chemicals and/or be unable to walk.

- Patients with lung conditions may get asthmatic reaction to Persantine® or adenosine. Dobutamine is suggested in those cases.

Patient History *(or use complete patient history in reference section)*

The patient should answer the following questions.

Do you have a history of or family history of heart disease?	Y	N
Do you have a history of heart attacks?	Y	N
Have you had any chest pain?	Y	N
If so, when, and are you having chest pain now?		
Have you been short of breath, had trouble breathing, or do you have asthma?	Y	N

Do you or did you smoke? How much?
   When did you quit?   Y   N

Do you have a pacemaker?   Y   N

Do you have a nitro patch or are you taking
   nitroglycerin?   Y   N

Have you had any recent surgery?   Y   N

Have you had any recent chemotherapy?   Y   N

Do you have high blood pressure or diabetes?   Y   N

Are you allergic to any medications?   Y   N

What medications are you presently taking?

Have you had any prior ECG tests or related
   tests (e.g., echocardiography, stress tests, etc.)? Y   N

Other department-specific questions.

Patient Preparation

- Identify the patient. Verify physician's order. Explain the procedure.
- Instruct patient to be NPO for 4–12 hours. Clear liquids and crackers only for sestamibi and tetrofosmin, nothing at all for thallium. Orange juice allowed for diabetics; may need to monitor blood sugar and adjust.
- Instruct patient to ingest no caffeine, dairy products, or sugar.
- Obtain a signed consent form.
- Shave and wipe chest with alcohol (as necessary).
- Prepare patient with a 10- or 12-lead ECG setup, run standing and lying or sitting test sheets.
- Start IV setup, flush IV, ensure patency.
- Triage patient for treadmill, Persantine® (dipyridamole), adenosine, or dobutamine. (If stress is dobutamine, have available atropine to boost heart rate and propranolol to lower heart rate. If Persantine® or adenosine, have available aminophylline to counter the effect.)
- Obtain a baseline blood pressure and record (some take both sitting and standing blood pressures).

Equipment

Camera

• Large field of view

Collimator

• Low energy, all purpose, or low energy, high resolution

Computer Set-up

• ^{99m}Tc window at 140 keV, ^{201}Tl windows at (minimum) Hg k x-rays (68–80 keV) and 167 keV at 20%

Static

• Timed for 300 seconds

Single Photon Emission Computed Tomography (SPECT)

• 180°, 32 or 64 projections at 20–40 sec/frame, 8 frames/cycle if gated, matrix at 64 × 64, runs ~25 minutes

Procedure *(time: exercise, ~10 minutes; image, ~15–30 minutes)*

Stress (many protocols)

• Patient prepared with 10- or 12-lead ECG. Run baseline ECG, with patient standing on the treadmill.

• Position patient on treadmill or supine for pharmacologic stress.

• Perform stress test by exercise or pharmacology in the presence of a physician. Heart rate should be between 85% and 100% of maximum (220 − age of patient).

  • Treadmill: Monitor heart rate, blood pressure, ECG changes, and patient (closely). Inject and flush on physician's order (when target heart rate is obtained or about 1 minute before patient gives out). Maintain exercise for 60–90 seconds after injection. Have crash cart handy. Some require a stretcher in proximity.

  • Dobutamine: Connect patient to pump. Begin first of five levels of drip on physician's order. Infusion changes by protocol. Inject and flush on physician's order. Used if there are known allergies, asthma, or pulmonary problems. Antidote: Inderal®.

  • Persantine®: Push or pump over 4 minutes on physician's order. Wait 3–4 minutes more, then inject and flush (ask physician). Antidote: aminophylline.

  • Adenosine: Connect patient to pump. Infuse drug for 6 minutes. Inject at 3 or 4 minutes (ask physician). Continue infusion and patient monitoring until done. Antidote: aminophylline.

    • Some protocols ask that, if possible, the patient is walked on the treadmill for a few minutes after the infusion to aid the perfusion process.

  • Treadmill

    • Sestamibi: have patient get down, remove IV setup (unless resting study is pending or it is an inpatient who may need the IV site) after proper monitoring time (~6–10 minutes), give patient glass of cold water, wait 35–45 minutes to image (some are imaging much sooner).

- Tetrofosmin: same, but can image 5 minutes to 4 hours after injection.
- Thallium: same, but image as soon as possible; some wait 15 minutes to eliminate heart creep. Redistribution images taken in 3–4 hours if a 1-day protocol.
- Chemical: Persantine, adenosine, and dobutamine
  - Sestamibi: monitor, disconnect, give water, wait 45–90 minutes to image.
  - Tetrofosmin: same, wait 5 minutes to 4 hours.
  - Thallium: image as soon as possible. Redistribution images taken in 3–4 hours if a 1-day protocol, some with a reinjection of 1 mCi. (Adenosine note: some image after 11 minutes for sestamibi or thallium. Most however, for sestamibi; wait 45–60 minutes to image; thallium, image as soon as possible.)

Imaging

- Remove ECG electrodes if necessary unless it is a gated study (for gated study, connect three-lead ECG, check for good R-R interval).
- Position patient supine with heart in center field of view and left arm up over head (if possible). If patient has shoulder problems or will have surgery that necessitates leaving the arm down, do both resting and stress images the same way.
- Images may include a static anterior picture first (300 seconds) for heart:lung ratio, e.g., for thallium studies.
- Start SPECT images at appropriate time (RAO to LPO). Some cameras allow mapping, noncircular orbits, or circular with setting the radius.
- Processing: Images are processed to show myocardium of left ventricle in vertical long axis, horizontal long axis, and short axis views. Also, polar or bull's eye images. Some software allows ejection fraction information. The films obtained vary greatly from hospital to hospital and from cardiologist to cardiologist.

Normal Results

- Heterogeneous uptake throughout the myocardium of the left ventricle.
- Normal left ventricular end-diastolic volume is ~70 mL, end-systolic volume is ~25 mL.
- Normal heart:lung ratio is 70:30. Some consider 50:50 within normal limits.

Abnormal Results

- If a defect (area of little to no uptake shown by a less or no uptake) is evident in stress but not with rest, the myocardium is ischemic and reversible.
- If the defect occurs in both tests in the same area, it is most likely infarcted and considered a fixed defect.
- Left ventricle walls of interest and supply arteries:
  - Apical: left anterior descending, distal end, and/or right coronary artery, posterior descending
  - Septal: left anterior descending
  - Anterior: left anterior descending
  - Lateral: left circumflex
  - Inferior: right coronary artery

- Transverse (transaxial) is horizontal long axis (slices, superior to inferior; image, left is septal wall, top is apex, right is lateral wall).

- Sagittal is vertical long axis (slices, right side of heart to left; image, top is anterior wall, right is apex, bottom is inferior wall).

- Coronal is short axis (slices, apex to base; image, top is anterior wall, right is lateral wall, bottom is inferior wall, left is septal wall).

- Heart:lung ratios greater than 30% in the lungs are considered abnormal. Some would say anything greater than 50% in the lungs. Abnormal heart:lung ratios indicate heart disease, e.g., congestive heart failure.

Artifacts

- Patient may not be NPO for 12 hours.

- Patient may not reach 85% maximum heart rate.

- Articles in pockets, medallions, necklaces, metal buttons, or ECG electrodes may cause artifacts.

- If patient has left arm down to side, it may cause unwanted attenuation.

- Patient may be on Theo-Dur®, theophylline, Elixophyllin®, Quibron®, Slo-phyllin®, or areolate, disallowing Persantine® stress, or may be allergic to pharmacology.

- With sestamibi, possibly shield gall bladder because of uptake.

- Test should be discontinued if patient experiences angina, severe shortness of breath, fall in blood pressure, ischemic ECG changes, arrhythmias, exhaustion, or reaches the 85% maximum heart rate.

- Risks involve adverse drug-related events and a mortality rate of 1 in 2000 (0.05%).

- Always look for focal uptake in thorax for possible tumor uptake.

Protocols

One day

- Thallium (only): The stress is performed first, imaged immediately, then 3-4 hours later the rest is completed using its ability to redistribute often with a 1 mCi booster shot. Some do a 24-hour delay rest study with a 1 mCi reinjection (wait 5-20 minutes to image) looking for viable or hibernating stunned tissue. Also performed with sublingual nitroglycerin dose.

- Thallium-Sestamibi (dual energy-dual isotope): The thallium rest study (3 mCi) is done first (inject, wait ~20 minutes, image), followed fairly quickly (within the hour) by the stress test using sestamibi. A 24-hour delay rest study with a 1 mCi reinjection (wait 5-20 minutes to image), looking for viable or hibernating stunned tissue, can also be performed with this study.

- Sestamibi-Sestamibi: Both tests are done on the same day. Either rest or stress can be done first; however, most prefer to do resting pictures first (e.g., in the morning), then set up for the stress (treadmill or chemical). The first study is done with a low dose, ~8 mCi, followed by the second (an hour or more later) with a high dose, ~25-30 mCi. Gated pictures are usually taken with whichever study used the higher dose.

- Tetrofosmin-Tetrofosmin: Same as sestamibi.

Two day

- Thallium–Thallium: Both tests are done with thallium but on different days.

- Thallium–Sestamibi: Thallium rest on first day with a redistribution and even a 24-hour delay looking for hibernating tissue; sestamibi or tetrofosmin stress on second day.

- Sestamibi–Sestamibi: Both tests are done with sestamibi but on different days. Some do the stress test first. If no defects are observed, there is no need for the rest study. Others do both tests, regardless.

- Tetrofosmin–Tetrofosmin: Same as sestamibi.

Note
· · · · · ·

Myoview® (^{99m}Tc-tetrofosmin) is similar in some characteristics to Cardiolite® (sestamibi). Preliminary research indicated that they both localize in the mitochondria of the myocytes of the myocardium and elicit the same-quality pictures; however, ^{99m}Tc-tetrofosmin has a faster clearance rate from the liver and gallbladder (within 5 minutes on stress and 15 minutes on rest) than sestamibi, making the agent a consideration for busy nuclear cardiac departments. The clearance has been disputed, and different departments have had a variety of results.

PDR®: Cardiovascular Preparations (has full list of drugs).

Beta Blockers:	Calcium-Channel Blockers:
Blocadren®	Adalat®
Brevibloc®	Calan®
Cartrol®	Cardene®
Corgard®	Cardizem®
Inderal®	DynaCirc®
Inderide®	Isoptin®
Kerlone®	Nimotop®
Levatol®	Plendil®
Lopressor®	Procardia®
Normozide®	Vascor®
Sectral®	
Tenoretic Tablets®	
Tenormin®	
Timolide Tablets®	
Visken®	

SUGGESTED READINGS

Datz FL. Handbook of Nuclear Medicine. 2nd ed. St. Louis: Mosby, 1993.

Early PJ, Sodee DB. Principles and Practice of Nuclear Medicine. 2nd ed. St. Louis: Mosby, 1995.

Murray IPC, Ell PJ, eds. Nuclear Medicine in Clinical Diagnosis and Treatment. Vols. 1 and 2. New York: Churchill Livingstone, 1994.

Wilson, MA. Textbook of Nuclear Medicine. Philadelphia: Lippincott-Raven, 1998.

Adalat® is a registered trademark of Miles, Inc., West Haven, CT.
Blocadren® is a registered trademark of Merck, Sharp, & Dohme, West Point, PA.
Brevibloc® is a registered trademark of DuPont Pharmaceuticals, Wilmington, DE.
Calan® is a registered trademark of GD Searle & Co., Chicago, IL.
Cardene® is a registered trademark of Syntex Laboratories, Inc., Palo Alto, CA.
Cardiolite® is a registered trademark of DuPont Pharmaceuticals, Wilmington, DE.
Cardizem® is a registered trademark of Marion Merrell Dow Inc., Kansas City, MO.
Cartrol® is a registered trademark of Abbott Laboratories, North Chicago, IL.
Corgard® is a registered trademark of Bristol Laboratories, Evansville, IN.
DynaCirc® is a registered trademark of Sandoz Pharmaceuticals, East Hanover, NJ.
Elixophyllin® is a registered trademark of Forest Pharmaceuticals, Inc., St. Louis, MO.
Inderal® is a registered trademark of Wyeth-Ayerst Laboratories, Philadelphia, PA.
Inderide® is a registered trademark of Wyeth-Ayerst Laboratories, Philadelphia, PA.
Isoptin® is a registered trademark of Knoll Pharmaceuticals, Whippany, NJ.
Kerlone® is a registered trademark of GD Searle & Co., Chicago, IL.
Levatol® is a registered trademark of Reed & Carnrick, Jersey City, NJ.
Lopressor® is a registered trademark of Geigy Pharmaceuticals, Ardsley, NY.
Myoview® is a registered trademark of Amersham International Plc, Amersham, UK.
Nimotop® is a registered trademark of Miles, Inc., West Haven, CT.
Normozide® is a registered trademark of Schering Corporation, Kenilworth, NJ.
PDR® is a registered trademark of Medical Economics Company, Montvale, NJ.
Persantine® is a registered trademark of Boehringer Ingelheim Pharmaceuticals, Inc., Ridgefield, CT.
Plendil® is a registered trademark of Merck, Sharp, & Dohme, West Point, PA.
Procardia® is a registered trademark of Pfizer Labs Division, New York, NY.
Quibron® is a registered trademark of Bristol Laboratories, Evansville, IN.
Sectral® is a registered trademark of Wyeth-Ayerst Laboratories, Philadelphia, PA.
Slo-phyllin® is a registered trademark of Rhône-Poulenc Rorer Pharmaceuticals, Inc., Collegeville, PA.
Tenoretic Tablets® is a registered trademark of ICI Pharma, Wilmington, DE.
Tenormin® is a registered trademark of ICI Pharma, Wilmington, DE.
Timolide Tablets® is a registered trademark of Merck, Sharp, & Dohme, West Point, PA.
Theo-Dur® is a registered trademark of Key Pharmaceuticals, Inc., Kenilworth, NJ.
Vascor® is a registered trademark of Wallace Laboratories, Cranbury, NJ.
Visken® is a registered trademark of Sandoz Pharmaceuticals, East Hanover, NJ.

Notes

· · · · · · · ·

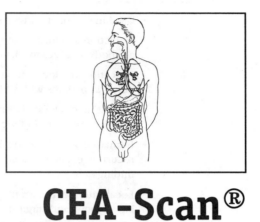

CHAPTER 14

CEA-Scan®

(Radioimmunoscintigraphy [RIS])

Radiopharmacy

Radionuclide

- ^{99m}Tc $t_{1/2}$: 6 hours

  Energies: 140 keV

  Type: IT, γ, generator

Radiopharmaceutical

- ^{99m}Tc-arcitumomab (murine monoclonal antibody [Moab] fragments [Fabs]). Generated from IMMU-4, a murine IgG_10; binds to carcinoembryonic antigen (CEA) on cell membrane. Fab fragments minimize the induction of HAMA (human anti-mouse antibody) reaction.

Localization

- Compartmental, blood flow; dose dependent, antibody binding

Quality Control

- From kit, chromatography, > 90% radiochemical purity

Adult Dose Range

- 20–30 mCi (740–1110 MBq)

Method of Administration

- IV butterfly (large bore, 18–22 gauge) for 5–20 minutes in up to 30 mL of saline.
- 10 mL of saline flush.
- Should have physician or nurse available for possible allergic reaction (1 mg of epinephrine available).
- Follow vital signs: baseline, 5, 15, 30, 60 minutes after injection (some simply observe patient for 15–30 minutes, looking for redness at injection site or signs of nausea and vomiting).

Indications

- Used in conjunction with standard diagnostic evaluations.
- Detection and localization of recurrent or metastatic colorectal carcinoma. The antibody localizes to CEA on cell.
- Detection and localization of antigen expression in liver, extrahepatic abdomen, and pelvis in patients with a histologically confirmed diagnosis of colorectal carcinoma.
- Evaluation of elevated or rising serum CEA, liver enzymes, or symptoms with no radiologic evidence of recurrence.
- Evaluation and detection of extent of regional lesions, occult metastases, and recurrence; detect occult metastases by clarifying equivocal diagnostic modality findings.
- Localization of recurrent disease in surgical candidate patients (biopsy, exploratory laparotomy, and surgical resection).

Contraindications

- Should not be administered to patients who are hypersensitive to murine products.
- Not indicated for differential diagnosis of colorectal carcinoma.
- Not indicated as a screening tool for colorectal cancer.
- Not intended for readministration or for assessment of treatment.

Patient History *(or use complete patient history in reference section)*

The patient should answer the following questions.

Do you have a history or a family history of cancer?	Y	N
If so, what type and since when?		
Do you have any pain?	Y	N
If so, where and since when?		
Do you have a history of allergies?	Y	N
Have you had any recent surgery?	Y	N

Have you had any recent radiation therapy or chemotherapy?	Y	N
Have you had any recent murine examinations?	Y	N
Have you had any recent or planned nuclear medicine (NM), CT, MRI, x-ray, or ultrasonography (US) examinations?	Y	N
Have you had any recent abnormal laboratory results?	Y	N

If so, please list (CEA, CA-19–9, HAMA, other).

Other department-specific questions.

Patient Preparation

- Identify the patient. Verify doctor's order. Explain the procedure.
- Obtain a signed consent form from patient.
- Obtain a history of allergies and prior examinations from patient.
- Instruct patient to void before imaging.

Equipment

Camera
- Large field of view

Collimator
- Low energy, all purpose, or low energy, high resolution

Computer Set-up
Statics
- 600 seconds or more per view (> 1,000,000 counts)

Whole Body
- 10 cm/min or slower; 30-minute sweep is recommended, e.g., patient length in cm ÷ 30 (minutes) = speed in cm/min.

Single Photon Emission Computed Tomography (SPECT)
- Rotation, 360° step and shoot; projections, 60, 30 sec/frame (single head), 45–60 sec/frame (dual head); matrix, 64 × 64 or 128 × 128 word mode; axis/COR (center of rotation), < 2 mm or 0.5 pixels; uniformity correction, yes (± 1%).

Procedure *(2–5 hours after injection, time: ~1–2 hours)*

- Instruct patient to void; check clothing for possible artifacts.
- Position patient supine on imaging table, no movement during imaging.
- Obtain static images or whole body sweep 2–5 hours after injection, obtain 24-hour delays if requested (advisable because of reduced target to background ratios, especially for questionable areas or suspect normal bowel activity).
- Acquire statics: 10 minutes (600 seconds) per view; anterior/posterior; pelvis, abdomen, chest. Static views often provide the best diagnostic pictures.
- Acquire whole-body sweep: 30 minutes (1800 seconds) or greater, anterior/posterior, at least head to mid-thigh.
- Acquire SPECT if requested. Center area(s) or suspected area(s) of interest. Processing: slice thickness to 2 mm. Using a low-pass filter, e.g., Butterworth, 0.4 Nyquist cutoff, and order 7 (or 0.5/5 order) has produced acceptable images.

Normal Results

- Activity in liver, spleen, bone marrow, and blood pool (heart and vessels).
- Activity in kidneys, bladder, male genitalia, and female nipples.
- Activity in gallbladder and intestines.
- Bowel activity may be present because of radiotracer in stool (ask patient if they bowel-cleansed the night before).
- 24-hour delay: activity in liver, gallbladder, spleen, kidneys, bladder, heart, and some major vessels.
- Background diminished and diffuse.

Abnormal Results

- Focal areas of increased extrahepatic uptake (equal to liver) in tumors.
- Focal areas of increased activity that remain persistent and stationary over time with delayed images, particularly over lymph nodes and/or organ of interest.
- Large lesions may present as cold spots and remain cold because of poor vascularization or central necrosis.

Artifacts

- Watch patient for allergic reaction, e.g., anaphylactic shock, nausea, redness or rash at injection site, bursitis, headache, itching, upset stomach, fever, and, if blood tests are run, transient eosinophilia.
- Patient motion will blur image, perhaps obscuring site.

SUGGESTED READINGS

Datz FL. Handbook of Nuclear Medicine. 2nd ed. St. Louis: Mosby, 1993.

Early PJ, Sodee DB. Principles and Practice of Nuclear Medicine. 2nd ed. St. Louis: Mosby, 1995.

Murray IPC, Ell PJ, eds. Nuclear Medicine in Clinical Diagnosis and Treatment. Vols. 1 and 2. New York: Churchill Livingstone, 1994.

Wilson, MA. Textbook of Nuclear Medicine. Philadelphia: Lippincott-Raven, 1998.

CEA-Scan® is a registered trademark of Immunomedics, Inc., Morris Plains, NJ.

Notes

CHAPTER 15

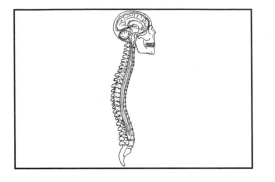

Cisternography

Radiopharmacy

Radionuclide

- ^{111}In t$_{1/2}$: 2.8 days

  Energies: 173, 247 keV

  Type: EC, γ, accelerator

- ^{99m}Tc t$_{1/2}$: 6 hours

  Energies: 140 keV

  Type: IT, γ, generator

Radiopharmaceutical

- ^{111}In-DTPA (diethylenetriaminepentaacetic acid)
- ^{99m}Tc-DTPA (diethylenetriaminepentaacetic acid)

Localization

- Compartmental, cerebrospinal fluid

Quality Control

- Test for radiochemical purity, chromatography for DTPA tag

Adult Dose Range

- ^{111}In: 0.5–1.5 mCi (18.5–55.5 MBq)
- ^{99m}Tc: 0.4–12 mCi (14.8–444 MBq) depending on scan

Method of Administration

- Spinal needle, intrathecal injection (slowly into the subarachnoid space of lumbar spine, usually performed by radiologist).

Indications

- Evaluation of cerebrospinal fluid (CSF) flow in the spinal column and brain.
- Detection of CSF leak (rhinorrhea or otorrhea).
- Evaluation for normal-pressure hydrocephalus. Patients should have clinical evidence of dementia, dyspraxia (disturbance in programming, control, and execution of conscious movement), and incontinence.
- Evaluation and detection of ventriculoperitoneal or ventriculoatrial shunt obstruction or patency.
- Evaluation of dispersal of intrathecally injected chemotherapy (Ommaya shunt)

Contraindications

- None

Patient History

The patient or caretaker should answer the following questions.

Do you have a history of hydrocephalus?	Y	N
Have you had any seizures?	Y	N
Do you have urinary incontinence?	Y	N
Do you have balance problems?	Y	N
Do you have memory problems?	Y	N
Do you feel any head pressure or pain?	Y	N
Do you have a shunt or have you had any other neurologic procedures?	Y	N
Do you have any ear or nasal discharge?	Y	N
Have you had any other related tests?	Y	N
Do you have a history or family history of cancer?	Y	N

If so, what type and since when?

_____

Other department-specific questions.
_____

Patient Preparation

- Identify the patient. Verify doctor's order. Explain the procedure.
- Obtain a signed consent from patient.
- Prepare patient for spinal injection by physician.
- Instruct patient to remain horizontal for 2 hours after injection to minimize headache from CSF leakage.

Equipment

Camera

- Large field of view

Collimator

- ^{111}In: medium energy, parallel hole
- ^{99m}Tc: low energy, all purpose, or low energy, high resolution

Computer Set-up
Statics

- 50,000–200,000 counts each

Procedure *(time: ~30 minutes each set of images)*

- Patient is injected by a physician with patient in left or right lateral decubitus or Sims' position.
- Position patient supine with camera anterior (generally). To image the injection site if extravasation is suspected, place patient in a lateral decubitus, Sims', or prone position. Obtain an image at injection site at 5–30 minutes after injection.
- Obtain images for study within 1–2 hours after injection.
- Obtain images of anterior head, and lateral and vertex views. Other views can include posterior images of the spinal column and skull. Optional: turn patient prone for lumbar spine images.
- Obtain repeat delayed images at 4, 24, 48, and 72 hours according to protocol.
- Obtain image of injection site if there is little or no activity in cranium at 2 hours after injection. This is to confirm injection extravasation, at which time, if confirmed, the study may be terminated.
- Obtain delayed anterior abdominal images (particularly at 48 and 72 hours after injection) to detect and/or confirm progress of CSF for shunt patency. Some use 10 mCi (370 MBq) ^{99m}Tc-DTPA.

- CSF leaks (otorrhea and rhinorrhea)

    - Pledgets (cotton, 1.5 × 1.5 cm) bilaterally inserted by otolaryngologist (ENT) either before injection or within an hour after. Some use 10 mCi (370 MBq) ^{99m}Tc-DTPA. Suggested placements are at both cribriform plates, at each sphenoethmoid recess under the middle turbinate, and one in the buccal mucosa (underside of tongue) for a control (counted to use for background).

    - Image injection site shortly after injection to confirm success. Place patient with head flexed forward and downward or in position known to exacerbate leakage. Image skull (anterior and laterals) at 2, 4, and 6 hours.

    - Remove pledgets after 6 hours; place in separate, labeled, preweighed tubes; separately weigh (subtract tube weight); and count in a well counter. Count all tubes the same amount of time, up to 10 minutes each.

    - Draw enough blood at this time so that after centrifuging, there is 0.5 mL of serum. Count the serum (with the buccal mucosa pledget, this is also used for background). Count for same amount of time as others.

    - If a leak is suspected, 24-hour images can be performed with or without new pledget placement and counting.

    - Posterior images should be added if a leak presents in other images.

Normal Results

- Activity appears in basal cisterns by 3 hours after injection, then enters interhemispheric and sylvian fissures forming Neptune's triumvirate or "Viking helmet."

- Flow over convexities by 24 hours.

- No reflux into ventricles is seen, although transient reflux at 12–24 hours not considered of significance.

- Shunt patency, e.g., to the abdomen, will show an area of increased activity particularly on the side of the shunt and more identifiable in 48- and 72-hour delays as there is an increase in target to background ratio and more time for movement to that area. Some studies use ^{99m}Tc-DTPA.

- Leakage (otorrhea or rhinorrhea): less than three times background (buccal mucosa pledget and/or serum counts).

Abnormal Results

- Persistence of activity in lateral ventricles is abnormal.

- Hydrocephalus: increase in CSF volume caused by overproduction, decreased absorption, blockage of flow, or cerebral atrophy.

- Nonobstructive: cerebral atrophy.

- Obstructive: caused by obstruction of outflow from

    1. Noncommunicating hydrocephalus caused by blockage of CSF motion.

    2. Communicating obstructive hydrocephalus caused by extraventricular blockage, e.g., cisterns or villi.

- Normal-pressure hydrocephalus (look for dementia, gait disorder, urinary incontinence); ventricle reflux that persists on 24-, 48-, and perhaps 72-hour images; delayed or lack of flow to convexities.

- Shunt patency: activity not reaching the vascular system or peritoneal cavity.
- Porencephalic cysts (meninges dilated), rhinorrhea (leaking out of meninges through nose), otorrhea (leaking out of ears).
- For leakage (otorrhea or rhinorrhea), it is considered significant leakage and positive if the activity is three to four times that of background (serum or buccal mucosa); the leak should have corroborating images. The pledgets should help localize the leak.

Artifacts

- Injection into spinal fluid is difficult and often missed.
- Patient motion to a minimum.
- Necklaces, metal plates in head, or metal glasses may give artifacts.
- Correct collimator, peaks, and windows must be used.

Note

CSF leak can be performed with 8–12 mCi (296–444 MBq) with ^{99m}Tc-DTPA. Intrathecal injection followed by 15–20 mL of fresh nonbacteriostatic sterile saline to accelerate time of study by quickly moving activity into region of suspected leak. Pledgets placed in area of suspected leak, removed, weighed, and counted at 5 hours after injection.

Shunt patency can be performed with 0.4–0.8 mCi (14.8–29.6 MBq) ^{99m}Tc-DTPA in 0.3–0.5 mL. Needle is inserted into shunt reservoir by physician. With needle in place, position patient for best view. Start camera, inject tracer. Take 2-minute immediate view, 2-minute orthogonal (oblique to first image) view, 2-minute thorax view, and 2-minute abdominal view. Repeat series at 20 minutes and 2–6 hours.

SUGGESTED READINGS

Datz FL. Handbook of Nuclear Medicine. 2nd ed. St. Louis: Mosby, 1993.

Early PJ, Sodee DB. Principles and Practice of Nuclear Medicine. 2nd ed. St. Louis: Mosby, 1995.

Murray IPC, Ell PJ, eds. Nuclear Medicine in Clinical Diagnosis and Treatment. Vols. 1 and 2. New York: Churchill Livingstone, 1994.

Wilson, MA. Textbook of Nuclear Medicine. Philadelphia: Lippincott-Raven, 1998.

Notes

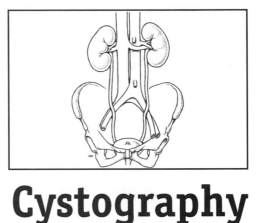

CHAPTER 16

Cystography

(Voiding Cystourethrogram): Direct and Indirect

Radiopharmacy

Radionuclide

- ^{99m}Tc t$_{1/2}$: 6 hours

  Energies: 140 keV

  Type: IT, γ, generator, or

- ^{131}I t$_{1/2}$: 8.1 days

  Energies: 364 keV

  Type: β^-, γ, fission product

Radiopharmaceutical

- Na ^{99m}TcO$_4^-$ (pertechnetate), ^{99m}Tc-SC (sulfur colloid), Microlite® (albumin colloid, temporarily off the market), ^{99m}Tc-DTPA (diethylenetriaminepentaacetic acid), ^{99m}Tc-MAG$_3$® (mercaptoacetyltriglycine), ^{131}I-OIH (orthoiodohippurate)

Localization

- Direct: compartmental, flows with saline and urine
- Indirect: compartmental, blood (bound to protein and some red blood cells)

Quality Control

- ^{99m}Tc: chromatography; ^{99m}Tc-SC, > 90%; particle size, < 1 µm; Microlite®: > 92% tagging. Use either within 6 hours. DTPA, > 90%, use within 1 hour.
- ^{131}I: chemical purity test for ^{131}I iodide (< 1.5%) and ^{131}I orthoiodobenzoic acid; radionuclide purity for anything other than ^{131}I, spectrometer test for tracer tag.

Adult Dose Range

- Direct: ^{99m}Tc, 1 mCi (37 MBq)
- Indirect: ^{99m}Tc, 3–10 mCi (111–370 MBq); ^{131}I, 150–300 µCi (5.55–11.1MBq)

Method of Administration

- Indirect: IV injection
- Direct: injection into Foley catheter by injection port or needle puncture of tube

Indications

- Evaluation and detection of vesicoureteral reflux.
- Evaluation of management and continuing assessment of patients with reflux.
- Evaluation for surgical intervention or other to prevent subsequent impairment of renal function.

Contraindications

- Indirect method not recommended in patients with known significant renal dysfunction.

Patient History

The patient should answer the following questions.

Do you have a history of or family history of renal obstruction or disease?	Y	N
Do you have a history of or family history of cancer?	Y	N
Do you have a history of ureter, bladder, or urethra infections or obstructions?	Y	N
Do you have any pain or problems with micturition?	Y	N

Other department-specific questions.

Patient Preparation

- Identify the patient. Verify doctor's order. Explain the procedure.
- Patients are usually children and require special attention to relieve apprehension. Most institutions require a consent to do the procedure.
- Instruct patient to void completely just before exam.
- Catheterize patient for direct cystography (see note).

Equipment

Camera

- Large field of view

Collimator

- Low energy, all purpose, or low energy, high sensitivity

Computer Set-up

Direct

- Flow: 1 or 2 sec/frame for 30 seconds to 1 minute during filling and voiding segments.
- Statics: 120-second images, bladder at full capacity and after voiding.

Indirect

- Flow and static images during void and after voiding.

Procedure *(time: ~45 minutes)*

Direct

- Usually with $^{99m}TcO_4^-$, ^{99m}Tc-SC, or ^{99m}Tc-DTPA.
- Cover camera and table area with disposable pads ("chucks") to absorb leakage or contamination.
- Hang 50–1500 mL (depending on size of patient) normal saline (tubing clamped) for gravity-feed infusion (no higher than 100 cm above table).
- For pediatric patients (normal ~250 mL): expected bladder capacity (oz) = age (in years) + 2 (30 mL = 1 oz).
- Note amount at start and finish.
- Position catheterized patient supine with camera posterior (or patient sitting with back and pelvis against camera), the dome of the bladder in lower field of view (FOV), kidneys in upper. This can be done before imaging if radiotracer is injected into catheter before filling starts, or "eyeball" position if radiotracer is to be injected after patency is established and while filling.
- Start camera for flow; fill bladder completely with radiotracer/saline mixture (this is usually verified by patient's urgency to micturate, leakage around the catheter, or cessation of flow into bladder).
- Monitor p-scope closely for signs of reflux. If reflux (activity just above bladder) is visualized, record amount of saline infused at time (see Note).
- When bladder is full, stop flow images and take 120-second immediate static of posterior and left and right posterior oblique images. Record the amount of saline used to fill bladder and the count rate (cpm) during posterior view.
- Instruct patient to resist the urge to micturate.
- Some remove catheter at this point, others do not. Position patient sitting, camera behind, or lateral decubitus, camera behind.
- Start second flow study, instruct patient to void into empty urinal or bedpan. Some take only a static while patient voids.
- Take a 120-second immediate postvoid posterior static. Record count rate (cpm).

- Measure and determine volume (in mL) voided by patient.
- To determine bladder retention (mL)

$$\frac{\text{Postvoid cpm} \times \text{vol. of voided urine (mL)}}{\text{(Prevoid cpm} - \text{Postvoid cpm)}} = \text{Bladder retention}$$

- Review images for signs of reflux.

Indirect

- Usually with ^{99m}Tc-DTPA, ^{131}I-OIH, or ^{99m}Tc-MAG$_3$®
- Patient is injected and must not void for 2 hours.
- At 2 hours after injection, when the radiotracer has cleared the kidneys and filled the bladder, the patient is positioned sitting with back and pelvis toward camera, bladder and kidneys in FOV, and told to void.
- Obtain dynamic images as patient voids.
- Obtain statics (120 seconds) when completely voided.
- Carefully monitor p-scope when patient is voiding for reflux.

Normal Results

- No visualization of reflux of solution and tracer past bladder during filling and/or voiding. (Normal valve action at ureterovesical junction depends on oblique entry of ureter into bladder, adequate length of intramural ureter, contraction of ureterotrigonal muscles, and active ureteral peristalsis.)
- All or nearly all solution is voided from bladder.

Abnormal Results

- Significant activity in upper urinary tracts during filling, at full capacity, and/or while voiding. This will visualize as a spot or elongated activity in one or both of the ureters just above the bladder.
- Reflux is associated with causing urinary tract infections (UTIs), particularly in pediatric patients. Reflux usually resolves itself. Reflux is potentially damaging to the kidneys.
- Reflux nephropathy usually develops in infancy or early childhood; low-grade reflux more likely to resolve than high-grade reflux.
- Bacterial infection of the kidney(s) may present with fever, leukocytosis, and bacteremia. Bacterial nephritis may present with only fever and leukocytosis. This test could help distinguish between lower and the more serious upper tract urinary infections.

Artifacts

- Recent contrast radiographic studies may interfere with results.
- Contamination of area by infusion leakage, etc.
- Indirect method: Reflux may be missed during filling phase, which is not imaged. Kidneys may retain radiotracer. Patient may not be able to hold contents of bladder for 2 hours until imaging or void on command.

Note
· · · · · · ·

Suggested Catheterization

- Boys under 1 year old, number 5-8 infant feeding tube.

- 1-3 years old, number 8 Foley catheter.

- 3 years and older boys, number 8 Foley catheter or greater.

- Girls under 1 year old, number 8 Foley catheter.

- 1-3 years old, number 10 Foley catheter.

- 3 years and older girls, number 12 Foley catheter.

Bladder volume at reflux helps predict which patients may experience spontaneous resolution of the problem. Children who have progressively larger volumes at reflux on follow-up studies tend to resolve the reflux naturally with no surgery.

SUGGESTED READINGS

Datz FL. Handbook of Nuclear Medicine. 2nd ed. St. Louis: Mosby, 1993.

Early PJ, Sodee DB. Principles and Practice of Nuclear Medicine. 2nd ed. St. Louis: Mosby, 1995.

Murray IPC, Ell PJ, eds. Nuclear Medicine in Clinical Diagnosis and Treatment. Vols. 1 and 2. New York: Churchill Livingstone, 1994.

Wilson, MA. Textbook of Nuclear Medicine. Philadelphia: Lippincott-Raven, 1998.

MAG$_3$® is a registered trademark of Mallinckrodt Medical, Inc., St. Louis, MO.
Microlite® is a registered trademark of DuPont Merck, Wilmington, DE.

Notes
· · · · · · ·

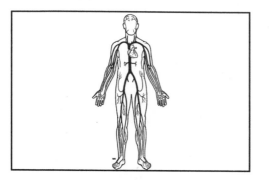

CHAPTER 17

DVT: AcuTect™

(Deep Venous Thrombosis)

Radiopharmacy

Radionuclide

- ^{99m}Tc $t_{1/2}$: 6 hours

  Energies: 140 keV

  Type: IT, γ, generator

Radiopharmaceutical

- ^{99m}Tc-apcitide (AcuTect™), a synthetic peptide

Localization

- Compartmental, blood flow. AcuTect™ binds to the glycoprotein GpIIb/IIIa ($\alpha_2\beta_3$) adhesion-molecule receptors (of the integrin family) found on activated platelets. During thrombus formation, platelets receive signals causing activation and subsequent aggregation. Platelet aggregation is dependent on the GPIIb/IIIa receptors expressed on these activated platelets. The peptide binds less avidly to the β_3 chain of the vitronectin receptor found on endothelial cells.

Quality Control

- Chromatography, ≥ 90% chemical tag

Adult Dose Range

- 20 mCi (740 MBq)

Method of Administration

- IV, butterfly, or venous catheter with flush in an upper extremity

Indications

- Detection and localization of acute venous thrombosis in the lower extremities.
- Differentiation of acute venous thrombosis from chronic venous thrombosis or postphlebitic syndrome.
- Assessment of patients with a probable suggestion of DVT and a negative Doppler ultrasound.

Contraindications

- None known

Patient History

The patient should answer the following questions.

Do you have a history or family history of cancer?	Y	N
If so, what type and for how long?		
Do you have any of the following symptoms in your extremities: edema or swelling, warmth, redness, and pain?	Y	N
If so, for how long?		
Do you have a history of deep vein thrombosis (DVT)?	Y	N
Is there a family history of DVT?	Y	N
Have you had any recent pelvic, hip, or knee operations?	Y	N
Have you had any recent trauma or fractures?	Y	N
Do you have cellulitis or arthritis?	Y	N

Do you have a history of phlebitis?	Y	N
Do you have varicose veins?	Y	N
Do you have a history of congestive heart failure?	Y	N
Have you had other tests, e.g., ultrasound, D-dimer test, contrast venography?	Y	N
If so, what type, where, and when?		
Have you been on any recent long trips or remained in the same position for extended periods of time?	Y	N
Are you on estrogen therapy?	Y	N
Other department-specific questions.		

Patient Preparation

- Identify the patient. Verify doctor's order. Explain the procedure.
- Remove tight clothing, stockings, or lower extremity vascular compression devices (with the exception of a cast, which should be noted).
- Instruct patient to hydrate well unless contraindicated and to void often.
- Instruct patient to void just before examination and to do so before each imaging session.

Equipment

Camera
- Large field of view

Collimator
- Low energy, all purpose, or low energy, high resolution

Computer Set-up
- 128 × 128 matrix, 15–20% window

Statics
- Pelvis: 750,000 counts or 300 sec/image
- Extremities: 500,000 counts or 300 sec/image

Procedure *(time: 20-40 min/session)*

- Instruct patient to void (before each set of images).
- Administer injection to patient. Wait 10 minutes to image.
- Position patient supine on table.
- Position camera anterior from pelvis to thighs (from the lower edge of the bladder to just above the knees), or anterior/posterior dual head.

  Note: Patient positioning is important.

  - Ensure limbs are straight, symmetrically positioned, and flat to bed (no knee cushion) with feet bound together so that legs are not rotated.
  - Ensure urinary catheters drain freely and are out of the field of view (FOV).
  - Shield the bladder.
  - Mark the right side of all views.
  - Ensure patient comfort and remind patient of no movement during acquisitions.
  - This is performed on all sets of imaging. Patient alignment is maintained for all sets of imaging.
- Obtain image at 10 minutes for 300 seconds or 750,000 counts.
- Reposition camera mid-thigh to mid-calf.
- Obtain image for 300 seconds or 500,000 counts.
- Reposition camera knees to ankles.
- Obtain image for 300 seconds or 500,000 counts.
- If using a single-head camera, image same series in posterior projection.
- Repeat same sequence of images at 60-90 minutes after injection. Ensure patient positioning is the same as early images. Remind patient of no motion during acquisitions.
- Repeat same sequence of images at 120 minutes after injection if requested.
- Images may be repeated up to 180 minutes as requested, without repeat injection.

Normal Results

- Lower extremities show symmetric (right/left) uptake in the deep and superficial veins.
- Symmetric and low soft tissue uptake.
- Bilaterally symmetric limb sizes.
- A "halo" of uptake may present in the soft tissue of the knees.
- Persistent intensity in a popliteal vein compared with the immediately proximal and distal segments of the same vein.
- Bladder uptake, bowel uptake especially in the delayed images.

Abnormal Results

- Acute DVT presents as an asymmetric linear uptake in a deep vein segment (greater uptake than is observed in the corresponding contralateral deep vein segment) that persists, or becomes apparent on delayed images. It will present as increased uptake after the course of a deep vein.

- Asymmetric vascular linear uptake (with or without superimposed diffuse uptake) in both anterior and posterior projections of one or both lower extremities.

- If asymmetry presents only after extreme contrast enhancement by computer manipulation, then diffuse asymmetry must also be present for scoring an image as positive.

Artifacts

- Repeat views if patient moves.

- Superficial increased uptake is not to be interpreted as acute DVT.

- Varicose veins will contribute to superficial uptake.

- Cellulitis or arthritis will contribute to soft tissue tracer uptake.

- Postsurgical uptake may present a false-positive result.

- The best candidates for this study are patients with the clinical indicators for acute DVT.

- The study may be most useful when used in conjunction with correlative clinical information and other modalities, e.g., contrast venography, duplex ultrasonography, or impedance plethysmography (IPG).

- Any patient with a history of drug reactions, allergies, or immune system disorders should be observed for up to several hours after injection.

Processing

- The use of image contrast and intensity is a must to visualize veins.

- The use of color scale may facilitate visualization.

- Images for each session should be shown in the same pattern and orientation for comparison.

Note

AcuTect™ is a peptide, not an antibody, and hence will not illicit the HAMA reaction. Acu-Tect™ appears to detect acute and not chronic venous thrombosis (from animal data, not confirmed clinically), whereas venography detects the presence of any clot. Agreement between venography and AcuTect™ of 100% is not expected. The manufacturer suggests that with patients who show signs and symptoms of acute venous thrombosis, a clinical management decision to withhold treatment with anticoagulants should not be based on a negative AcuTect™ study alone.

SUGGESTED READINGS

AcuTect™ Image Atlas. Londonderry, NH: Diatide, Inc., 1998.
Wilson, MA. Textbook of Nuclear Medicine. Philadelphia: Lippincott-Raven, 1998.

AcuTect™ is a trademark of Diatide, Inc., Londonderry, NH.

Notes

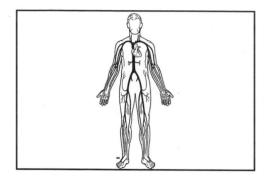

CHAPTER 18

DVT: Venography

(Deep Venous Thrombosis)

Radiopharmacy

Radionuclide

- ^{99m}Tc $t_{1/2}$: 6 hours

  Energies: 140 keV

  Type: IT, γ, generator

Radiopharmaceutical

- ^{99m}Tc-MAA (macroaggregated albumin). Tagged red blood cells by pyrophosphate or stannous chloride to ^{99m}TcO$_4^-$ (pertechnatate) by in vivo, in vitro, or kit, e.g., UltraTag®.

Localization

- Compartmental to blood supply

Quality Control

- ^{99m}Tc-MAA: chromatography; 90–95% tagging
- ^{99m}TcO$_4^-$: chromatography; tagging; 90% in vivo, 95% in vitro

Adult Dose Range

- ^{9m}Tc-MAA: total of 6 mCi (222 MBq)
- ^{99m}TcO$_4^-$: 20–50 mCi (740–1850 MBq)

Method of Administration

- ^{99m}Tc-MAA: IV using butterfly needles in a dorsal vein of each foot; 3 mCi (111 MBq) in each of two syringes brought up to 3 mL with normal saline.
- ^{99m}TcO$_4^-$: IV injections, or drawing, tagging, and reinjection of tagged red blood cells.

Indications

- Evaluation of deep venous thrombosis (DVT), especially with patients who do not tolerate radiographic contrast material.
- Evaluation of acute-onset symptoms in patients who have had no prior DVT (acute versus chronic or old).

Contraindications

- Should not be performed on patients with pulmonary hypertension.

Patient History

The patient should answer the following questions.

Do you have a history or family history of cancer?	Y	N
If so, what type and for how long?		
Do you have a history of deep venous thrombosis?	Y	N
Do you have phlebitis or other leg problems?	Y	N
Have you had any recent operations?	Y	N
If so, what type and when?		
Do you have any leg pain or swelling?	Y	N
If so, where and for how long?		
Do you have any chest pain?	Y	N

Have you been coughing up any blood?	Y	N
Have you been short of breath?	Y	N
Are you taking blood thinners?	Y	N
Have you recently remained lying or seated for a long time, as in a hospital stay or long trip?	Y	N
Are there any planned or recent related examinations?	Y	N

If so, what and when, and do you have
the results with you?

Other department-specific questions.

Patient Preparation

- Identify the patient. Verify doctor's order. Explain the procedure.
- Instruct patient to bring all results of previous related examinations.
- Ensure leg(s) are horizontal if DVTs are already known or highly suspected.

Equipment

Camera

- Large field of view

Collimator

- Low energy, all purpose, or low energy, high resolution

Computer Set-up
Flow

- 60 frames at 1 sec/frame

Statics

- 30 seconds per image. Delays: 1,000,000 counts

Whole Body

- Variable cm/min, toe to abdomen. Delayed head to toe optional.

Procedure *(time: ~30 minutes)*

- Position patient supine on table.
- IV setup: for A and B.
  - Insert 23- to 25-gauge butterfly needles, one in each foot, into a dorsal vein.
  - Attach three-way stopcocks to tubing.
  - Attach 10-mL syringes of saline flush to each stopcock.
  - Attach two doses to stopcocks.

Procedure A: Statics

- Position camera anterior (and posterior, dual head) over knees and tibia/fibula.
- Inject 1 mL (containing 1 mCi) from each syringe.
- Obtain a 30-second image.
- Reposition camera to thighs.
- Inject another 1 mL from each syringe.
- Obtain a 30-second image.
- Reposition camera to pelvis/lower abdomen.
- Inject last 1 mL from each syringe.
- Obtain a 30-second image.
- Remove butterfly catheters, and, if patient is not already believed to have DVTs, allow patient to walk around for several minutes.
- Reposition patient and camera.
- Obtain delays in same sequence for same amount of time as initial images.

Procedure B: Whole Body

- Set camera to run at 64 cm/min and to cover from feet to mid-abdomen (about 130 cm).
- Apply tourniquets at both ankles and just below both knees (this forces radiotracer to seek deep venous routes up the legs).
- Start camera. Inject all of both doses and flush both (there is always a short delay after the camera is started before it actually begins imaging).
- When the camera reaches the knees, reduce the speed of the camera to 48 cm/min.
- Reduce the speed again, to 16 cm/min, when it reaches the pelvis/abdomen.
- Remove tourniquets when imaging is complete.
- Obtain a 1,000,000-count anterior image of the lungs while patient exercises lower extremities.
- Repeat the whole-body scan of legs at 120 cm/min.
- Optional lung perfusion study can be performed after venography. If both a ventilation and perfusion is indicated, ventilation should be performed before venography.

Procedure C: Tagged Red Blood Cell Study, No Dorsal Vein Injections

- Patient must sign consent form to take and return blood. It must also be signed by technologist and witness.

- Introduce a large-bore venous catheter.
- In vitro method: Extract ~2–2.5 mL of blood into heparinized syringe from patient and follow instructions to tag with UltraTag®. Inject under camera for flow.
- In vivo method: Inject cold pyrophosphate, then 20 minutes later, inject radiotracer under camera for flow.
- Modified in vivo method: Inject cold pyrophosphate and wait 20 minutes. Extract ~2–2.5 mL of blood into a heparinized shielded syringe containing ~30 mCi of $^{99m}TcO_4^-$. Mix for 5–10 minutes. Reinject under camera for flow.
- Position patient under camera with camera set up for flow. Field of view should be lower extremity including area having pain, inflammation, or redness.
- Depending on method of tagging, at proper time, inject $^{99m}TcO_4^-$ or tagged blood, wait 8 seconds, then start camera for flow.
- Obtain static images of 1,000,000 counts each of anterior/posterior femoral, popliteals, calves, and feet immediately after flow.
- Optional: Obtain whole-body anterior/posterior pelvis to feet at 15–20 cm/min.

Normal Results

Flow

- Veins appear with a cellular flush that dissipates with time.

Statics and Whole Body

- Deep veins and collateral circulation should present clearly, smoothly, well defined, and with bilaterally even uptake.

Abnormal Results

Flow

- Higher uptake in tissue and collateral circulation in area(s) of swelling or inflammation.
- Late and asymmetric arrival of activity on one side of the deep venous system. This is useful only if postphlebitic syndrome and deep or superficial varicose veins have been excluded. Soft-tissue induration, inflammation, and edema can also result in uneven arrival of radiotracer.

Statics and Whole Body

- Absence of blood flow (e.g., nonvisualization of a major vein) beyond a point in affected leg (segmental or total). May or may not be associated with the presence of whorled or medusa-like collaterals. Occlusions at the iliac levels are associated with rich collateral formations; popliteal levels are associated with a paucity or absence of collaterals.
- Larger uptake than usual in a localized area of vein as opposed to nonaffected leg in that area (a hot spot). Some consider the hot spot a reliable sign of acute DVT if they are segmental rather than focal, there is a smudgy backdrop, and they present with a network of collaterals.
- More collateral uptake in affected leg in edematous areas.
- Thrombi are not directly visualized. Decreased flow in the venous system or the

obstruction to the deep venous system is apparent and comparable to radiographic venography.

- Venography cannot distinguish between acute (newly formed) and chronic DVT. The newer scan with AcuTect™, included in this manual, is showing promise.

Other Methods

- MRI—can image all important venous channels, even proximal upper limb veins. Cost and availability is restrictive.

- CT—detection in complicated cases involving abdomen or pelvis should be considered; can be used in limbs, generally superior to conventional contrast venography for proximal disease.

- Ultrasonography (US)—duplex, triplex, or color Doppler ultrasonography is now the gold standard for initial screening. Real-time imaging with color Doppler produces a color map of flow within the vessels. Compressibility of a deep vein is one of the most sensitive and specific criteria for Doppler detection of DVT, although the method detected only a low percentage of actual DVTs in patients showing pulmonary emboli by angiography. For patients with prior DVTs or postphlebitic syndrome, other tests are needed to improve the diagnostic accuracy.

- Plethysmography—measures the capacity of the venous system to fill and empty. Best used in symptomatic patients with no prior history of DVT. Not reliable in patients with prior DVT, cord injuries, strokes, arterial vascular insufficiency, impaired venous return from right heart failure, or external compression of veins, and varies greatly with patient population types.

- ^{125}I-fibrinogen—poor results above mid-thigh because of bladder uptake and larger adjacent blood vessels. Fibrinogen is a part of clot formation. Radiolabeled fibrinogen incorporates into a freshly formed clot and is detected with hand-held scintillation detector. Injections of 100 μCi are used, and counts of the lower extremities are taken twice a day for 7 days.

- ^{111}In-platelets—sensitive and specific for active DVT. It requires 18- to 24-hour delayed imaging for diagnostic results, particularly with those patients having venous stasis or low-grade thrombosis. Many false-negative results with patients receiving heparin or warfarin therapy. False-positive results are also seen from venous trauma, venipuncture, or persistent asymmetric increased blood pool activity in popliteal or inguinal regions.

- ^{99m}Tc-hexamethylpropyleneamine oxime-platelets—perhaps a useful alternative to the expense and time consumption of indium-oxine.

- ^{99m}Tc-T$_2$G$_1$ antifibrin—2- to 4-minute images of immediate up to 6 hours is an advantage localizing at sites of active thrombus formation in patients receiving anticoagulants. Dissociation and lysis of labeled antibody from the clot, poor binding to chronic thrombi, and cost limit use.

Artifacts

- MAA can trap behind a venous valve presenting a false-positive result.

- The ipsilateral saphenous vein, a main collateral, can easily be mistaken for an occluded main vein.

- DVT may appear to be the diagnosis in extraluminal causes, e.g., non-Hodgkin's lymphoma.

Note

The lower extremities hold the majority of the blood volume. The large deep venous system includes the iliacs, femorals, popliteals, and saphenous veins along with the smaller deep venous system of the calf.

Even in the absence of clinical suggestion of pulmonary emboli (PE), 35–51% of patients with clots detected above the knee have evidence of pulmonary emboli. All lower limb thrombi do not pose the same threat. Most clots arise in the soleal sinuses of the calf or near a venous valve, and 20–45% propagate to the iliofemoral veins which greatly enhances the possibility of pulmonary emboli. Pulmonary embolism is not the only medical concern. There is high correlation between distal vein (popliteal and below the knee) DVT and postphlebitic syndrome, skin pigmentation, and leg ulcers.

SUGGESTED READINGS

Early PJ, Sodee DB. Principles and Practice of Nuclear Medicine. 2nd ed. St. Louis: Mosby, 1995.

Murray IPC, Ell PJ, eds. Nuclear Medicine in Clinical Diagnosis and Treatment. Vols. 1 and 2. New York: Churchill Livingstone, 1994.

Wilson, MA. Textbook of Nuclear Medicine. Philadelphia: Lippincott-Raven, 1998.

AcuTect™ is a trademark of Diatide, Inc., Londonderry, NH.
UltraTag® is a registered trademark of Mallinckrodt Medical, Inc., St. Louis, MO.

Notes

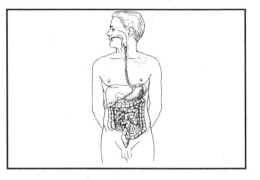

Esophageal Transit Time

Radiopharmacy

Radionuclide

- ^{99m}Tc $t_{1/2}$: 6 hours

  Energies: 140 keV

  Type: IT, γ, generator

Radiopharmaceutical

- ^{99m}Tc-SC (sulfur colloid)

Localization

- Compartmental; esophagus to gastrointestinal tract

Quality Control

- Chromatography, > 90%; particle size, < 1 μm

Adult Dose Range

- 150–300 μCi (5.55–11.1 MBq)

Method of Administration

- PO in 15 mL of water, one bolus swallow.
- Alternative: PO using 1.35 mCi (50 MBq) of ^{99m}Tc-SC in 50 mL of apple sauce.

Indications

- Evaluation of esophageal sphincter dysfunction.
- Evaluation of dysphagia and decreased esophageal motility attributed to achalasia (delay in peristalsis and marked esophageal retention), strictures, obstruction, retention, scleroderma, diffuse esophageal spasm (multiple uncoordinated peaks), or hiatal hernia.

- Evaluation of patients who cannot tolerate manometry or with equivocal or negative manometry results having reasonable suggestion of disease.
- Evaluation of clinical management by monitoring for serial changes or response to therapy.
- Evaluation of esophageal dysmotility in systemic sclerosis and Raynaud's phenomenon (episodic digital ischemia manifested by development of digital blanching, cyanosis, and rubor of the fingers or toes after cold exposure and subsequent rewarming). It is classified as primary (occurring in an otherwise healthy subject) or secondary (associated with a disease process, e.g., connective tissue disease such as systemic sclerosis; fibroblast proliferation, and collagen deposition frequently with esophageal involvement).

Contraindications

- None

Patient History

The patient should answer the following questions.

Do you have a history or family history of cancer?	Y	N
If so, what type and for how long?		
Do you have a history of esophageal motility dysfunction?	Y	N
Do you have trouble swallowing?	Y	N
Do you have any pain when swallowing?	Y	N
Do you feel that you must swallow many times to get food down?	Y	N
Do you have any abdominal pain?	Y	N
Do you have a history of Raynaud's phenomenon?	Y	N

Do you have a history of systemic sclerosis?	Y	N
Do you have a history of reflux esophagitis?	Y	N
Is there a recent or planned esophageal manometry study?	Y	N
Other department-specific questions.		

Patient Preparation

- Identify the patient. Verify doctor's order. Explain the procedure.
- Ensure patient has fasted for 8 hours or overnight.
- Instruct patient as to cooperation with swallowing.

Equipment

Camera
- Large field of view

Collimator
- Low energy, all purpose, or low energy, high sensitivity

Computer Set-up
Flow
- .25 sec/15 sec for 1 minute

  Or 1–2 sec/frame for 1 minute

Dynamic
- 15 sec/frame for 9 minutes

Procedure *(time: ~30 minutes)*

- Patient supine, camera anterior over thorax, mouth to stomach.
- Patient draws dose into mouth with straw and holds.
- On command, patient swallows once in a single bolus; camera is started.
- Patient dry-swallows once every 15 seconds for 10 minutes.
- For processing
  - Regions of interest (ROIs) are drawn around bolus dose, then entire esophagus, to calculate remaining activity at various times.
  - ROIs can be drawn around upper, middle, and lower regions of esophagus to evaluate regional esophageal dysfunction.

$$\% \text{ remaining esophageal activity} = \frac{A - B}{A} \times 100$$

where *A* is total activity of bolus dose, and *B* is activity of bolus during any one image.

Normal Results

- Low count rates or none detectable 5-10 seconds after first swallow.
- Transit rates > 90% after one to eight swallows.
- < 4% of the maximal activity in esophagus by 10 minutes.

Abnormal Results

- Transit rates 5-40% after eight swallows.
- Diffuse esophageal spasm has significantly reduced transit rate for first half of study, then normal after 20 swallows.

Artifacts

- Inability to swallow or aspiration of dose.
- Regurgitation with or without aspiration.
- Attenuating articles or clothing.

Note

Some definitions:

Transit time: the time from the entry of 50% of radioactivity into the upper esophagus until the clearance of 50% of the bolus from the whole esophagus.

Emptying time: the time from the entry of 50% of radioactivity into the upper esophagus until the clearance of 100% of the bolus from the whole esophagus.

Integral value: the total counts beneath the curve normalized to the maximum value.

Radionuclide stagnation: an esophageal emptying time >300 seconds.

SUGGESTED READINGS

Datz FL. Handbook of Nuclear Medicine. 2nd ed. St. Louis: Mosby, 1993.

Early PJ, Sodee DB. Principles and Practice of Nuclear Medicine. 2nd ed. St. Louis: Mosby, 1995.

Murray IPC, Ell PJ, eds. Nuclear Medicine in Clinical Diagnosis and Treatment. Vols. 1 and 2. New York: Churchill Livingstone, 1994.

Wilson, MA. Textbook of Nuclear Medicine. Philadelphia: Lippincott-Raven, 1998.

Notes

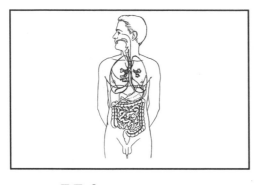

CHAPTER 20

Gallium Scan

Radiopharmacy

Radionuclide

- ^{67}Ga $t_{1/2}$: 78 hours

    Energies: 93, 185, 300 keV

    Type: EC, γ, accelerator

Radiopharmaceutical

- Gallium citrate (isotonic citrate solution)

Localization

- Competes for iron sites in transferrin and is absorbed by lysosomes of white blood cells (WBCs). Also has an affinity for lactoferrin. Distributes through plasma and body tissue with a T_b of 25 days.

Quality Control

- Chromatography, $> 95\%$; use within 2 weeks

Adult Dose Range

- 3-6 mCi (111–222 MBq) for inflammation; 10 mCi (370 MBq) for tumors

Method of Administration

- IV straight stick, Hep-Lock, or reseal (with saline flush), or because of the amount, a butterfly and three-way stopcock with flush.

Indications

- Evaluation of chronic inflammations (abscesses).
- Detection of myocardial or pericardial inflammation.
- Detection and localization of lymphomas, tumors, Hodgkin's disease, hepatomas, bronchogenic carcinomas, and osteomyelitis.

- Evaluation of pulmonary disorders.
- Detection and localization of osteomyelitis.
- Evaluation of fever of unknown origin.
- Evaluation of patients with acquired immunodeficiency syndrome (AIDS).

Contraindications

- Patients having other nuclear medicine studies during the time period needed for the gallium scan.
- Patients cannot have contrast studies during the time period needed for the gallium scan.

Patient History *(or use complete patient history in reference section)*

The patient should answer the following questions.

Do you have a history or family history of cancer?	Y	N
If so, what type and when?		
Do you have any pain?	Y	N
If so, where and for how long?		
Have you had any infections?	Y	N
Have you had any surgery?	Y	N
Have you had any recent trauma?	Y	N
Are you a diabetic?	Y	N
Do you have any bowel disease?	Y	N
Do you have a fever?	Y	N

Have you had any previous or planned related scans, x-rays, biopsies, or antibiotic therapy?	Y	N

Have you had any chemotherapy or radiation therapy?	Y	N

Other department-specific questions.

Patient Preparation

- Identify the patient. Verify doctor's order. Explain the procedure.
- Administer injection to patient.
- Instruct patient to return for images at designated hours from injection (e.g., 6, 24, 48, 72, 96, 120 hours) in accordance with purpose of diagnosis.
- Instruct patient to return home or send back to hospital room to await images.

Equipment

Camera
- Large field of vision

Collimator
- Medium to high energy, parallel hole

Computer Set-up
Statics
- Peak for gallium, windows at 25%, 1,000,000 counts/image

Whole Body
- 10 cm/min

Single Photon Emission Computed Tomography (SPECT)
- Circular or noncircular, 360°, 64 stops, 20–25 sec/stop; region-of-interest (ROI) centered.

Procedure *(time: ~20–60 minutes)*

- Instruct patient to void on return to department.
- Place patient in supine position; check for attenuating material.
- Obtain statics: anterior and posterior of head, thorax, abdomen, pelvis, and mid-femur; also anterior of extremities, obliques of ROI, axillas for history of lymphoma.
- Collect 600,000 to 1,000,000 counts according to protocol.
- Whole-body sweep: head to at least mid-femur.
- SPECT: center ROI(s).

Normal Results

- Soft-tissue activity at 6 and 24 hours, renal activity at 24 hours.

- Some bowel activity that will move over time.

- Lactoferrin content visualizes lacrimal glands, salivary glands, external genitalia, breasts, nasopharynx, bone marrow, spleen, and liver (most prominent).

- Some early activity in sternum, lung, thymus, surgical wounds, and epiphyseal plates; thymus and spleen in children.

- At 48 hours and beyond, renal and lung activity light; lacrimals and salivaries dimly; some nasal activity present; liver, transverse colon, thoracic spine, sternum, scapula tips, skeleton, and genitalia still present.

Abnormal Results

- Inflammations show up as hot spots within 6 hours.

- Also 6-hour scan for abdominal abscess.

- Any bowel activity in the 4- to 6-hour scan is significant in patients with AIDS having a fever.

- Large hematomas present as cold spots.

- Benign sarcoidosis present as intense uptake in organs.

- Tumors are usually scanned at 24–48 hours and beyond.

- Can show AIDS-related pulmonary infections, neoplasia associated with Hodgkin's disease, hepatomas from alcoholic cirrhosis, and malignant melanomas of bone, brain, and lung.

- Persistent renal activity at 48 hours may indicate hypertension pyelonephritis or interstitial nephritis.

- Continued renal activity at 72 hours may indicate inflammation, infection, acute tubular necrosis, acute pyelonephritis, interstitial nephritis, amyloidosis, or impaired renal function.

Artifacts

- Articles in pockets, medallions, necklaces, metal buttons on shirts and blouses, belt buckles, and prostheses may cause attenuation.

- Patient not voiding before scan. Bladder activity could mask ROI.

- Wrong collimator will burn out film.

- Care must be taken for analog cameras to have proper anatomy in view as pictures are hard to visualize on standard p-scopes.

- False-positive results possible from intestinal, spleen, spine, or bladder activity.

SUGGESTED READINGS

Datz FL. Handbook of Nuclear Medicine. 2nd ed. St. Louis: Mosby, 1993.

Early PJ, Sodee DB. Principles and Practice of Nuclear Medicine. 2nd ed. St. Louis: Mosby, 1995.

Murray IPC, Ell PJ, eds. Nuclear Medicine in Clinical Diagnosis and Treatment. Vols. 1 and 2. New York: Churchill Livingstone, 1994.

Wilson, MA. Textbook of Nuclear Medicine. Philadelphia: Lippincott-Raven, 1998.

Notes
. . . .

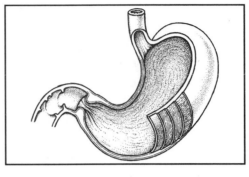

CHAPTER 21

Gastric Empty

(Solid and Liquid)

Radiopharmacy

Radionuclide

- ^{99m}Tc t$_{1/2}$: 6 hours

  Energies: 140 keV

  Type: IT, γ, generator

Radiopharmaceutical

- Solid: ^{99m}Tc-SC (sulfur colloid), Microlite® (temporarily off the market), ^{99m}Tc-albumin colloid

- Liquid: ^{99m}Tc-DTPA (diethylenetriaminepentaacetic acid)

Localization

- Compartmental; moved along with food through gastrointestinal tract

Quality Control

- Chromatography: SC, > 90%; particle size, < 1 μm; Microlite®, > 92% tagging. Use either within 6 hours. DTPA, > 90%; use within 1 hour.

Adult Dose Range

- 200 μCi to 1 mCi (7.4–37 MBq)

Method of Administration

- Radiotracer usually mixed with 1 or 2 whole eggs or egg whites for solid study (type of meal and amounts vary)

- Radiotracer mixed into 120 mL of water or other for liquid and ingested orally.

Indications

- Determination of delayed gastric emptying with quantitation of gastric emptying rate.
- Evaluation of mechanical obstruction.
- Evaluation of anatomic obstruction (pyloric, postsurgical, postradiotherapy).
- Evaluation for altered function, e.g., gastroparesis (diabetic and idiopathic), scleroderma, amyloidosis, or anorexia nervosa.
- Evaluation of suspected tumors or surgery.
- Evaluation of nausea, vomiting, and early satiety.
- Evaluation of weight loss.
- Evaluation of gastric therapy, e.g., Reglan®.

Contraindications

- Allergy to eggs; use oatmeal, baby food, sweet potatoes, or chicken or beef livers.

Patient History *(or use complete patient history in reference section)*

The patient should answer the following questions.

Do you have a history of or family history of cancer?   Y   N

If so, what type and when?

Are you diabetic?   Y   N

Do you have abdominal pain?   Y   N

If so, where and since when?

Do you feel bloated or have acid burning after eating?   Y   N

Do you have nausea and vomiting?   Y   N

Do you have a history of ulcers?   Y   N

Have you had any gastric surgery?	Y	N
Are you on any medications, especially like Reglan® or domperidone?	Y	N
Have you had any previous related tests?	Y	N

Other department-specific questions.

Patient Preparation

- Identify the patient. Verify doctor's order. Explain the procedure.
- Ensure that diabetics receive orange juice 2 hours before test if necessary.
- Ensure patient to be NPO 4–12 hours before examination.
- Physician to discontinue sedatives 12 hours before examination.

Equipment

Camera
- Large or small field of view

Collimator
- Low energy, all purpose, or low energy, high resolution

Computer Set-up
Statics
- Preset for 60–120 seconds or 50,000 counts

Dynamic
- Preset for 60 sec/image, 60–90 minutes

Procedure *(time: ~1.5 hours liquid, up to 3 hours solid)*

Baseline Solid Study
- Prepare one or two eggs and mix in radiotracer.
- Stir and scramble.
- Or prepare choice of gastronomic vehicle with radiotracer.
- Administer to patient PO with 30–120 mL of water. Encourage patient to eat quickly.

Patient Supine
- Place patient in supine position. Acquisition should be started as quickly as possible after ingestion of food.
- Position camera anterior or LAO.
- Instruct patient to remain motionless during imaging.

- Obtain static images every 5 minutes up to 30 minutes, then every 15 minutes thereafter, allowing patient to ambulate between images. If camera or patient moves between images, reposition patient for subsequent imaging by using a small marker at a specific point on the patient and circling the spot on the p-scope for ease of processing. Realign marker and circle, then remove marker for subsequent images.

- Or preset dynamic images for 60-90 minutes. Patient remains motionless under camera.

- Supine is good for checking esophageal reflux.

Patient Standing

- Position patient standing or sitting, one image facing camera. Optional: one image with back to camera.

- Use patient realignment technique described above.

- Obtain immediate image(s), then every 10 minutes.

- Standing, sitting, then standing uses normal movement and gravity to aid realism in study.

Baseline Liquid Study

- Add 500 µCi of ^{99m}Tc-DTPA to 120 mL of water or orange juice.

- Administer to patient PO. Encourage patient to drink quickly.

- Images same as solid study, although only imaged for 1.5 hours.

Additional Testing

- If emptying is slow or nonexistent, Reglan® (metoclopramide) may be administered (standard adult dose, 10 mg IV slowly during 2 minutes) to cause stomach contractions; check with radiologist. Reglan® IV should show movement within 3 minutes after injection, oral Reglan® may take up to 60 minutes for a response.

- Continue with protocol for 60 minutes.

Normal Results

- Liquid (e.g., radiolabeled water or orange juice): $t_{1/2}$ (50%) at 10-45 minutes or 80% in 1 hour.

- Solid (type and size of meals and population varies): $t_{1/2}$ (50%) movement out of stomach within a lower limit of 32 minutes to an upper limit of 120 minutes with an adult mean of 90 minutes. Others suggest 63% by 1 hour.

- Terminate study before 60 minutes if gastric emptying becomes ≥ 95%.

Abnormal Results

- Very little or no movement from stomach after 60 minutes. Causes of delayed gastric emptying are mechanical obstruction or altered function (e.g., diabetic gastroparesis, diabetes mellitus, surgery, drugs, gastric outlet obstruction, scleroderma, chronic idiopathic intestinal pseudoobstruction [CIIP], idiopathic gastroparesis, amyloidosis, anorexia nervosa).

- Rapid emptying may occur in cases of "dumping syndrome."

Processing

- Either study, calculate percent emptying by following methods:
  - Computer program.
  - Generate regions of interest (ROIs) around stomach.
  - Manual: Use counts taken in ROI, correct counts by following decay factors:

Start Time (x_0)	1.00
10 min	0.981
20 min	0.962
30 min	0.944
40 min	0.926
50 min	0.909
60 min	0.891

- Divide gastric counts by decay factor to obtain corrected counts.
- This is performed on each frame, plotted on a semilogarithmic graph, and compared with a normal curve. Obtain the $t_{1/2}$ emptying time from graph.

Artifacts

- Burn eggs; nonuniform mixing of radiotracer and eggs.
- Too little or too much food or water.
- Patient allergies or intolerance to eggs or to food.
- Patient unable to eat or may vomit or aspirate food and dose.
- Belt buckles or buttons.
- Camera or patient position changes, which affects the number of counts. Patient must be placed exactly in same position for each picture. To help, for supine/anterior pictures, place camera as close as possible, reposition patient for subsequent imaging by using a small marker at a specific point on the patient and circling the spot on the p-scope, realign marker and circle, then remove marker before imaging, especially if going for counts. Or draw outline of initial activity in stomach on p-scope to reposition patient for next picture. The same can be performed for standing pictures. Draw outline on p-scope; realign in p-scope for next picture.

Note

Drugs that promote motility are Reglan® (not to be confused with diabetic insulin medication referred to as "regular"), domperidone, cisapride, erythromycin. These cause the stomach to be more sensitive to nervous stimulation and increase motility of solid foods in the stomach.

SUGGESTED READINGS

Datz FL. Handbook of Nuclear Medicine. 2nd ed. St. Louis: Mosby, 1993.

Early PJ, Sodee DB. Principles and Practice of Nuclear Medicine. 2nd ed. St. Louis: Mosby, 1995.

Murray IPC, Ell PJ, eds. Nuclear Medicine in Clinical Diagnosis and Treatment. Vols. 1 and 2. New York: Churchill Livingstone, 1994.

Wilson, MA. Textbook of Nuclear Medicine. Philadelphia: Lippincott-Raven, 1998.

Microlite® is a registered trademark of DuPont Merck, Wilmington, DE.
Reglan® is a registered trademark of AH Robbins Company, Richmond, VA.

Notes
. . . .

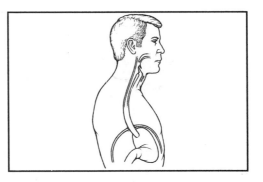

CHAPTER 22

Gastroesophageal Reflux

Radiopharmacy

Radionuclide

- ^{99m}Tc $t_{1/2}$: 6 hours

  Energies: 140 keV

  Type: IT, γ, generator

Radiopharmaceutical

- ^{99m}Tc-SC (sulfur colloid)

Localization

- Compartmental, esophagus to gastrointestinal tract

Quality Control

- Chromatography, > 90%; particle size, < 1 μm

Adult Dose Range

- 300 μCi to 2 mCi (11.1–74 MBq); 1 mCi or more if acidified orange juice is used.

Method of Administration

- PO in water, orange juice, milk, oatmeal, or saline.
- PO with acidified orange juice (150 mL of 0.1 normal HCl) to delay gastric emptying time and predispose the patient to reflux.
- Ingested through a nasogastric tube if patient has a history of esophageal motility dysfunction.

Indications

- Detection and quantitation of gastroesophageal reflux.
- Evaluation of patients with diaphragmatic hernia.
- Evaluation of children with asthma, chronic lung disease, or aspiration pneumonia.

Contraindications

- None

Patient History

The patient should answer the following questions.

Do you have a history or family history of cancer?	Y	N
If so, what type and for how long?		

Do you have a history of esophageal motility dysfunction?	Y	N
Do you feel burning or have pain in upper abdomen or lower chest after eating?	Y	N
Do you have any liver diseases?	Y	N
Do you have any stomach diseases or problems?	Y	N
After a meal, does it taste like gastric juices when you belch (as in a mini-vomit)?	Y	N
Other department-specific questions.		

Patient Preparation

- Identify the patient. Verify doctor's order. Explain the procedure.
- Ensure patient has fasted for 4 hours or overnight.

Equipment

Camera

- Large field of view

Collimator

- Low energy, all purpose, or low energy, high resolution

Computer Set-up

Statics

- 30 sec/image; some go for 300,000–500,000 counts

Procedure *(time: ~30 minutes)*

- At 15 minutes after ingestion, position patient sitting or standing in front of camera, anterior projection.
- Acquire 30-second image.
    - From this baseline image before abdominal binding, a region of interest (ROI) of the esophagus will be drawn to use as esophageal background subtraction.
    - From this image, the ROI around the stomach is also drawn to obtain total counts of dose ingested for quantitation of reflux.
    - If there are significant counts remaining in the esophagus, administer more fluid and image again. If the counts remain, consider rescheduling the test at a later date using a nasogastric tube.
- Place patient in supine position on table.
- Place an abdominal binder around lower abdomen below the rib cage.
- Attach a sphygmomanometer anterior, under the binder (or use manual pressure). This can also be accomplished by using a plastic block used for IV pyelograms, for example, placed beneath the binder and a blood pressure cuff folded underneath the plastic block.
- Acquire 30-second images with pressures in the abdominal binder at 0, 20, 40, 60, 80, and 100 mm Hg.
- Processing: to obtain percent gastroesophageal reflux
    - Draw ROIs around lower esophagus, stomach, and lower left lung (for background).
    - Calculate reflux at each pressure with the following equation using counts from each ROI.

$$\% \text{ Gastroesophageal reflux} = \frac{A - B}{C} \times 100$$

where A is esophageal counts (minus the prebinder esophageal ROI counts), B is background counts (lung ROI), and C is gastric counts from prebinder gastric ROI image.

- To be extremely accurate, correct the prebinder counts (esophageal and gastric counts) for each image by a decay factor.

Normal Results

- ≤ 4–5% refluxed radiotracer at any pressure level.
- Dose should present brightly in stomach with very little or no residual activity in esophagus.
- The activity should remain in the stomach (and perhaps begin to move out toward the duodenum as in a gastric empty study) with no reflux at any pressure level.

Abnormal Results

- > 4–5% refluxed radiotracer.
- Activity will appear to be refluxing up the esophagus toward the mouth.

Artifacts

- Inability to swallow or aspiration of dose.
- Esophageal retention.
- Regurgitation with or without aspiration.
- Attenuating articles or clothing.
- Patient with known esophageal varices (potentially life-threatening condition involving dilation of distal esophageal blood vessels usually associated with chronic obstruction of venous drainage from esophageal veins into the hepatic portal system caused by cirrhosis of the liver and alcoholism); perhaps not enough for a contraindication, but consideration may be given to this condition.

SUGGESTED READINGS

Datz FL. Handbook of Nuclear Medicine. 2nd ed. St. Louis: Mosby, 1993.

Early PJ, Sodee DB. Principles and Practice of Nuclear Medicine. 2nd ed. St. Louis: Mosby, 1995.

Murray IPC, Ell PJ, eds. Nuclear Medicine in Clinical Diagnosis and Treatment. Vols. 1 and 2. New York: Churchill Livingstone, 1994.

Wilson, MA. Textbook of Nuclear Medicine. Philadelphia: Lippincott-Raven, 1998.

Notes

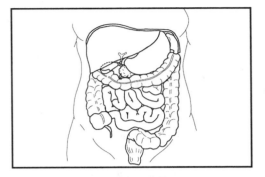

Gastrointestinal Bleed

Radiopharmacy

Radionuclide

- ^{99m}Tc $t_{1/2}$: 6 hours

  Energies: 140 keV

  Type: IT, γ, generator

Radiopharmaceutical

- Tagged red blood cells by pyrophosphate or stannous chloride to ^{99m}TcO$_4^-$ (pertechnate) by in vivo, in vitro, or kit, e.g., UltraTag®. For active bleeding, ^{99m}Tc-SC (sulfur colloid).

Localization

- Compartmental, tagged to and circulating with blood

Quality Control

- ^{99m}TcO$_4^-$: chromatography; tagging, 90% in vivo, 95% in vitro
- ^{99m}Tc-SC: chromatography, > 90%

Adult Dose Range

- ^{99m}TcO$_4^-$: 20–50 mCi (740–1850 MBq)
- ^{99m}Tc-SC: 10–20 mCi (370–740 MBq)

Method of Administration

- IV injections, or drawing, tagging, and reinjection of tagged red blood cells

Indications

- Detection and localization of bleeding sites in patients with active or intermittent gastrointestinal bleeding. This could be caused by aspirin, ulcers, perforation, cancers, inflammation, diverticula, or angiodysplasia.

- Detection and localization of secondary blood loss as in blood pooling in peritoneal cavity or ruptured arterial or venous supplies.
- ^{99m}Tc-SC: Detection and localization of actively bleeding sites, for patients with portal hypertension (caused by obstruction of blood flow through the liver), and hypertension to abdominal collateral vessels.

Contraindications

- Patients with contrast studies under way.
- Patients receiving blood products.

Patient History *(or use complete patient history in reference section)*

The patient should answer the following questions.

Do you have a history or family history of cancer?	Y	N
If so, what type and for how long?		
Do you have a history of bleeding?	Y	N
Are you bleeding now?	Y	N
If so, for how long and what is the color of the stool?		
Are you taking aspirin?	Y	N
Do you have any pain?	Y	N
Do you have a history of diverticulitis, Crohn's disease, or other disease?	Y	N
Have you had a colostomy or other surgery?	Y	N

**Have you had any related studies, e.g.,
    endoscopy, CT, upper gastrointestinal,
    barium enema?**   Y   N

Other department-specific questions.

Patient Preparation

- Identify the patient. Verify doctor's order. Explain the procedure.
- Obtain a signed consent for blood work.
- Instruct patient to empty bowel and bladder before beginning procedure.
- If possible, have patient look for active signs of bleeding.

Equipment

Camera

- Large field of view

Collimator

- Low energy, all purpose, or low energy, high resolution

Computer Set-up

Flow

- 2–5 sec/frame, 60–180 seconds

Statics

- 500,000–2,000,000 counts

Procedure *(time: ~1 hour; delays, ~15 minutes)*

- Patient must sign consent form to take and return blood. It must also be signed by technologist and witness.
- In vitro method: extract ~2–2.5 mL of blood into heparinized syringe from patient and tagged with UltraTag®.
- In vivo method: inject cold pyrophosphate, then 20 minutes later, inject radiotracer under camera for flow.
- Modified in vivo method: inject cold pyrophosphate and wait 20 minutes. Extract ~2–2.5 mL of blood into a heparinized shielded syringe containing ~30 mCi of $^{99m}TcO_4^-$. Mix for 5–10 minutes.
- Place patient in supine position, camera anterior and if possible from bottom of heart to lower bowel in view. If patient is tall, upper and lower pictures may be taken.
- Inject under camera for initial flow if protocol.
- Acquire flow if active bleeding is suggested. ^{99m}Tc-SC is best used to present the

active bleeding site. Sulfur colloid is taken up and removed quickly by the reticuloendothelial system (RES), so careful positioning, injection, and computer start are important.

- Acquire statics anteriorly. Include immediately and at 5, 10, 15, 30, 45, and 60 minutes with RAOs and LAOs indicated if positive.

- Or acquire dynamic study for 60 minutes after flow study. Delayed images as necessary. Patients with melena (black, tarry feces because of intestinal chemical interaction with free blood) are candidates for prolonged studies with delays.

- Show study. Laterals and posteriors may be indicated with presentation of a positive scan. Four-hour and 24-hour delays may also be indicated.

- If a patient has a bowel movement after tagging, some hardy souls bag the bedpan and image it for activity, which would be signs of active bleeding.

Normal Results

- Heart and great vessels prominent.

- Bladder, bowel, and penile activity not unlikely.

Abnormal Results

- Flow: focal area of increased activity. Blood pooling in abdominal cavity may also be present.

- Statics: focal area peristalses with time. Blood pool may persist in abdominal cavity and may or may not move.

- If little or no movement, it may be vascular activity or pool in abdominal cavity. Typical focal areas of active bleeding include ascending, transverse, descending, and sigmoid colon, right colonic (hepatic) flexure, left colonic (splenic) flexure, and small bowel.

Artifacts

- Bad radiotracer tag could lead to poor results. Do a thyroid image to confirm a bad tag. Free ^{99m}Tc will go to thyroid, salivary glands, and gastric mucosa.

- Belt buckles, articles in clothing, necklaces, and so forth, may attenuate image.

- A full bladder may mask a bleeding area.

- Intermittence of bleeding compounds the problem of detection.

- ^{99m}Tc-SC (10–20 mCi or 370–740 MBq) may be indicated if there is known active bleeding. The drawback is the relatively quick removal by the reticuloendothelial system (RES) when intermittence is indicated. Do a flow at 1 sec/frame for 60 seconds to catch the bleed site. If positive, take full series of immediates (obliques, laterals, posterior) to localize, followed by timed images.

SUGGESTED READINGS

Datz FL. Handbook of Nuclear Medicine. 2nd ed. St. Louis: Mosby, 1993.

Early PJ, Sodee DB. Principles and Practice of Nuclear Medicine. 2nd ed. St. Louis: Mosby, 1995.

Murray IPC, Ell PJ, eds. Nuclear Medicine in Clinical Diagnosis and Treatment. Vols. 1 and 2. New York: Churchill Livingstone, 1994.

Wilson, MA. Textbook of Nuclear Medicine. Philadelphia: Lippincott-Raven, 1998.

UltraTag® is a registered trademark of Mallinckrodt Medical, Inc., St. Louis, MO.

Notes

CHAPTER 24

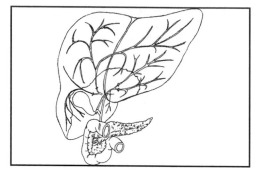

HIDA

(Hepatobiliary or Gallbladder Scan) With Ejection Fraction

Radiopharmacy

Radionuclide

- ^{99m}Tc t$_{1/2}$: 6 hours

  Energies: 140 keV

  Type: IT, γ, generator

Radiopharmaceutical

- IDA (iminodiacetic acid), disofenin (DISIDA), mebrofenin (e.g., Choletec®)

Localization

- Polygonal cell uptake and excretion, follows bile path

Quality Control

- Chromatography for ^{99m}Tc > 90%; 6-hour shelf life

Adult Dose Range

- 5–10 mCi (185–370 MBq), higher doses for patients with elevated bilirubin concentrations (> 30 mg/dL causes less hepatic uptake, more background activity, and greater renal excretion).

Method of Administration

- IV injection under camera. Some radiologists want to see how long the heart shadow remains after the injection and perform an immediate view.
- A flow study may be requested.

Indications

- Evaluation of cholecystitis; inflammation of gallbladder (GB), cystic, or common bile ducts.

- Evaluation of cholelithiasis; obstruction. Acute is caused by cystic duct obstruction, usually by stone; chronic is reoccurring gallstones and many other types of obstruction, e.g., stenosis, tumor, lack of ability to react to cholecystokinin (CCK), or sphincter failure.
- Detection of perforation of gallbladder; may occur in chronic cholecystitis, immunocompromised patients, and atherosclerotic disease.
- Evaluation for biliary dyskinesia (cystic duct syndrome [CDS], sphincter of Oddi spasm [SOS] [see Note], and congenital anomalies, e.g., biliary atresia).
- Evaluation after gallbladder surgery for suspected leakage.
- Evaluation of hepatic transplant.

Contraindications

- Person has just eaten a meal (affects liver uptake and gallbladder function).
- No CCK if recently positive for gallstones. Some will administer fatty meal or Pulmocare® instead as it is not so forceful in contracting the gallbladder.
- No morphine sulfate if allergic to morphine (there are alternative drugs) or has elevated amylase or other pancreatic enzymes indicating pancreatitis.

Patient History *(or use complete patient history in reference section)*

The patient should answer the following questions

When was your last solid meal?

Do you have a history or family history of cancer?   Y   N

If so, what type and for how long?

Do you have a history of gallbladder or liver disease (e.g., gallstones, hepatitis)?   Y   N

Have you had recent abdominal pain?   Y   N

If so, where, when (e.g., after eating), and for how long?

Do you experience nausea or vomiting?   Y   N

Are you running a fever?	Y	N
Have you had abnormal blood test results?	Y	N
Have you had any recent surgery?	Y	N
Have you had any recent CT, MRI, ultra-sonography (US), or nuclear medicine (NM) scans of abdomen?	Y	N

Assess for jaundice or signs of alcohol abuse (discern discreetly).

For inpatients, note laboratory results for serum glutamate pyruvate transaminase (SGPT), serum glutamic-oxaloacetic transaminase (SGOT), GGTP, alkaline phosphatase, lactate dehydrogenase (LDH), creatine phosphokinase (CPK), white blood cells (WBC), amylase, total bilirubin, creatinine/blood urea nitrogen (BUN).

Other department-specific questions.

Patient Preparation

- Identify the patient. Verify doctor's order.
- Ensure patient NPO 2–14 hours before exam (usually 4–6 hours).
- Explain the procedure; usually runs ~1 hour but baseline studies can go as long as 4 hours with up to 24-hour delays required in some instances.
- Some physicians require that a form of CCK such as Kinevac® is given 15 minutes before the injection of the radiotracer to ensure that the gallbladder is clear.

Equipment

Camera
- Large field of view

Collimator
- Low energy, all purpose, or low energy, high resolution

Computer Set-up
Static Images
- Peak for ^{99m}Tc, preset time 90–180 seconds, or for ~750,000 counts; correct orientation.

Flow Studies

- 2 sec/frame for 60 seconds, then immediate blood pool image

Procedure *(time: ~1 hour, possibly longer, delays ~15 minutes)*

- Place patient in supine position, camera anterior, liver in upper left quadrant of field of view (FOV). Position liver in middle FOV if taking immediate heart shadow image, then move camera to position liver in upper left quadrant for remaining images.

- Images: immediate, then every 5 minutes up to 30 minutes. Some take the time in seconds from the 5- or 10-minute view for the rest of the views in the study, giving a better visualization of the radiotracer washout from the liver.

- Gallbladder and bowel visualization: image RAO and RLAT. Some require LAO. The study is complete.

- No visualization: for baseline HIDA, image every 5–15 minutes up to 60 minutes, then images to protocol or ask radiologist, e.g., patient returns for 2- to 6-hour delays.

- No visualization with nonpharmacologic intervention:
    - If no visualization of gallbladder or bowel by 30–45 minutes and patient is supine, turn patient to right decubitus position.
    - If no visualization of gallbladder or bowel by 30–45 minutes and patient is ambulatory, let the patient walk around for a few minutes.

- No visualization with pharmacologic interventions (see Note).
    - Gallbladder but no bowel: CCK or fatty meal (e.g., Pulmocare®).
    - Bowel but no gallbladder: morphine sulfate. Check for contraindications, then obtain order from radiologist.

- Images: preinjection image, then postinjection images by protocol, usually every 5 minutes for 30 minutes. Check again with radiologist for continuance or delays before releasing patient.

- If patient has not eaten for a substantial amount of time (e.g., 24 hours or more), the gallbladder may be in "shock" or stasis and filled with "sludge." In these cases, the study may appear as gut with no gallbladder but may need a fatty meal to contract the gallbladder and empty the sludge before it can refill and present. Some physicians routinely require CCK administered 10–15 minutes before injection of radiotracer.

Normal Results

- Visualization of liver 5–15 seconds after injection, hepatic and common bile duct and gallbladder 5–20 minutes up to 60 minutes.

- Intestinal activity visualizing and moving within 10–60 minutes.

- A flow study will show the liver immediately but dimly from activity entering through the hepatic artery, then brightly with portal vein flow.

- The liver diminishes in activity as the gallbladder visualizes in its "bed" and grows brighter and bowel activity visualizes and moves with time. Bile ducts in the liver appear as lines leading to the bowel.

- For postgallbladder surgery, there should be no activity pooling around the liver or in abdomen.

Abnormal Results

- Nonvisualization of gallbladder within 1 hour with visualization of common bile duct and bowel (indicating possible cystic duct obstruction, acute cholecystitis).

- Nonvisualization of bowel within 1 hour with good hepatic uptake, visualization of gallbladder and common bile duct (indicating possible sphincter of Oddi dysfunction or obstruction).

- Nonvisualization of gallbladder or bowel within 1 hour with good hepatic uptake but no draining (indicating complete or near complete obstruction of hepatic ducts or hepatocyte dysfunction).

- For postgallbladder surgery, pooling of activity either in area of extracted gallbladder or in abdominal cavity adjacent to area. This should visualize quickly, but images should be taken for about 60 minutes.

Artifacts

- Breast attenuation (may need to tape or strap breast up out of the way or have patient help hold breast up), buttons or articles in shirt pockets.

- A meal too soon before study will deleteriously affect results.

- Elevated serum bilirubin levels may not allow uptake by hepatocytes causing radiotracer to excrete too quickly (use larger dose).

- If patient is already taking Demerol®, the action may occlude the images by obstructing normal radiotracer flow into the bowel.

Note

Pharmacologic Interventions

CCK (or fatty meal) is used to contract gallbladder so that visualization of bowel may occur. For CCK, 0.02 μg × patient weight in kilograms, IV (1 μg/mL) slow push for 3 minutes. With GB visualization and no common bile duct or gut, CCK squeezes activity out into system (this could be painful to patient depending on degree of obstruction). Also used to calculate gallbladder ejection fraction (EF). Note: If patient is NPO for many hours, GB is inactive (in shock) and may be full of bile or sludge and not visualizing. CCK empties GB to refill for visualization. Contraindicated if patient has recent positive ultrasound examination for gallstones. CCK relaxes the sphincter of Oddi. Nitroglycerin can be used for the same effect. Check with physician for dose. A fatty meal or preparation such as Pulmocare® may also produce the desired result.

Morphine sulfate is used to spasm (contract) the sphincter of Oddi forcing radiopharmaceutical (RP) back into gallbladder if cystic duct is patent (distinguishes between acute [no visualization] and chronic cholecystitis [eventual visualization]). Nonvisualization of gallbladder 30–150 minutes after morphine injection (cholecystitis). For morphine sulfate (MS), 0.04 mg × patient weight in kilograms, IV (diluted to 5–10 mL) slow push for 3 minutes. Some just administer 2.0 mg regardless of weight. Reverse the effects with naloxone hydrochloride. Contraindicated for patients allergic to morphine or history of pancreatitis (check for elevated amylase levels).

Other: Some literature indicates that if there is a known allergy to morphine sulfate, other controlled drugs are available to constrict the sphincter of Oddi. This would have to be discussed with the radiologist as the literature was not specifically in conjunction with an HIDA scan.

Fentanyl citrate: administered as 50 μg slowly for 3 minutes. Onset at 1 minute, peak at 5 minutes with a short pharmacologic half-life.

Hydromorphone hydrochloride (Dilaudid®): onset at 15 minutes, peak up to 30 minutes. Requires 1 mg or less for the desired result. Slow injection for 3 minutes.

Pentazocine hydrochloride: onset at 2–3 minutes, peaks at 15 minutes, 30 mg/mL IV.

Meperidine hydrochloride (Demerol®): onset at 1 minute, peak at 7 minutes, 1 mg/kg, 10 mg/mL IV, or 50 mg slow push for 2–3 minutes.

This approach and amounts given (the above are adult doses) would have to be discussed with the nuclear physician or radiologist. Demerol® was successfully substituted at Palms of Pasadena Hospital in St. Petersburg, FL. An adult male patient with a history of violence when given morphine sulfate presented with bowel visualization but no gallbladder after 60 minutes. After consultation with the radiologist, he was given 50 mg of Demerol® IV slow push for 3 minutes. The results were gallbladder visualization shortly after injection and no violent episodes.

Gallbladder EF: normal ~35%. Some literature indicates > 50% for men, > 20% for women.

Computer: using image just before CCK injection and post-CCK images, draw regions of interest, make note of counts, and then process if automatic. Find the image with lowest counts to get EF.

Manually, it is similar to MUGA:

$$EF = \frac{ED - ES}{ED} \times 100; \text{ or } \frac{\text{pre-CCK cts} - \text{lowest post-CCK cts}}{\text{pre-CCK cts}} \times 100$$

where ED is end-diastolic volume, ES is end-systolic volume, pre-CCK cts is counts before CCK, and post-CCK cts is counts after CCK.

Biliary Dyskinesia

Cystic duct syndrome (CDS) (chronic acalculous gallbladder disease or chronic acalculous cholecystitis): kinking, fibrosis, and thickening of the wall causing narrowing of the lumen of the cystic duct. Slow release of hepatic bile even with CCK.

Sphincter of Oddi spasm (SOS) (sphincter of Oddi dysfunction, papillary stenosis, and bile duct dyskinesia): sphincter of Oddi remains tightened or in spasm. Liver function laboratory tests and ultrasonography examination appear normal. Gallbladder or common bile duct may serve as compensatory reservoir. In these cases, CCK only serves to increase constriction.

Cholecystokinin

Release is stimulated by food from cells in mucosa of duodenum and upper jejunum only. Kinevac® (sincalide) are synthetics of the functional 8-amino acid chain.

Actions of CCK include the following:

Contraction and emptying of the gallbladder.

Relaxation of the sphincter of Oddi.

Increase in pancreatic enzyme secretion.

Increase in secretion of insulin, glucagon, and somatostatin by islet cells.

Inhibition of gastric emptying by contraction of the pyloric sphincter.

Increase in hepatic bile secretion.

Increase in intestinal peristalsis.

Increase in intestinal blood flow.

Suppression of appetite.

Decrease in systolic blood pressure.

CCK acts by attaching to CCK receptors in smooth muscle of gallbladder and sphincter of Oddi.

The sphincter of Oddi refers to three sphincters: the choledochal sphincter surrounding the intraduodenal part of the distal CBD, the pancreatic sphincter at the distal end of the pancreatic duct (of Wirsung), and the ampullary sphincter surrounding the common channel. This common channel or duct surrounded by the ampullary sphincter opens into the duodenum at the ampulla of Vater.

SUGGESTED READINGS

Datz FL. Handbook of Nuclear Medicine. 2nd ed. St. Louis: Mosby, 1993.

Early PJ, Sodee DB. Principles and Practice of Nuclear Medicine. 2nd ed. St. Louis: Mosby, 1995.

Klingensmith W, Eshima D, Goddard J. Nuclear Medicine Procedure Manual 1997–98. Englewood, CO: Wick, 1998.

Murray IPC, Ell PJ, eds. Nuclear Medicine in Clinical Diagnosis and Treatment. Vols. 1 and 2. New York: Churchill Livingstone, 1994.

Wilson, MA. Textbook of Nuclear Medicine. Philadelphia: Lippincott-Raven, 1998.

Choletec® is a registered trademark of Bracco Diagnostics, Inc., Princeton, NJ.
Demerol® is a registered trademark of Sanofi Winthrop Pharmaceuticals, New York, NY.
Dilaudid® is a registered trademark of Knoll Pharmaceuticals, Whippany, NJ.
Kinevac® is a registered trademark of Bracco Diagnostics, Inc., Princeton, NJ.
Pulmocare® is a registered trademark of Ross Laboratories, Columbus, OH.

Notes

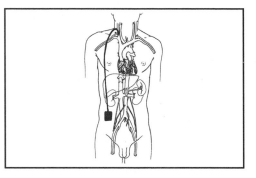

CHAPTER 25

LeVeen or Denver Shunt Patency

Radiopharmacy

Radionuclide

- ^{99m}Tc t$_{1/2}$: 6 hours

  Energies: 140 keV

  Type: IT, γ, generator

Radiopharmaceutical

- ^{99m}Tc-MAA (macroaggregated albumin) or HAM (human albumin microspheres)

- ^{99m}Tc-SC (sulfur colloid)

Localization

- Compartmental, peritoneal to blood circulation

Quality Control

- ^{99m}Tc-MAA: particle size, 10–90 μm; 75,000–700,000 particles/injection. Chromatography (MAA and SC), 90–95% tagging.

Adult Dose Range

- ^{99m}Tc-MAA; 1.5–5 mCi (55.5–187 MBq)

- ^{99m}Tc-SC; 3 mCi (111 MBq)

Method of Administration

- Intraperitoneal injection with local anesthetic by physician.

- Typically, lower left quadrant. Can be guided by ultrasonography (US) to location of ascites.

- Usually administered in 7–10 mL of normal saline solution.

Indications

- Evaluation of LeVeen shunt (peritoneovenous) patency (shunts ascitic fluid from the peritoneal cavity to the venous circulation using a low-pressure valve activated by breathing exercises, inserted into the abdominal wall with collection tube inserted through the jugular vein into the superior vena cava).
- Evaluation of Denver shunt (peritoneovenous) patency (shunts ascitic fluid from the peritoneal cavity to the venous circulation using a mechanical pumping device inserted into the abdominal wall with collection tube inserted through the jugular vein into the superior vena cava).
- Evaluation of increasing ascites secondary to the use of implanted shunt, e.g., increased sodium consumption, inadequate diuretic agents, or worsening liver (hepatic cirrhosis) or heart failure.

Contraindications

- Patient with pulmonary hypertension may be a consideration with ^{99m}Tc-MAA.

Patient History

The patient should answer the following questions.

Do you have a history or family history of cancer?	**Y**	**N**
If so, what type and for how long?		

Do you have abdominal pain?	**Y**	**N**
Do you have abdominal distention?	**Y**	**N**
If so, more so than before or after surgery?	**Y**	**N**

Other department-specific questions.

Patient Preparation

- Identify the patient. Verify doctor's order. Explain the procedure.
- Prepare patient for intraperitoneal injection.

Equipment

Camera
- Large field of view

Collimator
- Low energy, all purpose, or low energy, high resolution

Computer Set-up
Flow
- Denver shunt; 3 sec/frame for 60 seconds. Injection directly into pump.

Statics
- 180–300 sec/image or 500,000 counts

Whole Body Sweep
- Check length of patient, patient orientation, 8–10 cm/min

Procedure *(time: ~1 hour)*
- Place patient on table in supine position. Ensure that there are no objects on patient or in clothing to cause attenuation.
- Flow: Position camera anterior over abdomen/thorax to visualize as much of the pump and tubing as possible. Start camera on injection.
- Injection (usually into lower left quadrant of abdomen) performed by physician.
- LeVeen: Perform ballottement (abdominal palpation) to distribute radiotracer or roll the patient from side to side.
- Denver: Instruct patient to pump system vigorously after injection as in normal operation.
- Obtain images
  - Immediate anterior abdominal image after injection.
  - Anterior abdomen and thorax at 15, 30, 45, and 60 minutes after injection.
  - Option: whole-body sweep from head to pelvis.
- Obtain 2- to 4-hour delays if no lung (or liver) visualization within 60 minutes.

Normal Results
- Lungs present within 60 minutes. Usually this is a rapid visualization (within 10–30 minutes of injection).
- If ^{99m}Tc-SC is used, liver is the target organ within 60 minutes. This method is not presently used as much because of the difficulty of separating the liver from the ascites.

Abnormal Results
- ^{99m}Tc-MAA: no activity in the lungs after 4-hour delays, indicating obstruction.

- ^{99m}Tc-SC: no activity in the liver after 4-hour delays, indicating obstruction.
- Activity stops at abdominal pump; very little or no activity in tubing (indicating valve failure or obstruction in tubing).

Artifacts

- Risk of infection with injection. Patient should be monitored.
- Jewelry, medallions, buttons, items in shirt pockets, or belt buckles can cause artifacts. Also note any surgically implanted devices.
- ^{99m}Tc-MAA: Test should be performed with reduced amounts of radiotracer (and hence reduced number of injected particles) on patients with known compromised pulmonary function (known disease, shunting, arteriole malformation, liver disease) or one lung, and considerations should be made as to whether to perform the test on patients with pulmonary hypertension.
- If little or no visualization of lungs with visualization of superior vena cava and right heart, check patient history for compromising diseases, operations, and cancers.
- If no visualization of radiotracer in abdomen, check needle and radiotracer tag.

SUGGESTED READINGS

Early PJ, Sodee DB. Principles and Practice of Nuclear Medicine. 2nd ed. St. Louis: Mosby, 1995.
Wilson, MA. Textbook of Nuclear Medicine. Philadelphia: Lippincott-Raven, 1998.

Notes

CHAPTER 26

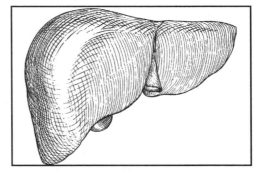

Liver SPECT

(Hepatic Hemangioma)

Radiopharmacy

Radionuclide

- ^{99m}Tc $t_{1/2}$: 6 hours

  Energies: 140 keV

  Type: IT, γ, generator

Radiopharmaceutical

- Tagged red blood cells by pyrophosphate (pyp) or stannous chloride to ^{99m}Tc O_4^- by in vivo, in vitro, or kit, e.g., UltraTag®.

Localization

- Compartmental, tagged to and circulating with blood

Quality Control

- ^{99m}Tc O_4^-: chromatography; tagging, 90% in vivo, 95% in vitro

Adult Dose Range

- ^{99m}Tc O_4^-: 20–50 mCi (740–1850 MBq)

Method of Administration

- IV injections, or drawing, tagging, and reinjection of tagged red blood cells

Indications

- Detection and localization of hepatic hemangiomas.

- Detection and localization of vascularized primary and metastatic tumors.

- Detection and localization of cysts, space-occupying lesions, necrosis, or abnormal focal areas (marked increased or decreased activity) considered for biopsy.

Contraindications

- Patients with contrast studies under way.
- Patient receiving blood products.

Patient History *(or use complete patient history in reference section)*

The patient should answer the following questions.

**Do you have a history or family history
of cancer?**   Y   N

If so, what type and for how long?

Do you have a history of liver disease?   Y   N

Have you had any recent abdominal pain?   Y   N

If so, where and for how long?

Have you had any recent trauma?   Y   N

Have you had any recent surgery?   Y   N

If so, where?

**Have you had any recent related studies
(US, MRI, CT, NM)?**   Y   N

**Have you had any recent laboratory tests
performed?**   Y   N

Other department-specific questions.

Patient Preparation

- Identify the patient. Verify doctor's order. Explain the procedure.
- Obtain a signed consent form for blood return if required.

Equipment

Camera

- Large field of view

Collimator

- Low energy, all purpose, or low energy, high resolution

Computer Set-up
Flow

- 1-5 sec/frame, 60-120 seconds

Statics

- 500,000-2,000,000 counts

Single Photon Emission Computed Tomography (SPECT)

- 1.4-1.5 magnification, noncircular or elliptical orbit, 64 × 64 or 128 × 128 matrix, 360°, 64 stops, 20-30 sec/stop, Butterworth filter with 0.3 cutoff or Hanning with 0.8 cutoff, slice thickness 6-12 mm.

Procedure *(time: ~40 minutes for flow and statics; ~30-45 minutes for SPECT)*

- Obtain a signed consent form from patient to take and return blood. It must also be signed by technologist and witness.
- In vitro method: ~2-2.5 mL of blood is extracted into heparinized syringe from patient and tagged with UltraTag®
- Or in vivo method: inject cold pyp, then 20 minutes later, inject radiotracer under camera for flow if required.
- Place patient in supine position, camera anterior for flow if required, liver and spleen centered in field of view (FOV), or preload setup for SPECT orbit. Camera posterior if that is what is determined for best view from other imaging techniques.
- Flow: Obtain images of early blood supply from hepatic artery to primary and metastatic tumors and hemangiomas.
- Statics: Obtain immediate anterior with marker, anterior, right anterior oblique, right lateral, posterior, and more as to protocol.
- SPECT: Obtain images 1-2 hours (recommended) after injection. Set proper patient orientation, set camera.
- Process transverse, sagittal, and coronal slices. Use 0.11-0.12 attenuation correction.

Normal Results

- Heart, great vessels, spleen, and kidneys prominent.
- Heterogeneous light uptake of liver within seconds of injection from hepatic artery.
- Heterogeneous brighter uptake from portal system.
- SPECT: Heterogeneous uptake of liver parenchyma. Hepatic vessels prominent in various slices. Organs and great vessels prominent.

Abnormal Results

- Initially (typically), hemangiomas are hypovascular, filling with time. They become hypervascular with delays. A differential diagnosis is a solitary hepatoma that is typically hypervascular. Although there are some hemangiomas that do not present with early hypovascularity, typically they increase with time.
- Flow: Focal area(s) of increased or decreased activity. Hemangiomas, because they are benign tumors of dilated blood vessels, will show markedly increased activity that increases with time.
- Statics: Focal area(s) persist in relative positions from different views.
- SPECT: Focal areas of an overabundance of vascularity (e.g., hemangiomas) will present as hot spots; focal areas of less than normal or lacking vascularity will present as cold spots. Although flow and statics can establish the existence of a suspected hemangioma, SPECT images can aid in the presentation of added unsuspected sites that were hidden in other diagnostic techniques.

Artifacts

- Bad radiotracer tag could lead to poor results. Do a thyroid image to confirm a bad tag as ^{99m}Tc will go to thyroid, salivary glands, and gastric mucosa.
- Belt buckles, articles in clothing, necklaces, and so forth may attenuate image.
- Different slice orientations of SPECT images may allow liver vessels to present as possible hot or cold spots.

SUGGESTED READINGS

Datz FL. Handbook of Nuclear Medicine. 2nd ed. St. Louis: Mosby, 1993.

Early PJ, Sodee DB. Principles and Practice of Nuclear Medicine. 2nd ed. St. Louis: Mosby, 1995.

Murray IPC, Ell PJ, eds. Nuclear Medicine in Clinical Diagnosis and Treatment. Vols. 1 and 2. New York: Churchill Livingstone, 1994.

Wilson, MA. Textbook of Nuclear Medicine. Philadelphia: Lippincott-Raven, 1998.

UltraTag® is a registered trademark of Mallinckrodt Medical, Inc., St. Louis.

Notes

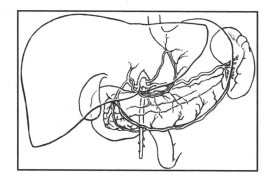

Liver/Spleen Scan

Radiopharmacy

Radionuclide

- ^{99m}Tc t$_{1/2}$: 6 hours

  Energies: 140 keV

  Type: IT, γ, generator

Radiopharmaceutical

- ^{99m}Tc-SC (sulfur colloid)

Localization

- Phagocytosis by reticular cells of liver, spleen, bone marrow, and lungs

Quality Control

- Chromatography, > 90%; particle size, 0.1–1.0 μm; use within 6 hours

Adult Dose Range

- 2–7 mCi (74–259 MBq)

Method of Administration

- IV straight stick or IV catheter and flush

Indications

- Assessment of anatomy, size, and relative position of liver and spleen.
- Assessment of hepatomegaly, splenomegaly, splenic infarcts, accessory spleen or splenosis, or situs inversus.
- Assessment of benign mesenchymal (Kupffer cells) focal lesions (hemangioma, hamartoma) and hepatocellular focal nodular hyperplasia.
- Assessment of chronic liver or spleen disease including primary liver tumors and metastasis, jaundice, cirrhosis, hepatocellular disease, hepatitis, hepatic abscess, or elevated laboratory results.

- Detection and assessment of hepatic or splenic trauma.
- Evaluation for liver disease, chronic anemia, leukemia or other blood disorders, thrombocytopenia, white blood cell (WBC) sequestration, tumors, abscesses, cysts, hemangiomas, hematomas, and trauma.
- Evaluation of hepatic infections, e.g., amebic abscess, hydatid cyst, pyogenic abscess.
- Evaluation of relative splenic function by liver:spleen ratio.

Contraindications

- None.

Patient History *(or use complete patient history in reference section)*

The patient should answer the following questions.

Do you have a history or family history of cancer?	Y	N
If so, what type and for how long?		
Do you have a history of liver or spleen disease?	Y	N
Do you have a history of malaria or tropical diseases?	Y	N
Do you have any abdominal pain?	Y	N
Have you had any recent trauma?	Y	N
Are you diabetic?	Y	N
Have you been feeling lethargic?	Y	N
Do you have high blood pressure?	Y	N
Have you had any previous related scans, x-rays, or recent barium studies?	Y	N

**Have you had any surgery on the liver
or spleen?**   Y   N

**Assess patient for jaundice and possible
alcohol abuse (discern discreetly).**

Other department-specific questions.

Patient Preparation

- Identify the patient. Verify doctor's order. Explain the procedure.
- If available, write concentrations of serum glutamate pyruvate transaminase (SGPT), serum glutamic-oxaloacetic transaminase (SGOT), lactate dehydrogenase (LDH), and total bilirubin on history sheet.

Equipment

Camera
- Large field of view

Collimator
- Low energy, all purpose, or low energy, high resolution

Computer Set-up
Flow
- 1–3 sec/frame for 1 minute followed by immediate static blood pool (60 seconds or 500,000 counts)

Statics
- 600,000–1,000,000 counts

Single Photon Emission Computed Tomography (SPECT)
- 360° rotation, 128 × 128 matrix, 120 stops at 30 sec/stop

Procedure *(time: ~30-60 minutes)*

- Place patient in supine position, camera anterior over lower thorax-abdomen.
- Flow: Position using point source on xiphoid process at top of camera field of view (FOV).
  - Inject, wait a couple of seconds, and start camera.
  - Take immediate blood pool image.
- Statics: Without flow, inject and wait 15 minutes. Position liver and spleen in upper left and right quadrants of FOV.
- Obtain images: anterior with marker(s) over last costal margin for liver (and spleen if

splenomegaly indicated), anterior, RAO, RLAT, (RPO if protocol), posterior, LLAT, and LAO.

- Optional: Posterior with marker on spleen, anterior inspiration and expiration (10 seconds each) to show viability of organs, and standing to reduce motion and improve resolution.

- SPECT: center region of interest (ROI) in FOV. Set parameters and start camera. Contoured or noncircular.

- Processing may include centering liver and spleen, getting ROIs, and doing some combination of computer generated regional ratios of spleen:liver, vertebrae:liver, and vertebrae:spleen uptakes (vertebrae ROI taken from center just below organs). Try Hanning filter, 0.8 cutoff, uniformity correction, 1–2 pixel thickness.

Normal Results

- Flow: Because liver is fed 75% by portal system, there should be ~6-second delay from aorta showing to liver showing. Liver will show dimly at first from aortic (hepatic artery) flush, then brightly from the portal venous system of the superior mesenteric vein (small intestine) and splenic vein (including the stomach, large intestine, and pancreatic veins).

- Statics: Liver and spleen should have equal heterogeneous distribution with little or no bone marrow uptake.

- Relative radiotracer uptake is 85% liver, 10% spleen, and 5% bone marrow.

Abnormal Results

- Flow:

    - Fast uptake: tumors or hepatitis.

    - Increased uptake: hepatomas, hemangiomas.

    - Slow uptake: congestive heart failure, severe cirrhosis.

- Statics:

    - Hepatomegaly: fatty infiltration, chronic passive congestion. Splenomegaly: leukemia, myelofibrosis, malaria, visceral leishmaniasis.

    - Splenic dominance: compromised liver function.

    - Splenic absence: functional asplenia (sickle cell).

    - Bone marrow shifting (shunting): hepatitis, cirrhosis, anemia, leukemia, infection, tumor, diabetes, chronic heart failure.

    - Hot spots: tumors, superior vena cava obstruction because of lung cancer, and focal nodular hyperplasia.

    - Cold spots: metastatic tumors (primary), hepatomas, adenomas, abscess, cyst, infarction, hematoma, trauma, hemangioma.

    - Patchy areas: lacerations, advanced cirrhosis.

Artifacts

- Tape marker to camera to prevent movement and distortion of holes.

- For women, breasts may cause attenuation. Patient can hold them up out of FOV. Also, obese skin folds may cause attenuation; standing will help eliminate these.

- Lung uptake may indicate colloid clumping within radiopharmaceutical (caused by aluminum contamination).

- Deep lesions may be missed.

- Reversible rectangular area (usually liver) of decreased activity from radiation therapy.

SUGGESTED READINGS

Datz FL. Handbook of Nuclear Medicine. 2nd ed. St. Louis: Mosby, 1993.

Early PJ, Sodee DB. Principles and Practice of Nuclear Medicine. 2nd ed. St. Louis: Mosby, 1995.

Murray IPC, Ell PJ, eds. Nuclear Medicine in Clinical Diagnosis and Treatment. Vols. 1 and 2. New York: Churchill Livingstone, 1994.

Wilson, MA. Textbook of Nuclear Medicine. Philadelphia: Lippincott-Raven, 1998.

Notes
. . . .

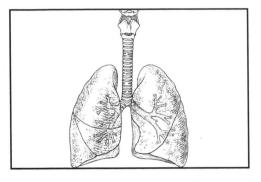

Lung Perfusion

(usually performed with lung ventilation) and Quantitation

Radiopharmacy

Radionuclide

- ^{99m}Tc T$_{1/2}$: 6 hours

  Energies: 140 keV

  Type: IT, γ, generator

Radiopharmaceutical

- MAA (macroaggregated albumin) or HAM (human albumin microspheres)

Localization

- Blood flow to pulmonary capillary or arteriolar embolism

Quality Control

- Particle size, 10-90 μm, 75,000-700,000 particles/injection; chromatography, 90-95% tagging

Adult Dose Range

- 2-6 mCi (74-222 MBq); T$_b$ = ~4-6 hours

Method of Administration

- Patient supine. IV straight stick, or if existing IV catheter, flush heavily with saline only (MAA and heparin do not mix, flush well).
- No reblush. Lift injected arm momentarily to assist in circulation of radiotracer.

Indications

- Usually performed in conjunction with the lung ventilation or aerosol scan and recent (taken within 24 hours) chest x-ray.

- Evaluation for pulmonary embolism (PE), the main cause being deep vein thromboses (DVTs), clots from recent surgery, or trauma. If perfusion defects match with same areas as ventilation defects, chronic obstructive pulmonary disease (COPD) is the diagnosis. If defects mismatch, PE is the diagnosis.
- Evaluation of pulmonary perfusion.
- Evaluation of chest pain.
- Evaluation of shortness of breath.
- Evaluation of low blood oxygen saturation.
- Evaluation and management of carcinoma of the bronchus.
- Evaluation of perfusion affected by emphysema, chronic bronchitis, asthma, inflammatory disease, and cardiac disease.
- Detection of right to left cardiac shunt. Primarily for pediatrics patients; dose must be adjusted.

Contraindications

- Should not be performed on patients with pulmonary hypertension.
- Studies on patients with known active pneumonia or other known debilitating lung disease will yield a nondeterminable result for PE.

Patient History *(or use complete patient history in reference section)*

The patient should answer the following questions.

Do you have a history or family history of cancer?   Y   N

If so, what type and for how long?

Do you have any difficulty or pain with breathing?   Y   N

If so, where?

Do you have shortness of breath?   Y   N

If so, for how long?

Are you coughing up blood?	Y	N
Do you have a history of any lung diseases, e.g., pulmonary emboli, asthma, emphysema, chronic bronchitis, COPD?	Y	N
Do you now or have you ever smoked?	Y	N
If so, how much and for how long?		
Are you running a fever?	Y	N
Do you have fainting spells?	Y	N
Are you taking any oral contraceptives?	Y	N
Do you have a history of heart problems (tachycardia, atrial fibrillation, clots)?	Y	N
Do you have a history of DVTs or phlebitis?	Y	N
Have you had any recent long-distance travel?	Y	N
Have you had any recent surgery?	Y	N
Have you had any recent related scans or x-rays?	Y	N
Are you on heparin, warfarin, aspirin, or other blood-thinning drugs?	Y	N
Other department-specific questions.		

Patient Preparation

- Identify the patient. Verify doctor's order. Explain the procedure.
- Obtain a recent (within 24 hours) chest x-ray or have one ordered.

Equipment

Camera

- Large field of view

Collimator

- Low energy, all purpose, or low energy, high resolution

Computer Set-up

Perfusion

Flow

- Dynamic, 1–3 sec/frame, 60–120 seconds

Statics

- 500,000–1,000,000 counts or as per protocol

Procedure *(time: ~15–30 minutes)*

- Flow:
    - Place patient in supine position with camera posterior.
    - Start computer just before injection.
- Static:
    - Administer injection to patient in supine position.
    - Acquire series of static images in supine or upright (sitting) position for 500,000–1,000,000 counts each.
    - Images (typically): anterior, RAO, RLAT, RPO, posterior, LPO, LLAT, and LAO, or as per protocol. A lung transmission ("nuclear x-ray") picture may also be taken but should precede ventilation or perfusion study.
- Right to left shunt:
    - Acquire anterior, posterior, and right and left laterals of head to verify shunt.
    - Acquire whole-body sweep if quantitation is desired.

Normal Results

- Homogeneous uptake except for normal attenuation by skeletal structures, breasts, and heart.
- Upright position allows for better lung base visualization.

Abnormal Results

- Segmental or wedge-shaped areas of decreased activity, sometimes involving much of the lung, shows high probability of PE especially with mismatch or filled-in areas on ventilation scan.
- Stripe sign of activity may indicate COPD.

- Matching defects with ventilation scan can indicate COPD, lung dysfunction, or tumors.
- Emphysema presents as increased size of lungs.
- Bronchogenic carcinoma can present as complete absence of activity in affected lung or as "edge sign."
- Pleural effusion is indicated by decreased or lack of activity at the base of affected lung(s) or the "fissure sign" (decreased interlobar activity).
- Reverse mismatch, i.e., missing areas on ventilation scan that are filled in on perfusion scan, indicates pneumonia.
- Bacterial pneumonia presents as slightly decreased perfusion and markedly decreased ventilation.
- Radiation causes vasculitis and obliteration of small blood vessels.
- One lung not presenting or presenting very poorly on ventilation scan and presently lightly on perfusion scan indicates collapsed lung, complete or partial bronchial obstruction, e.g., tumor, mucus, or surgery to lung on that side, e.g., complete or partial removal.
- Right to left cardiac shunt: activity in the cerebral hemispheres. Quantitation can be performed by drawing regions of interest (ROIs) on whole-body sweep (around lungs, then around whole body).

$$\% \text{ shunt} = \frac{\text{total body counts} - \text{lung counts}}{\text{total body counts}} \times 100$$

Quantitation

- Lung perfusion quantitation is used to evaluate high-risk patients preoperatively for surgical candidacy. The normal right:left ratio is 55:45.
- Obtain results from pulmonary function test if available.
- Quantitation obtained with the computer software.
- Usually uses the posterior lung perfusion view for analysis although when study is requested, a full perfusion study (all views) is usually performed.
- Most software is set up to draw ROIs in a specific order around areas of the lung, e.g., upper left lung, lower left lung, upper right lung, lower right lung.
- The computer then calculates percent uptake of the two lungs.
- Other calculations (one method):
  - Add the counts of both lungs together for total counts.
  - Divide each lung counts by the total counts and multiply by 100 to give percent function of each lung.
  - From the pulmonary function test, record the actual results (e.g., 1.46 L). Convert to milliliters (e.g., 1.46 L = 1460 mL).
  - Multiply the 1460 mL by the percent of each lung for predicted postsurgical expiratory volume.
  - If this method is used for the decision, the patient is approved for surgery if the volume is greater than 800 mL in the good lung.

Artifacts

- Turn syringe before injection to mix MAA in dose. Do not pull blush back and reinject as hot spots may occur because of radioactive clots injected into system. Patient should be injected while in supine position to avoid gravity-fill of lower lobes.

- Jewelry, medallions, buttons, or items in shirt pockets can cause artifacts.

- Test on patients with known compromised pulmonary function (known disease, shunting, arteriole malformation, liver disease) or one lung should be performed with reduced amounts of radiotracer (and hence reduced number of injected particles) and not performed at all on patients with pulmonary hypertension.

- If little or no visualization of lungs occurs, check patient history for compromising diseases, operations, or cancers, and check syringe for radiotracer retention in hub or needle (sometimes carefully redrawing about 0.5 mL of saline and reinjecting will yield results).

- At least 75,000 particles per injected adult dose. Too few injected will yield "quantum mottled" views.

- Particles in MAA cause microemboli in the 350 million arterioles and 2 billion small capillaries of lungs. Because of the 10- to 90-μm size of the particles, the total particle numbers injected have upper limits so as not to compromise patient. Please refer to Kit Preparation in the Reference Section. When making kits, check the insert for manufacturer's suggestions. Some make sure that the millicuries (megabecquerels) are within normal kit ranges and that not more than 1 mL total quantity of radiotracer is drawn from the kit. This is particularly important with patients who already have a compromising pulmonary condition.

- Patients receiving lung scans can be critically compromised without showing it. If at all possible, never take your eyes off the patient or leave them unattended in a room; things can "go bad" very quickly.

- Serious PE involvement may present with no symptoms of chest pain, shortness of breath, hemoptysis, history of recent long trips, or history of DVT. Tachycardia is a classic symptom of PE and, together with low O_2 saturation and distension of the vessels in the neck, could mean cardiac tamponade (ruled out with an echocardiograph) or PE (ruled out with a lung scan). Tachycardia may arise because the brain perceives the diminished supply of oxygen, causing an increase in beats per minute to compensate. There may be other mechanisms.

Note

Some other agents and modalities for lung scans include [186]Re, [117m]Sn, and ^{99m}Tc-antibodies or peptides (chemically bond to PE and DVTs), or CT scans.

SUGGESTED READINGS

Datz FL. Handbook of Nuclear Medicine. 2nd ed. St. Louis: Mosby, 1993.

Early PJ, Sodee DB. Principles and Practice of Nuclear Medicine. 2nd ed. St. Louis: Mosby, 1995.

Klingensmith W, Eshima D, Goddard J. Nuclear Medicine Procedure Manual 1997–98. Englewood, CO: Wick, 1998.

Murray IPC, Ell PJ, eds. Nuclear Medicine in Clinical Diagnosis and Treatment. Vols. 1 and 2. New York: Churchill Livingstone, 1994.

Wilson, MA. Textbook of Nuclear Medicine. Philadelphia: Lippincott-Raven, 1998.

Notes

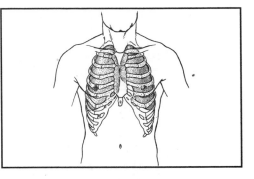

Lung Transmission

(usually performed with lung ventilation and perfusion)

Radiopharmacy

Radionuclide

- ^{99m}Tc t$_{1/2}$: 6 hours

  Energies: 140 keV

  Type: IT, γ, generator

Radiopharmaceutical

- Na ^{99m}TcO$_4{}^-$ (pertechnetate)

Localization

- N/A

Quality Control

- Moly breakthrough, Al breakthrough, chromatography

Adult Dose Range

- 50 mCi (1850 MBq)

Method of Administration

- Exposed to, not administered

Indications

- Detection of gross anatomy and relative position of lungs.
- Detection and localization of major lesions, constrictions, or gross physical deformities.
- Evaluation of thorax in conjunction with lung ventilation and lung perfusion tests. Test is used as a type of nuclear medicine x-ray.

Contraindications

- None

Patient History *(or use complete patient history in reference section)*

The patient should answer the following questions.

**Do you have a history or family history
of cancer?**   Y   N

If so, what type and for how long?

**Do you have any difficulty or pain with
breathing?**   Y   N

If so, where?

Do you have shortness of breath?   Y   N

If so, for how long?

Are you coughing up blood?   Y   N

**Do you have a history of any lung diseases,
e.g., pulmonary emboli, asthma,
emphysema, chronic bronchitis,
COPD?**   Y   N

Do you now or have you ever smoked?   Y   N

If so, how much and for how long?

Are you running a fever?	Y	N
Do you have fainting spells?	Y	N
Are you taking any oral contraceptives?	Y	N
Do you have a history of heart problems (tachycardia, atrial fibrillation, clots)?	Y	N
Do you have a history of deep vein thrombosis (DVT), phlebitis?	Y	N
Have you had any recent long-distance travel?	Y	N
Have you had any recent surgery?	Y	N
Have you had any recent related scans or x-rays?	Y	N
Are you on heparin, warfarin, aspirin, or other blood-thinning drugs?	Y	N
Other department-specific questions.		

Patient Preparation

- Identify the patient. Verify doctor's order. Explain the procedure.

Equipment

Camera
- Large field of view

Collimator
- Low energy, all purpose, or low energy, high resolution

Computer Set-up
- One static picture, 3,000,000 counts

Procedure (time: ~15 minutes)

- Place patient in supine position on scanning bed, camera anterior, thorax.
- Roll container, e.g., large drum, holding $^{99m}TcO_4^-$ directly under patient.

- Position container and patient such that lungs are centered in camera field of view.
- Take one static image for 3 million counts.

Normal Results

- Both lungs will present fully, uniform, and symmetric.

Abnormal Results

- Lung does not present.
- Lung(s) appears deformed, portions missing or containing light or dark areas depending on defect.

Other Types of Transmission Scans

- Outlining patient: Using ^{57}Co "cookie sheet," place opposite side of patient to camera. Image acquired has outline of patient that can be useful for relative positioning of region of interest (ROI).
- Lung ventilation positioning: Using the syringe containing ^{133}Xe, as patient lies supine with camera posterior, wave syringe over anterior thorax and check p-scope to make sure lungs are fully in camera view. This allows proper positioning before ^{133}Xe gas is administered and dynamic pictures are started. This method, if used, should be done quickly to reduce exposure, or tape into dose lead-container (pig) using opening toward patient. It also works well in the seated position with camera behind patient.

Artifacts

- Jewelry, medallions, buttons, pacemakers, and prostheses may attenuate the picture.

SUGGESTED READINGS

There isn't much in the literature about these techniques. These techniques were taken from the Nuclear Medicine Departments of the following institutions:

Bayfront Medical Center, St. Petersburg, FL: ^{133}Xe lung positioning.

Columbia Doctor's Hospital, Sarasota, FL: ^{57}Co torso outlining.

H. Lee Moffitt Cancer Center, Tampa, FL: ^{57}Co torso outlining.

James A. Haley Veterans Hospital, Tampa, FL: ^{99m}Tc lung transmission scan.

Notes

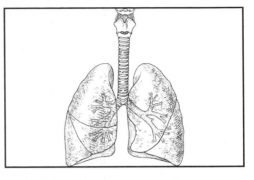

CHAPTER 30

Lung Ventilation: Gas and Aerosol

(usually performed with lung perfusion)

Radiopharmacy

Radionuclide

- ^{133}Xe $t_{1/2}$: 5.3 days

  Energies: 32 x-ray, 81 keV

  Type: β^-, γ, fission product

- or: ^{99m}Tc $t_{1/2}$: 6 hours

  Energies: 140 keV

  Type: IT, γ, generator

Radiopharmaceutical

- ^{133}Xe: gas

- ^{99m}Tc-DTPA (diethylenetriaminepentaacetic acid)

- ^{99m}Tc-HAMM (human albumin mini-microspheres)

Localization

- Compartmental by inhalation into lung space

Quality Control

- ^{133}Xe: dose calibrate vial before use

- ^{99m}Tc-DTPA: chromatography > 95%

Adult Dose Range

- ^{133}Xe: 10–20 mCi (370–740 MBq); $T_b = \sim 30$ seconds

- ^{99m}Tc-DTPA: 25–40 mCi (925–1480 MBq)

Method of Administration

- Inhalation through mask or mouth apparatus, PO.

Indications

- Usually done in conjunction with lung perfusion study and recent (taken within 24 hours) chest x-ray.
- Evaluation and detection of pulmonary embolism (PE) in conjunction with lung perfusion (mismatching defects).
- Evaluation of chronic obstructive pulmonary disease (COPD) in conjunction with lung perfusion (matching defects).
- Evaluation of obstructed or constricted airways, alveolar spaces, and air distribution resulting in shortness of breath.
- Evaluation of pulmonary retention.
- Evaluation of chest pain.
- Evaluation of low blood oxygen saturation.
- Evaluation of adult respiratory distress syndrome (ARDS), emphysema, inflammation, chronic bronchitis, or pneumonia.
- Evaluation of tracheobronchial epithelium function (aerosol).
- Evaluation and staging of patients with COPD, lung carcinoma, and bronchial obstruction (aerosol).
- Evaluation of pulmonary permeability in restrictive lung disease or pulmonary edema by observing clearance rates using submicrometer aerosols (DTPA).

Contraindications

- Studies on patients with known active pneumonia or other known debilitating lung disease will yield a nondeterminable result for PE.

Patient History *(or use complete patient history in reference section)*

The patient should answer the following questions.

Do you have a history or family history of cancer? Y   N

If so, what type and for how long?

Do you have any difficulty or pain with breathing?   **Y   N**

If so, where?

Do you have shortness of breath?   Y   N

   If so, for how long?

_____

Are you coughing up blood?   Y   N
_____

Do you have a history of any lung diseases,
   e.g., pulmonary emboli, asthma,
   emphysema, chronic bronchitis, COPD?   Y   N
_____

Do you now or have you ever smoked?   Y   N

   If so, how much and for how long?

_____

Are you running a fever?   Y   N
_____

Do you have fainting spells?   Y   N
_____

Are you taking any oral contraceptives?   Y   N
_____

Do you have a history of heart problems
   (tachycardia, atrial fibrillation, clots)?   Y   N
_____

Do you have a history of deep vein thrombosis
   (DVT), phlebitis?   Y   N
_____

Have you had any recent long-distance travel?   Y   N
_____

Have you had any recent surgery?   Y   N
_____

Have you had any recent related scans or
   x-rays?   Y   N
_____

Are you on heparin, warfarin, aspirin, or
   other blood-thinning drugs?   Y   N
_____

Other department-specific questions.
_____

Patient Preparation

- Identify the patient. Verify doctor's order. Explain the procedure.
- Obtain recent (within 24 hours) chest x-ray or have one ordered.

Equipment

Camera

- Large field of view

Collimator

- ^{133}Xe: low energy, all purpose, or low energy, high sensitivity
- ^{99m}Tc-DTPA: low energy, all purpose, or low energy, high resolution

Computer Set-up

- ^{133}Xe: dynamic, flow study, 20–60 sec/frame for 6–8 minutes
- ^{99m}Tc-DTPA: static images (500,000–1,000,000 counts) usually same views as perfusion

Procedure *(time: ~15–30 minutes)*

^{133}Xe: gas

- Place patient in sitting position with camera on back, or in supine position, camera posterior.
- If ventilation scan is first, position patient using the dose as a marker on the suprasternal notch or top of shoulders for the upper field of view (FOV), along sides of patient to ensure sides are in FOV, xiphoid process just below center. Lungs must be fully in FOV. If the dose is in a syringe, wave over thorax for a transmission-type view. Lungs will visualize on p-scope.
- Explain and apply mask, ready apparatus depending on type and protocol.
- Inject or pump in gas as deep breath is taken (and held, if protocol), start computer simultaneously. Adjust apparatus, e.g., Pulmonex®, as necessary if used.
- Acquire dynamic images for inspiration, equilibrium, and wash-out. Mask stays on for at least 60 seconds or longer as per protocol (if acquisition is for eight frames, some leave mask on for four frames or until count rate falls to a low level).
- Remove mask and allow patient to breath room air. Remind patient to remain still.

^{99m}Tc-DTPA: aerosol

- Place patient in supine position on bed, or upright (sitting or standing).
- Inject ^{99m}Tc-DTPA into canister or aerosol dispenser (nebulizer). Place mouthpiece in patient's mouth. Attach nose clamp. A mask can also be used. Hook up nebulizer to ~10 L/min of air from wall. Only about 1 mCi (37 MBq) makes it into the lungs.
- Instruct patient to breath normally for 5 minutes.
- Remove equipment.
- Obtain images as to protocol, the usual eight as in the perfusion although some only require six in both (anterior, posterior, LLATs and RLATs, and LPOs and RPOs).

Normal Results

- ^{133}Xe gas: Uniform and symmetric wash-in, equilibrium, and wash-out pictures in both lungs with the left lung having the typically light cardiac notch. Wash-out fairly complete with no retention of gas.

- Aerosol (e.g., ^{99m}Tc-DTPA): The pharynx shows bright from inhalation, the stomach and gut may show from swallowed contaminated saliva (have patient expectorate into a facial tissue as soon as the mouthpiece is removed and dispose to reduce this phenomenon). Trachea and bronchi show branching nicely with this method.

Abnormal Results

^{133}Xe gas

- Areas of decreased activity occur where lung was not ventilated.

- Ventilation study usually presents as normal (uniform and symmetrical uptake and washout in all three phases) in cases of pulmonary embolism (PE). Mismatching areas of activity (usually two or more segmental defects) in the perfusion study is the indicator for PE.

- COPD presents as inhomogeneous wash-in, patchy equilibrium, and areas of trapping delaying wash-out (especially lower lobes).

- Bacterial pneumonia presents as markedly decreased ventilation and slightly decreased perfusion.

- Localization and retention in liver with ventilation indicates liver fatty infiltrates prevalent with alcoholics and obese patients.

- One lung not presenting or presenting very poorly indicates collapsed lung or complete or partial bronchial obstruction, e.g., tumor, mucus, or surgery to lung on that side (removal).

Aerosol (^{99m}Tc-DTPA)

- Areas of decreased activity occur where lung was not ventilated.

- Ventilation study usually presents as normal (uniform and symmetrical uptake) in cases of pulmonary emoblism (PE). Mismatching areas of activity (usually two or more segmental defects) in the perfusion study is the indicator for PE.

- Obstruction presents with bronchial branching missing or noticeably not as well ventilated distal to obstruction.

- Accelerated clearance of aerosols may present in patients with chronic interstitial lung disease or with inflammation of the lung such as ARDS and pneumocystic pneumonia.

- One lung not presenting or presenting very poorly indicates collapsed lung or complete or partial bronchial obstruction, e.g., tumor or surgery to lung on that side (removal).

Artifacts

- Some computers must be manually peaked for ^{133}Xe.

- Mask not fitting tightly over face, allowing gas to escape. This is more possible with very thin faces, facial hair, noncoherent patients.

- Patient disrupting mask or mouthpiece by coughing or removing.

- Lungs not properly positioned before start of ventilation.
- Injection of gas made on patient's exhale.
- Missing proper start time on computer.
- Patient not breathing well using aerosol apparatus.
- Patient movement.

SUGGESTED READINGS

Datz FL. Handbook of Nuclear Medicine. 2nd ed. St. Louis: Mosby, 1993.

Early PJ, Sodee DB. Principles and Practice of Nuclear Medicine. 2nd ed. St. Louis: Mosby, 1995.

Murray IPC, Ell PJ, eds. Nuclear Medicine in Clinical Diagnosis and Treatment. Vols. 1 and 2. New York: Churchill Livingstone, 1994.

Wilson, MA. Textbook of Nuclear Medicine. Philadelphia: Lippincott-Raven, 1998.

Pulmonex® is a registered trademark of Atomic Products, Center Moriches, NY.

Notes

CHAPTER 31

· · · · · · · ·

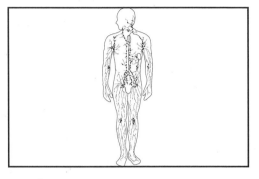

Lymphoscintigraphy

(Lymphangiogram)

Radiopharmacy

Radionuclide

- ^{99m}Tc t$_{1/2}$: 6 hours

  Energies: 140 keV

  Type: IT, γ, generator

Radiopharmaceutical

- ^{99m}Tc-SC (sulfur colloid, antimony sulfide is out of production)

Localization

- Compartmental, phagocytosis

Quality Control

- ^{99m}Tc, chromatography > 90%; sulfur colloid filtered to < 0.10 μm

Adult Dose Range

- 200 μCi to 2 mCi (7.4-74 MBq), 450 μCi to 1 mCi (16.65-37 MBq)
  is typical, two to six injections. Some use up to 7 mCi (259 MBq) total.

Method of Administration

- For melanoma: IV injection, two or six subcutaneous and/or intradermal, producing
  a wheal, placed around cancer site, surgery, or region of interest (within 5 mm).
  Other routes are intradermal into the web of hand or foot. Volume should not
  exceed 0.25 mL per injection site (tuberculin syringe).

- For breast lesions: IV injection, four placed in tissue surrounding lesion (within 2-3
  mm), as much as 4 mL per syringe at 3-, 6-, 9-, and 12-o'clock positions around tumor
  site. Injections may be done under ultrasound. Some include lidocaine or sedation to
  reduce pain of injections. Some include hyaluronidase, a testicular enzyme, to limit

time of pain with injection and increase radiotracer clearance time (distributes radiotracer faster).

- For lymphedema: IV injection, two sites per limb, subcutaneous, producing a wheal, placed into the web between fingers or toes depending on the area of interest.

Indications

- Evaluation of staging (spread) of cancers (e.g., lymphatic leukemia, reticulum cell carcinoma, Hodgkin's disease, and melanomas) into the lymph system.
- Evaluation of lymphatic kinetics, particularly for cancers.
- Detection of metastatic invasion of the lymph nodes.
- Evaluation of node resection as an alternative to removing an entire bed of lymph nodes, which may cause edema of that area and other related complications. It is designed to find the few sentinel nodes to which the cancer may drain.
- Evaluation of pelvic or periaortic lymphatic drainage for blockage by trauma or tumor (e.g., rectal, prostatic, or vulvar cancer).
- Evaluation for endolymphatic radiotherapy and radical surgery candidates.
- Evaluation of chronic lymphedema of swollen extremity.
- Differentiation of primary (neither lymphatic nor proximal lymph node visualization) and secondary (interstitial lymphatic uptake but poor visualization of proximal lymph vessels and nodes) lymphedema.
- Evaluation of lymph vessel patency before lymphovenous anastomosis (connecting of vessels).

Contraindications

- None

Patient History

The patient should answer the following questions.

Do you have a history or family history of cancer?   Y   N

   If so, what type and for how long?

Is this study for before or after surgery?

Have you had any surgery in area of interest?   Y   N

Where is the site (or sites) under scrutiny?

Have you had any recent biopsies?	Y	N

Have you had any past or recent related scans (mammography, CT, NM, MRI, x-rays)?	Y	N

Do you have a history of lymphedema?	Y	N

Other department-specific questions.

Patient Preparation

- Identify the patient. Verify doctor's order. Explain the procedure.
- Wipe area with alcohol pad, shave if necessary; clean area with Betadine®.
- For breast study, patient is to bring mammograms and any related studies with her (outpatient) or make previous related studies available (inpatient).
- For breast study, patient is instructed to massage area of injection after injections and between imaging sessions.
- For lymphedema, physician to instruct patient to wear elastic stockings. These should be removed 3–4 hours before study.

Equipment

Camera

- Large field of view

Collimator

- Low energy, all purpose, or low energy, high resolution

Computer Set-up

Flow

- 30–60 sec/frame, 10–15 minutes

Immediate Statics

- Collect for 5 minutes (300 seconds) every 5 minutes for up to 30 minutes; 256 × 256 × 16 matrix; try 10% window to reduce scatter

Delays

- 40,000–200,000 counts or 5 minutes each; try 10% window

Whole Body

- Set for 10–15 cm/min

Procedure *(procedures vary greatly [see Sample Protocols]; time: ~1-6 hours)*

- Prepare the area of interest for the patient (e.g., shave, alcohol wipe, Betadine®).
- Melanoma: Patient is injected around the region of interest (ROI) with two to six doses subcutaneously and/or intradermally.
- Breast lesion: Patient is injected with four to six injections around lesion.
- Lymphedema: Patient is injected subcutaneously in webs of feet or hands as indicated, two sites per limb.
- Place patient in prone, supine, or sitting position, depending on site to best obtain images of lymph drainage.
- Flow: position ROI under camera, image dynamic flow for 10-15 minutes.

  Immediate statics: 5-10 minutes per view, with or without markers or transmission images.
- Views: anterior, posterior, obliques, and/or laterals to best image the direction of lymph node drainage.
- Marker images: use a point source outlining the body and/or a transmission image using a ^{57}Co flood source (cookie sheet) placed behind the patient to help define the position of the nodes of interest.
- Extremities: the inguinals or axillas should visualize within 10-30 minutes depending on how distal the site is. In these cases and trunk-oriented cancers, delays of the whole body (1-2 hours) may be required to visualize secondary drainage.
- Abdominal lymph nodes: subcutaneous injection in the interdigital webs of the feet.
- Lymphatic internal mammary chain: injection into the space behind the rectus abdominal muscle.
- Presurgical patients: position patient as they will be in surgery, e.g., arm up or down. When all related nodes are believed to be exposed, their locations are marked on the patient's skin with indelible ink. The patient returns just before surgery to have the spots reconfirmed and tattooed for the surgeon.
- Delays: 1-4 hours after injection (see below), use same views as before.
- Whole body: sweep or statics to cover all drainage areas.
- Single photon emission computed tomography (SPECT): center area of interest, set parameters, and start camera.

Normal Results

- The radiotracer enters the lymphatic system through normal channels and proceeds through the system into the major lymphatic beds (e.g., retroperitoneal, the axillaries, inguinal, parasternal, and cervical lymph nodes).
- Visualizing the sentinel node or nodes is normal within the first half hour.
- After 4 hours, a chain of activity should visualize in the inguinal, iliac, and periaortic regions.
- Liver should also present.
- A biopsy of those nodes, once removed, will yield the result.

Abnormal Results

- None or only some of the expected nodes visualizing indicates malignant disease or blockage. Intervening surgical or trauma scars can block the normal progression of the lymph system.

- Continuity of a chain interrupted.

- Enlargement of a chain width because of lymphoma, congestion, or lymphadenitis.

- Unexpected intensity difference, reduced in malignant lymphoma or increased in congestion and lymphadenitis.

- Displacement of expected location by metastasis or collateral circulation.

- Missing liver activity may indicate insufficient movement of the extremities or lymphatic blockade.

Injection Sites for Visualization and Suggested Delayed Pictures

- Surface lesion: two to six injections around area of cancerous tissue or ROI. Delays 2–4 hours, 50,000–100,000 counts. Be sure to shield injection site or center counts on lymph nodes, not injection site.

- Retroperitoneal lymph nodes: injection into medial two interdigital webs of feet. Image at 4 hours with part of liver in view, lumbar lymph nodes are focal area, 100,000 counts.

- Axillary and apical lymph nodes: injection into medial two interdigital webs of the hands. Image at 2–4 hours, upper chest and neck in view, 40,000 counts. Axillary image, arm up, face turned away from ROI, 40,000 counts.

- Cervical nodes: injection into dorsum of the mastoid process.

- Internal mammary chain: injection into posterior rectus sheath below rib cage, angling toward diaphragm. Delays 2–4 hours, 50,000–100,000 counts.

- Iliopelvic lymph nodes: injection into perianal region just lateral to the anal margin at the 3- and 9-o'clock positions. Patient in knee-to-chest position. Delays 2–4 hours, 100,000 counts.

Sample Protocols

Protocol for Detecting Direction of Flow

- Set-up
  - Flow: 10 sec/image for 300 seconds.
  - Immediate dynamics: 6 images for 300 seconds each.
  - Static: immediate static (oblique for axilla) for 40,000 counts.
- Patient placed on imaging table to allow access to ROI. Obtain lead shield just big enough to shield injection sites.
- (Optional) With camera placed in approximate position making sure to include suspected drainage area of nodes, ^{57}Co sheet placed under patient with camera over top. One or more images obtained with anatomic markers included and outline of body contours with ^{99m}Tc source. These can be filmed separately in the same format as the flow for superimposition (statics for 40,000 counts).

Breast Lesions

- Inject four to six doses ~200–500 µCi each with patient in place on imaging table.

- Position ROI under camera, making certain to include closest suspected lymphatic bed. Shield injection sites. Start flow quickly as radiotracer begins migration quickly. Add anatomic markers if none have been done.

- Note migration. Adjust camera for dynamics if necessary (add anatomic markers to one or more if camera is moved).

- Immediate static, especially oblique with axilla, adding anatomic marker(s) (e.g., xiphoid process, umbilicus, suprasternal notch [SSN], etc.) for 150,000 counts.

- Delays: Static(s) at 1 or 2 hours; shield injection site, same position as dynamics and oblique if taken for 150,000 counts or 5 minutes each. Again at 3–4 hours.

- Alternative delays: If computer has a region-extraction program, take an image without a lead shield, increase counts to 500,000 or so, using earlier images as a guide. Using computer program, extract injection sites and increase intensity to visualize possible nodes.

Alternative for Breast Lesions

- After injection: flow 20 frames at 30 seconds each. Immediate static for 300 seconds with ^{57}Co cookie sheet behind patient and/or markers. Optional additional with shield and ^{57}Co behind patient.

- At 1–2 hours with ^{57}Co: one 300-second image without shield, one with shield (anterior, posterior, obliques, laterals, or combination to get best picture of drainage).

- At 3–4 hours with ^{57}Co: same images.

- Processing: if you have region-extraction program or something similar, choose image without shield and extract injection sites (careful of not extracting possible proximal nodes) and increase intensity. Show films for possibility of performing more delays using same protocol.

Easiest Protocol for Breast Lesions

- After injection: obtain flow and immediates (e.g., anterior and oblique) with cookie sheet for patient outline.

- Patient returns at 1.5–2 hours for repeat statics.

- If no visualization, patient returns in 3–4 hours for repeat statics.

Role of Technologist in Operating Room (OR)

- Many institutions are using these studies to localize and resect lymph nodes. The role of the technologist differs with the institution, but they generally perform the following tasks.

- Draw up doses and bring them to physician doing injections. For melanomas, some institutions allow technologists to inject.

- Images taken as suggested above, patient and images are brought to preoperative area to prepare for surgery.

- In OR

  - Technologist uses gamma probe to locate "hot" node(s). (Only in some institutions, others hire a company to manipulate the probe.)

  - Technologist takes resected nodes and material to pathology for inspection.

- Technologist may have to take material to radiology for x-ray if requested for "needle loc (localization)" specimen.
- Technologist assays material for storage (10 half-lives) if > 0.05 mR at 1 m or disposal if background ≤ 0.05 mR at 1 m.
- Technologist assays pathology room and equipment for contamination.
- Technologist assays OR for contamination after removal of patient.

Artifacts

- A "star" artifact, caused by the intensity of the injection site(s), may obscure nodes in the proximity from presenting properly.
- Injection sites that are too distant from the area of interest may obscure primary nodes close to the lesion.
- The injection(s) may not migrate as expected if there is intervening scar tissue from a prior surgery or injury.
- One view of the lighted nodes may not be enough to properly locate the node or nodes. Multiple views including anterior, posterior, oblique, and laterals may be needed.
- Some nodes will be small or weak in intensity. Enough counts and care must be taken to locate all that may be present.
- If whole-body static images are necessary, there may be no visual clues on the p-scope to position by, so careful eyeballing may be required.
- Care must be taken when marking the affected nodes for presurgical candidates because that is where the surgeon will make the excisions.

Note

Variables that can alter the image outcome include the total amount of radiotracer, volume of each injection, number of sites, distance of injections from lesion or ROI, depth of injections, flow, delay times, length of acquisitions, markers, silhouette, and region extraction or lead shields or both. Always check with physicians as to preferences.

SUGGESTED READINGS

Datz FL. Handbook of Nuclear Medicine. 2nd ed. St. Louis: Mosby, 1993.

Early PJ, Sodee DB. Principles and Practice of Nuclear Medicine. 2nd ed. St. Louis: Mosby, 1995.

Murray IPC, Ell PJ, eds. Nuclear Medicine in Clinical Diagnosis and Treatment. Vols. 1 and 2. New York: Churchill Livingstone, 1994.

Wilson, MA. Textbook of Nuclear Medicine. Philadelphia: Lippincott-Raven, 1998.

Betadine® is a registered trademark of Purdue Fredrick Co., Norwalk, CT.

Notes

CHAPTER 32

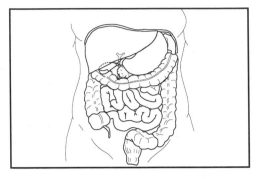

Meckel's Diverticulum

Radiopharmacy

Radionuclide

- ^{99m}Tc $t_{1/2}$: 6 hours

  Energies: 140 keV

  Type: IT, γ, generator

Radiopharmaceutical

- Na $^{99m}TcO_4^-$ (pertechnetate)

Localization

- Active transport, concentrated and rapidly secreted by the epithelial tissue of the (ectopic) gastric mucosa

Quality Control

- Moly breakthrough, Al breakthrough, chromatography

Adult Dose Range

- 10-15 mCi (370–555 MBq); 200 µCi/kg in pediatrics

Method of Administration

- IV injection

Indications

- Localization of a Meckel's diverticulum with functioning gastric mucosa.
- Detection of gastrointestinal bleeding.
- Evaluation of positive guaiac test (blood in feces).
- Evaluation of abdominal pain (especially in children). Usually early age onset from abnormal development of fetal intestine from yolk sac. Meckel's is formed from

incomplete closure of yolk duct and usually within 18 inches of the ileocecal valve. It may contain ileal, duodenal, colonic, pancreatic, or gastric tissue.

- Evaluation of bleeding, diverticulitis, or intestinal obstruction caused by intussusception (intestinal invagination) and volvulus (twisting of bowel causing obstruction).

Contraindications

- Patients with barium or contrast studies under way

Patient History *(or use complete patient history in reference section)*

The patient should answer the following questions.

Do you have a history or family history of cancer?   Y   N

If so, what type and for how long?

Do you have any pain?   Y   N

If so, where and for how long?

Are you actively bleeding?   Y   N

Do you have blood in your stool?   Y   N

If so, is it dark or bright red?

Have you had any recent related examinations or contrast radiographic examinations?   Y   N

Do you have any recent laboratory results with you?

Other department-specific questions.

Patient Preparation

- Identify the patient. Verify doctor's order. Explain the procedure.

- Ensure patient to be NPO for 4–12 hours. Infants: NPO equal to normal feeding time minus 30 minutes (study time).

- Physician to discontinue thyroid blocking agents, e.g., perchlorate or saturated solution of potassium iodide 48 hours before study.

- Instruct patient to void before procedure.

- Ensure patient has no radiographic barium studies on same day or 48 hours before study.

- If pentagastrin is to be used, ensure patient to be NPO for 8 hours. It must be ordered from pharmacy 24 hours in advance. Inject 15 minutes before $^{99m}TcO_4^-$ injection.

- Cimetidine suggested in difficult cases; 300 mg adjusted for age, qid up to 6 times hourly for 24 hours.

Equipment

Camera

- Large field of view

Collimator

- Low energy, all purpose, or low energy, high resolution

Computer Set-up
Flow

- 1–5 sec/frame for 1 minute

Dynamic

- 15 sec/frame for 29 minutes or 1 min/frame for 15 minutes

Statics

- Acquire ~500,000–1,000,000 counts per image

Procedure *(time: ~60 minutes)*

- Place patient in supine position with camera anterior covering xiphoid to pubis.

- Inject and start camera for flow and dynamic study.

- Statics: Obtain immediate image(s) and, depending on length of dynamic, one image every 5 minutes up to 30 minutes after injection. Image posterior, laterals, and obliques as per protocol if possible area is visualized.

- Drug interventions may be included.

  - Pentagastrin: (Peptavlon®) ~6 µg/kg, stimulates ectopic gastric mucosal uptake of pertechnetate by 30–60% while decreasing emptying time into small bowel and decreasing background. Administered intramuscularly in children, subcutaneously in adults. Administer 15 minutes before $^{99m}TcO_4^-$ injection.

- Glucagon: ~50 μg, decreases peristalsis and increases persistence of activity in the ectopic mucosa.

- Cimetidine: ~300 mg qid, decreases release of pertechnetate from the ectopic mucosa into the bowel lumen and increases gastric uptake (or ranitidine).

- Potassium perchlorate: blocks uptake of pertechnetate by thyroid and salivary glands.

- If delays are required, instruct patient to void between images (in the bathroom, not in the formatter).

Normal Results

- Increased gastric uptake and renal activity in first 10–20 minutes of study, decreasing as study progresses.

- Bladder uptake increases with time.

Abnormal Results

- Focally increased activity not associated with normal structures, particularly in lower right quadrant.

- Activity in Meckel's will appear at the same time normal gastric mucosa presents and remains in same position despite peristalsis.

"Rule of Two's" for Meckel's

- Occurs in 2% of population

- Occurs within 2 feet of the ileocecal valve

- Average length of 2 inches

- Usually symptomatic by age of 2

Artifacts

- Radiographic study before scan for Meckel's may mask activity.

- Barium studies and proctoscopy may present as false-positive results.

- Early renal activity, unassociated ectopic gastric mucosa, or blood pooling from inflammation or tumors may give false-positive reading (for Meckel's).

- Radiotracer may present in renal pelvis and duodenum, which are difficult to separate. This is done by lateral views.

- False-negative results could be caused by small Meckel's, no gastric mucosa (no activity), rapid radiotracer wash-out, or obscured by normal activity.

SUGGESTED READINGS

Datz FL. Handbook of Nuclear Medicine. 2nd ed. St. Louis: Mosby, 1993.

Early PJ, Sodee DB. Principles and Practice of Nuclear Medicine. 2nd ed. St. Louis: Mosby, 1995.

Murray IPC, Ell PJ, eds. Nuclear Medicine in Clinical Diagnosis and Treatment. Vols. 1 and 2. New York: Churchill Livingstone, 1994.

Wilson, MA. Textbook of Nuclear Medicine. Philadelphia: Lippincott-Raven, 1998.

Peptavlon® is a registered trademark of Wyeth-Ayerst Laboratories, Philadelphia, PA.

Notes

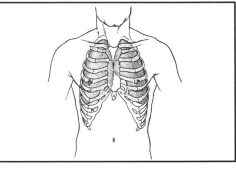

CHAPTER 33

NeoTect™

(Lung Mass)

Radiopharmacy

Radionuclide

- ^{99m}Tc T$_{1/2}$: 6 hrs

  Energies: 140 keV

  Type: IT, γ, generator

Radiopharmaceutical

- ^{99m}Tc-depreotide (NeoTect™); ~ 50 µg depreotide

Localization

- Blood flow; depreotide is a synthetic peptide that binds to somatostatin receptor-bearing normal and abnormal tissue (e.g., pulmonary mass tissue)

Quality Control

- Chromatography, ≥ 90% radiochemical purity

Adult Dose Range

- 15–20 mCi (555–740 MBq)

Method of Administration

- Peripheral intravenous injection; IV catheter or butterfly with saline flush (monitor patient 5–10 minutes for possible reaction)

Indications

- Identification and localization of malignant, somatostatin receptor-bearing pulmonary masses.

- Verification of pulmonary lesions presented on CT and/or chest x-ray. Study should be performed with correlating recent CT scan and/or chest x-ray.
- Detection and evaluation of masses in patients who have known malignancy or highly suspect for malignancy.

Contraindications

- No known medical contraindications.
- Not to be used as an alternative to CT or biopsy.

Patient History

The patient should answer the following questions.

Do you have a history or family history of cancer? Y N

If so, what type and for how long?

Do you have any difficulty or pain with breathing? Y N

If so, where and for how long?

Do you have shortness of breath? Y N

If so, for how long?

Are you coughing up blood? Y N

Do you have a history of any lung diseases (e.g., pulmonary emboli, asthma, emphysema, chronic bronchitis, COPD)? Y N

Do you have a history of or now have a lung infection (e.g., pneumonia)? Y N

Do you now or have you ever smoked?	Y	N

If so, how much and for how long?

Are you running a fever?	Y	N
Do you have fainting spells?	Y	N
Have you had any recent surgery?	Y	N
Have you had a recent CT, chest x-ray, biopsy, or previous nuc-med scans?	Y	N

Other department-specific questions.

Patient Preparation

- Identify the patient. Verify doctor's order. Explain the procedure.
- Instruct patient to be well hydrated unless contraindicated.
- Instruct patient to drink at least 8 ounces of fluid prior to injection.
- Instruct patient to void several times during the first few hours post injection.

Equipment

Camera

- Large field of view

Collimator

- Low energy, all purpose, or low energy, high resolution or ultra-high resolution, parallel hole

Computer Set-up

- Window 20% at 140 keV

Statics

- 500,000–1,000,000 counts or as per protocol

Single Photon Emission Computed Tomography (SPECT)

- Non-circular, elliptical, or body contour, 64×64 matrix, continuous or step and shoot, 360°, 60 stops (single head) or 120 stops (dual head), 30–40 sec/step (30,000–50,000 counts/step)

Procedure *(time: ~30–40 minutes)*

- Ensure patient is well hydrated or has had at least 8 ounces of fluid.
- Inject patient with radiopharmaceutical.
- Wait 2–4 hours post injection to image patient; instruct patient to void often before imaging begins.
- Place patient in supine position on table, with arms extended over head if possible.
- Ensure patient is straight on table and comfortable.
- Remind patient to be still during acquisition.
- Ensure that both entire lungs are in the field-of-view (FOV) of camera.
  - SSN not less than 1″ from top of FOV.
  - Xiphoid process and 10th rib within the lower third of FOV.
- Acquire SPECT images of chest.
- Acquire static images of chest (anterior, posterior, obliques, laterals) as per protocol as an option.
- SPECT processing suggestions:
  - Reconstruction filter—Ramp.
  - Post-reconstruction filter—Butterworth or equivalent or 3-D restoration.
  - Slice thickness—1 cm.
  - Ensure with filter selection that small lesions in the chest remain visible.

Normal Results

- Homogeneous uptake in both lung areas.
- No localized and/or non-symmetric areas of uptake in either lung area.
- Increased uptake in the spine, sternum, and rib-ends.
- Bilateral, symmetric uptake in the hilum and/or mediastinum.

Abnormal Results

- Uptake that is localized and/or non-symmetric and increased compared to surrounding normal lung tissue.
- Abnormal uptake should be confirmed in at least two SPECT projections.
- Abnormal uptake should correspond to pulmonary lesions identified on the CT scan and/or chest x-ray.

Artifacts

- Possible false-negatives in patients with lesions ≤ 7 cm confirmed on CT and positive biopsy for adenocarcinomas, squamous cell, carcinoid, or non-small cell cancers.
- Possible false-positives in patients with biopsy results consistent with acute or chronic inflammation, infectious processes (e.g., abscess and pneumonia, hamartoma, fibrosis, or caseating ["cheesy"] degeneration as in certain types of necroses]), or non-caseating granulomas.

- Caution should be used when administering this drug to patients with insulinomas because of the possibility of hypoglycemic reaction.
- Small peptides such as this drug may induce hypersensitivity or anaphylactic reactions. Adequate treatment (e.g., epinephrine) should be made available.
- Patient movement will blur SPECT images.

Note

Information provided by Diatide, Inc., 9 Delta Drive, Londonderry, NH, 03053.

NeoTect™ is a trademark of Diatide, Inc., Londonderry, NH.

Notes

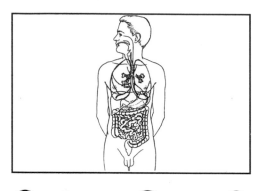

CHAPTER 34

OctreoScan®

Radiopharmacy

Radionuclide

- ^{111}In $t_{1/2}$: 2.8 days

  Energies: 173, 247 keV

  Type: EC, γ, accelerator

Radiopharmaceutical

- ^{111}In-pentetreotide, a DTPA (diethylenetriaminepentaacetic acid) conjugate, or octreotide (labeled peptides), a long-acting analog of the hormone somatostatin

Localization

- Extravasation and chemical bonding to somatostatin receptors, concentrating in tumor cells with a high density of receptors

Quality Control

- Chemical tag must be > 90%

Adult Dose Range

- 6 mCi (222 MBq)

Method of Administration

- IV using butterfly catheter and 10 mL of flush

Indications

- Detection and localization of somatostatin receptors on primary and metastatic neuroendocrine tumors, e.g., pheochromocytomas, incidentalomas, etc. (see Note).

- Detection and localization of endocrine pancreatic tumors, e.g., primary and metastatic gastrinomas, glucagonomas, insulinomas (less sensitive).

- Detection and localization of paragangliomas and neuroblastomas.

- Evaluation of elevated tumor markers, patients with a history of cancers, or known somatostatin receptor-type cancers.
- Evaluation of before or after surgery patients.

Contraindications

- Patients with severely impaired renal function.
- Do not inject through total parenteral nutrition (TPN) admixtures or into TPN IV catheters.

Patient History *(or use complete patient history in reference section)*

The patient should answer the following questions.

Do you have a history or family history of cancer?   Y   N

  If so, what type and for how long?

Do you have any pain?   Y   N

  If so, where and for how long?

Are you on TPN?   Y   N

Have you ever had any therapeutic doses of octreotide acetate?   Y   N

Do you have a history of insulinomas?   Y   N

Do you have impaired renal function?   Y   N

Female patients

Are you pregnant or nursing?   Y   N

When was your last menstrual period?

**Have you had a hysterectomy or are you
 in menopause?**   Y   N

Other department-specific questions.

Patient Preparation

- Identify the patient. Verify doctor's order. Explain the procedure.
- Instruct patient to hydrate well before and after injection.
- Physician to order mild laxative (cathartic) evening before injection and continued with light meals recommended and clear liquids until after all images are completed (refer to Patient Study Preparation).

Equipment

Camera

- Large field of view

Collimator

- Medium energy, general purpose, or medium energy, all purpose

Computer Set-up
Statics

- Abdomen; 500,000 counts or 15 min/image

Whole Body

- 512 × 1024 matrix, 10 cm/min or longer (minimum 30 minutes) head to pelvis

Single Photon Emission Computed Tomography (SPECT)

- 360°, 64 stops, 45–60 sec/stop, 64 × 64 word matrix

Procedure *(time: ~1–1.5 hours each scan day)*

- Instruct patient to void before scan.
- Place patient in supine position on table, check for attenuating items.
- Images: Obtain at 4 hours (whole-body sweep or statics or planar of abdomen), 24 hours (whole-body planar SPECT with liver, spleen, and kidneys in field of view [FOV]), 48 hours (same), and 72 hours (same as per radiologist).

Normal Results

- Excretion is almost exclusively renal: 50% at 6 hours, 85% at 24 hours, and 90% at 48 hours (hence the need for hydration).
- Uptake seen in liver, spleen, kidneys, and urinary bladder.
- Planar images at 4 and 24 hours can differentiate bowel contents from true uptake as there is seldom fecal contamination at 4 hours.

- Pituitary gland and thyroid present at 24 hours as background vascularity clears.
- Image at 48 hours may differentiate between radioactivity in a tumor and normal uptake in the bowel.

Abnormal Results

- Focal areas of uptake, particularly visible as time and biologic activity diminishes background distribution.

Patient Study Preparation

Day 1

1. Purchase four bottles of magnesium citrate at drug store.
2. Eat full breakfast on morning of injection and be well hydrated.
3. After injection, drink first bottle of magnesium citrate; drink plenty of clear liquids until after scan is completed.
4. Eat a light dinner that evening, followed by the second bottle of magnesium citrate.
5. Plenty of clear liquids until after the 24-hour scan.

Day 2

1. After the 24-hour scan, eat a light lunch and dinner.
2. After evening meal, drink third bottle of magnesium citrate; drink plenty of clear liquids until the 48-hour scan is completed.

Day 3 (72-hour scan if requested by radiologist)

1. After the 48-hour scan, eat a light lunch and dinner.
2. After the evening meal, drink the fourth bottle of magnesium citrate with plenty of clear liquids until the 72-hour scan is completed.

Processing

- Slice thickness to 2 mm.
- Use a low-pass filter, e.g., Butterworth, 0.4 Nyquist cutoff, and seventh-order (or 0.5 cutoff and fifth-order).

Artifacts

- Carefully monitor patients with impaired renal function.
- Pediatric patients or patients with insulinoma (tumor of the islets of Langerhans of the pancreas) must consult with clinician before bowel cleansing.
- *Do not* administer in TPN admixtures or inject into TPN IV catheters; an octreotide conjugate may form.
- Sensitivity to ^{111}In-pentetreotide may be reduced in patients receiving therapeutic doses of octreotide acetate and should consider suspending therapy before administering radiotracer.

- False-positive results, especially in the lungs, can occur possibly as a result of inflammatory reaction.

Note

Somatostatin is a linked, 14-amino acid, cyclic polypeptide neuropeptide that inhibits growth hormone secretion. In doing so, it slows the growth of neuroendocrine tumors. It unfortunately has a short biologic half-life, meaning when used as a therapy, constant infusion is needed for the effect, with a strong rebound effect (recurrence) once therapy is stopped. OctreoScan® (octreotide) is a somatostatin analog, binding to somatostatin receptors on tumor tissues to suppress hormonal hypersecretions from endocrine-secreting tumors, e.g., carcinoids, gastrinomas (VIPomas).

Neuroendocrine tumors with APUD (neuroendocrine) characteristics include the following:

Carcinoids

Islet cell tumors

Paragangliomas

Medullary thyroid carcinomas

Pheochromocytomas

Small cell lung cancers

Pituitary tumors

Others that possess somatostatin receptors include the following:

Meningiomas

Neuroblastomas

Astrocytomas

Lymphomas

Merkel cell tumors

Breast cancers

SUGGESTED READINGS

Early PJ, Sodee DB. Principles and Practice of Nuclear Medicine. 2nd ed. St. Louis: Mosby, 1995.

Murray IPC, Ell PJ, eds. Nuclear Medicine in Clinical Diagnosis and Treatment. Vols. 1 and 2. New York: Churchill Livingstone, 1994.

Wilson, MA. Textbook of Nuclear Medicine. Philadelphia: Lippincott-Raven, 1998.

OctreoScan® is a registered trademark of Mallinckrodt Medical, Inc., St. Louis, MO.

Notes

· · · · · · · ·

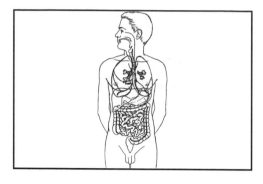

CHAPTER 35

OncoScint®

(Radioimmunoscintigraphy [RIS])

Radiopharmacy

Radionuclide

- ^{111}In t$_{\frac{1}{2}}$: 2.8 days

  Energies: 173, 247 keV

  Type: EC, γ, accelerator

Radiopharmaceutical

- ^{111}In chloride satumomab pendetide (murine monoclonal antibodies [Moabs] and fragments of antibodies [Fabs])

Localization

- Compartmental, blood flow; dose-dependent, antibody binding

Quality Control

- If made from kit, chromatography > 95% radiochemical purity

Adult Dose Range

- 4–6 mCi (148–222 MBq)

Method of Administration

- IV butterfly (large-bore, 18–22 gauge) for 5 minutes

- 10 mL saline flush

- Should have physician or nurse available for possible allergic reaction (1 mg epinephrine available).

- Follow vital signs: baseline, 5 minutes after injection, 15, 30, and 60 minutes (some simply observe patient for 15 minutes looking for redness at injection site or signs of nausea and vomiting).

Indications

- Detection of colorectal or ovarian carcinoma. The antibody localizes to the tumor-associated glycoprotein TAG-72.
  - Colorectal carcinoma: primary, detection of extent of regional lesions, occult metastases; recurrent, detection of occult metastases, clarify equivocal CT/MRI findings.
  - Ovarian carcinoma: detection and localization of extent of extrahepatic or occult disease, and evaluation for surgery approach. Detection of peritoneal "studding" (carcinomatosis).
- Detection of breast, non–small cell lung, pancreatic, gastric, and esophageal cancers.
- Evaluation of elevated serum CEA (carcinoembryonic antigen: respiratory and gastrointestinal tract), AFP (α-fetoprotein: hepatomas), CA-19–9 (colorectal), or CA-125 (ovarian) with no radiologic evidence of recurrence.
- Localization of recurrent disease in patients who are surgical candidates.
- Evaluation of presurgical and postsurgical recurrence of adenocarcinoma with equivocal CT/MRI studies.
- Differentiation of postoperative or postradiation therapy changes from disease recurrence.

Contraindications

- Patients with human anti-mouse antibody (HAMA) titer > 100 ng/mL. Fabs are being used to reduce the possibility of the HAMA reaction.

Patient History *(or use complete patient history in reference section)*

The patient should answer the following questions.

Do you have a history or family history of cancer?   Y   N

If so, what type and for how long?

Do you have any pain?   Y   N

If so, where and for how long?

Have you had any recent surgery?   Y   N

Have you had any recent chemotherapy or radiation therapy?	Y	N
Have you had any recent Moab-type examinations?	Y	N
Are there any recent or planned CT, MRI, x-ray, US, or NM examinations?	Y	N
Have you had any recent abnormal laboratory results (CEA, CA-125, HAMA, other)?	Y	N
Other department-specific questions.		

Patient Preparation

Before Day of Injection

- Identify the patient. Verify doctor's order. Explain the procedure.
- Obtain a signed consent form from patient.
- Ensure patient supplies list of history of allergies and prior examinations.
- Patients who have had a previous Moab test must have a HAMA titer performed before another injection.
- Physician to order Fleet® kit or laxative (cathartic) night before scan days.

Day of Injection

- Identify the patient. Verify doctor's order. Explain the procedure.
- No special preparation; bring all paperwork.

Equipment

Camera

- Large field of view

Collimator

- Medium energy, general purpose, or medium energy, all purpose

Computer Set-up

Statics

- Indium peaks, 15–20% windows, 128 × 128 or 256 × 256 matrix, 600 seconds or more per view (> 1,000,000 counts)

Whole Body

- Same, 10 cm/min or slower, check patient for length

Single Photon Emission Computed Tomography (SPECT)

- Rotation, 360°; projections, 60; 40 sec/frame; matrix, 64 × 64 or 128 × 128 word mode; axis/COR, < 2mm or 0.5 pixels; uniformity correction, yes (± 1%)

Procedure *(time: ~1–2 hours each scan day)*

- Instruct patient to void before imaging; check clothing for possible artifacts.

- Place patient on table in supine position, remind patient of no movement during imaging.

- Image at 72, 96, and 120 hours after injection (as per protocol). Some protocols image as soon as 48 hours.

- Statics: 10 minutes (600 seconds) per view. Anterior-posterior views of thorax, abdomen, and pelvis. Static views often provide the best diagnostic pictures.

- Whole body: 30 minutes (1800 seconds) anterior-posterior.

- SPECT at 72 hours or more (especially if planar appears normal).

Normal Results

- Activity in liver, spleen, bone marrow, and blood pool.

- Bowel activity may be present because of radiotracer in stool (ask patient if they cleansed their bowels the night before).

- Activity in kidneys, bladder, male genitalia, and female nipples.

Abnormal Results

- Increased extrahepatic uptake (equal to liver) in tumors.

- Persistent and stationary over time with delayed scans, particularly over lymph nodes or organ of interest.

- If trying to isolate hepatic tumors, a background subtraction technique with ^{99m}Tc-sulfur colloid (1 mCi) can be used.

- Background vascularity will decrease on 96- and 120-hour images except for liver, which shows lesions then as less activity than normal tissue.

Artifacts

- Observe patient for allergic reaction, e.g., anaphylactic shock, nausea, redness, or rash at injection site, particularly if not using the newer version of Fab.

- Some benign ovarian tumors express the antigen; therefore, cannot distinguish between benign and malignant disease.

- Check for surgical scars on patient; they may obscure positive results or provide false-positive results.

- Do not image before 48 hours and even that may be too soon.

- Must do HAMA titer if patient has had previous Moab test (results usually take 10–14 days and must be ≤ 100 ng/mL).

- Patients undergoing radiation therapy should wait ≥ 6 weeks before having an OncoScint® scan.

- Patient may not cleanse bowel (enema or cathartic) and give a false-positive result, or may be HAMA-positive and yield altered biodistribution.
- Check collimation and peaks.
- Patient motion may distort or obscure possible sites.
- Dose infiltration: increase acquisition times.

Processing

- Slice thickness to 2 mm.
- Using a low-pass filter, e.g., Butterworth, 0.4 Nyquist cutoff and seventh-order (or 0.5 and fifth-order) has produced acceptable images.

Note

The use of Fabs, or fragments of antibodies, is a new addition to the procedure designed to reduce or completely eliminate the HAMA reaction caused by using the entire Moab.

SUGGESTED READINGS

Early PJ, Sodee DB. Principles and Practice of Nuclear Medicine. 2nd ed. St. Louis: Mosby, 1995.

Murray IPC, Ell PJ, eds. Nuclear Medicine in Clinical Diagnosis and Treatment. Vols. 1 and 2. New York: Churchill Livingstone, 1994.

Wilson, MA. Textbook of Nuclear Medicine. Philadelphia: Lippincott-Raven, 1998.

Fleet® Kit is a registered trademark of CB Fleet Co., Inc., Lynchburg, VA.
OncoScint® is a registered trademark of Cytogen Corporation, Princeton, N.J.

Notes

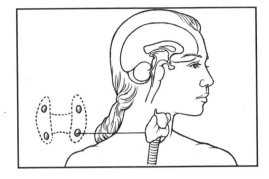

Parathyroid Scan

(dual-isotope subtraction technique and single-isotope two-phase)

Radiopharmacy

Radionuclide

- ^{99m}Tc $t_{1/2}$: 6 hours

  Energies: 140 keV

  Type: IT, γ, generator

- ^{201}Tl $t_{1/2}$: 73 hours

  Energies: 68–80 keV k x-ray, 135, 167 keV

  Type: EC, γ, accelerator

Radiopharmaceutical

- ^{99m}Tc as pertechnetate
- ^{201}Tl as thallous chloride
- ^{99m}Tc-sestamibi (hexakis[2-methoxyisobutylisonitril])
- ^{99m}Tc-1,2-bis (bis[2-ethoxyethyl]phosphino) ethane

Localization

- ^{99m}TcO$_4^-$: active transport into normal thyroid tissue
- ^{201}Tl-chloride: similar to potassium, distributes with Na/K pump and enters thyroid and parathyroid tissue with blood flow, as well as into adenomatous and hyperplastic tissue.
- ^{99m}Tc-sestamib/tetrofosmin: passive transport in proportion to blood flow into thyroid and normal and abnormal parathyroid tissue, remaining longer in adenomatous and hyperplastic tissue.

Quality Control

- ^{99m}TcO$_4^-$: chromatography, moly and Al breakthrough
- ^{201}Tl-chloride: chromatography > 95%, use within 7 days
- ^{99m}Tc-sestamibi/tetrofosmin: chromatography > 90%

Adult Dose Range

- $^{99m}TcO_4^-$: 5–12 mCi (185–444 MBq)
- ^{201}Tl-chloride: 2–3 mCi (74–111 MBq)
- ^{99m}Tc-sestamibi/tetrofosmin: 16–30 mCi (592–1110 MBq)

Method of Administration

- IV injection, some use butterfly for subtraction method for patient comfort (instead of two injections)

Indications

- Detection and localization of primary and secondary parathyroid cancer.
- Identification of single adenomas, multiple adenomas, or glandular hyperplasia in patients with newly diagnosed hypercalcemia and elevated parathyroid hormone (PTH) levels.
- Localization of cancer for surgery candidates. Some, using probe, localize and bring straight to surgery.
- Localization of parathyroid tissue after surgery for persistent or recurrent hyperparathyroidism (elevated serum calcium and PTH).

Contraindications

- Patient on calcium medications.
- Patient on thyroid medications.
- Patient too agitated or prone to movement or claustrophobia.

Patient History *(or use complete patient history in reference section)*

The patient should answer the following questions.

Do you have a history or family history of cancer?	Y	N
If so, what type and for how long?		
Do you have a history or family history of parathyroid disease?	Y	N
Do you have osteoporosis?	Y	N
Are you sensitive to pain?	Y	N

Do you have kidney disease or stones?	Y	N
Have you had recent thyroid surgery?	Y	N
Have you noticed any swelling or tenderness in your neck?	Y	N
Have you had any recent iodine contrast studies?	Y	N
Have you had any related studies?	Y	N
What medications are you taking?		
Do you have results of recent laboratory tests, particularly Ca^{2+} and PTH?	Y	N
Other department-specific questions.		

Patient Preparation

- Identify the patient. Verify doctor's order.
- Explain the procedure and the need to remain still during acquisitions.
- Palpate neck to localize any abnormal parathyroid or thyroid tissue.

Equipment

Camera

- Large field of view

Collimator

- Pinhole or low energy, all purpose, or low energy, high resolution

Computer Set-up
Planar

- $128 \times 128 \times 8$ or $64 \times 64 \times 16$ matrix, 1,000,000 counts or 300–900 sec/image, computer processing image subtraction, correct peak for radiotracer

Single Photon Emission Computed Tomography (SPECT)

- Circular or noncircular, 360°, 128×128 matrix, 64 stops, 20–25 sec/stop; centered for region of interest

Procedure *(time: subtraction: ~1.5 hours; sestamibi/tetrofosmin: ~30 minutes, then delays ~15–30 minutes)*

Dual-Isotope Subtraction Technique

- Place patient in supine position, pillow under shoulders, head back, neck extended.
- Position camera anterior over extended neck and mediastinum.
- Remove any attenuating necklaces or pendants. Immobilize head if necessary.
- Instruct patient to remain motionless during acquisitions.
- Inject ^{201}Tl.

Procedure A

- Within 2–3 minutes of injection, obtain a 300-second image, preferably with a pinhole collimator, looking for focal uptake between heart and thyroid.
- Immediately follow image with a 900-second image of thyroid centered in field of view (FOV).
- Immediately follow image with injection of 5–10 mCi of ^{99m}TcO$_4^-$. Wait 5 minutes.
- Obtain a 900-second image of thyroid.
- Run subtraction program, if necessary, to separate ^{201}Tl accumulation from ^{99m}TcO$_4^-$ trapping.

Procedure B

- Position camera anterior with thyroid near top of FOV, looking for focal uptake between heart and thyroid using a high-resolution collimator, 128 × 128 matrix, zoom 1.3.
- Obtain a 180-second image.
- Reposition camera to center thyroid.
- Obtain dynamic images; 1 frame/min for 15 minutes, zoom 2.6. No patient motion.
- Inject 5–10 mCi of ^{99m}TcO$_4^-$ and begin dynamic images; 1 frame/min for 15 minutes, zoom 2.6. No patient motion.
- Run subtraction program, if necessary, to separate ^{201}Tl accumulation from ^{99m}TcO$_4^-$ trapping.

Procedure C

- Wait 30 minutes after injection.
- Acquire anterior image of neck and mediastinum with LEHR collimator, 100,000 counts.
- Acquire anterior image of thyroid with pinhole if available, 100,000 counts.
- Inject ^{99m}TcO$_4^-$; wait 20 minutes. No patient motion.
- Acquire anterior image of thyroid, 100,000 counts.
- Run subtraction program, if necessary, to separate ^{201}Tl accumulation from ^{99m}TcO$_4^-$ trapping.

Single-Isotope Two-Phase: (thyroid phase, parathyroid phase)

- Inject patient. Wait 15 minutes to obtain image. Remove any attenuating necklaces or pendants.

- Place patient in supine position, pillow under shoulders, head back, neck extended.

- Position camera anterior over extended neck and mediastinum.

- Immobilize head if necessary.

- Using LEAP/LEHR collimator, acquire 300–600 second ($\geq$ 1,000,000 counts), anterior, RAO, and LAO 30° images. Obtain marker image: thyroid cartilage and suprasternal notch (SSN) if protocol. Be sure to include salivary glands to mediastinum with anterior images.

- Obtain repeat images after 15 more minutes if protocol. This may work depending on the size and weight of the suspected adenoma. If this accelerated method of imaging is to be used, give lemon to the patient on the day of procedure to reduce salivary uptake.

- Repeat images at 1.5–3 hours after injection (especially if preoperatively).

- Repeat images at 4–6 hours after injection if there are questionable areas.

- SPECT acquisition may also be a consideration. Acquire at 30 minutes after injection and delay at 2 hours. Reconstruct with Butterworth filter, cutoff 0.5, power 10. Check with physician.

Normal Results

- Dual-isotope subtraction technique:
  - No increased ^{201}Tl activity within or outside normal thyroid tissue.
  - Normal parathyroid tissue does not accumulate ^{201}Tl.
- Single-isotope two-phase:
  - Initially; heterogeneous uptake by thyroid, salivary glands, heart, gut.
  - Delays; heterogeneous washout, no focal points of lingering uptake.

Abnormal Results

- Dual-isotope subtraction technique: area(s) of increased ^{201}Tl within and outside normal thyroid tissue.

- Single-isotope two-phase: washout of thyroid tissue with focal area of increased activity on delayed images anywhere from salivary glands to mediastinum. Obliques help define position of abnormal uptake in neck area.

Role of Technologist in Operating Room (OR)

- Many institutions are using these studies to localize and resect adenomas within the parathyroid glands. The role of the technologist differs with the institution, but they generally perform the following tasks.

- Inject patient as per protocol of institution.

- Images taken as suggested above, patient and images are brought to preoperative area to prepare for surgery.

- In OR
  - Technologist uses gamma probe to locate "hot" gland(s). (Only in some institutions; others hire a company to manipulate the probe.)
  - Technologist takes resected gland(s) and material to pathology for inspection.

- Technologist assays material for storage (10 half-lives) if > 0.05 mR at 1 m or disposal if background ≤ 0.05 mR at 1 m.
- Technologist assays pathology room and equipment for contamination.
- Technologist assays OR for contamination after removal of patient.

Artifacts

- No patient movement is critical in subtraction method and with use of pinhole collimator.
- May not visualize ectopic parathyroid tissue.
- May not visualize abnormal tissue < 300 mg in size.

Note

The parathyroid glands synthesize, store, and secrete PTH. PTH regulates calcium and phosphorus levels in the blood stream by increasing osteoclastic activity in bone to release calcium and decrease calcium release from kidneys, which increases the release of phosphorus, potassium, and sodium, and acts with vitamin D to increase intestinal absorption of calcium.

SUGGESTED READINGS

Datz FL. Handbook of Nuclear Medicine. 2nd ed. St. Louis: Mosby, 1993.

Early PJ, Sodee DB. Principles and Practice of Nuclear Medicine. 2nd ed. St. Louis: Mosby, 1995.

Murray IPC, Ell PJ, eds. Nuclear Medicine in Clinical Diagnosis and Treatment. Vols. 1 and 2. New York: Churchill Livingstone, 1994.

Wilson, MA. Textbook of Nuclear Medicine. Philadelphia: Lippincott-Raven, 1998.

Notes

CHAPTER 37

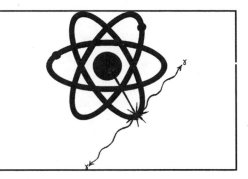

Positron Emission Tomography (PET)

(Coincidence Imaging: An Overview)

Radiopharmacy

- Positron emitters

Radionuclide

- ^{15}O $t_{1/2}$: 2.04 minutes

  Energies: 1.72 MeV

  Type: Cyclotron

- ^{13}N $t_{1/2}$: 9.96 minutes

  Energies: 1.19 MeV

  Type: Cyclotron

- ^{11}C $t_{1/2}$: 20.4 minutes

  Energies: 0.96 MeV

  Type: Cyclotron

- ^{18}F $t_{1/2}$: 110.0 minutes

  Energies: 0.64 MeV

  Type: Cyclotron

- ^{82}Rb $t_{1/2}$: 1.27 minutes

  Energies: 3.35 MeV

  Type: Generator

- ^{62}Cu $t_{1/2}$: 9.8 minutes

  Energies: 2.93 MeV

  Type: Generator

- ^{68}Ga $t_{1/2}$: 68.1 minutes

  Energies: 1.90 MeV

  Type: Generator

Radiopharmaceutical

- Radiolabeled biochemical compounds

Localization

- Biochemical metabolism within the cell

Quality Control

- Similar to standard radiopharmaceuticals, performed at plant

Adult Dose Range

- 5–15 mCi (185–555 MBq)

Method of Administration

- Standard IV injection, performed quickly because of the kiloelectron volts (KeVs) of the radiotracer. Time, distance, and shielding considerations are of particular importance, requiring special changes to the standard department (packages available).

Indications

Brain

- Imaged patterns of metabolic activity can change depending on input at the time of the study (e.g., eyes open or closed, sounds, smells, movement, thought).

- Evaluation of cerebrovascular disease: Physiologic effects of blood flow because of strokes and transient ischemic attacks (TIAs).

- Evaluation of epilepsy:
  - Localization of focus of epilepsy.
  - Findings are similar to single photon emission computed tomography (SPECT) except more sensitive interictally (between attacks).

- Evaluation of movement disorders:
  - Huntington: decreased metabolism in caudate nuclei, decreased D_2 dopamine receptor density.
  - Parkinson: reduced basal ganglia uptake of ^{18}F-dopa (3,4-dihydroxyphenylalanine).

- Evaluation of psychiatric disorders: findings are still highly debated. Localization of regional metabolic abnormalities and changes.
  - Schizophrenia:
    - Decreased perfusion and metabolism of frontal lobes.
    - Increased perfusion and metabolism in left hemisphere.
    - Increased subcortical:cortical ratio.
  - Mood disorders:
    - Globally diminished blood flow and metabolism in depressed patients.
    - Differences noted in scan appearance between patients with unipolar and bipolar depression.

- Evaluation of dementia: reveals regional metabolic patterns (e.g., Alzheimer's disease).

- Evaluation of tumors:
  - Evaluation of grade of glioma and true extent of brain tumor.
  - Differentiation of recurrent tumor from scar and radiation necrosis.
  - Evaluation of chemotherapy: effect on tumor metabolism.

Cardiac

- Detection and evaluation of coronary artery disease (CAD) (10–15% more sensitive than SPECT, specificity improved because of less soft tissue attenuation).
- Evaluation of intervention.
- Differentiation of ischemia (increased fluorodeoxyglucose [FDG] uptake) and infarction.
- Differentiation of hypoperfused viable tissue from infarction.
  - PET will show enhanced FDG uptake and glycolysis in affected region and decreased ^{13}N-NH$_3$ (blood flow) if viable.
  - Decreased FDG and decreased ^{13}N-NH$_3$ indicates scar tissue.

Oncology

- Evaluation of grade and true extent of brain tumor for therapeutic intervention.
- Differentiation of recurrent tumor from scar and radiation necrosis.
- Evaluation of chemotherapy; effect on tumor metabolism.

Contraindications

- Patient too agitated, uncooperative, or claustrophobic to remain still for acquisition.
- Because PET involves cellular metabolism, drug and food ingestion, or lack thereof, bears specific consideration for each study.

Patient History

- Patient histories vary with the scan and are basically the same as for standard nuclear medicine procedures.

Patient Preparation

- Identify the patient. Verify doctor's order. Explain the procedure.
- Instruct patient to remain NPO after midnight before examination.
- Instruct patient to refrain from caffeine or tobacco 12 hours before examination.
- Physician is to discontinue all medications on the morning of examination.
- Physician is to instruct diabetic patients to take a half-dose.
- Instruct patient to be fully hydrated for examination unless contraindicated for other reasons.
- Instruct patient to bring or make available all medical records and prior examinations.

- Instruct patient to arrive 3 hours in advance of scheduled examination time and to plan on a half day for entire examination.
- Instruct patient to notify department immediately if there is a change in plans because of elaborate scheduling and radiopharmaceutical quality control and delivery.
- Instruct patient to remain calm with no movement throughout imaging.
- Instruct patient that once injection is administered to be extremely careful about urine and body fluid contamination.

Equipment

Camera

- Special bismuth germinate (BGO) (or other) crystal cameras or normal NaI crystal cameras (optimum thickness is 0.75 inch)

Collimator

- Electronic collimation, high energy, high resolution (for 511 keV) for NaI cameras

Computer Set-up

- PET and coincidence counting software necessary. Cameras acquire similar to SPECT in that the cameras rotate around patient.

Procedure *(time: ~half day)*

- Administer injection to patient in advance of scan or as imaging is about to begin according to protocol for particular examination.
- Place patient in supine position on imaging table.
- Remind patient to remain motionless during acquisition.
- Position cameras centering area of interest. Set parameters and start cameras.
- Obtain one set of images or more as to protocol. Some require two sets of images of same area, then sum images. Some require multiple sets of images of various areas of interest.

PET Scanning

- PET imaging creates functional pictures of blood flow or metabolism. The isotopes used for tagging allow incorporation into the first step of cellular metabolism. It is more similar to the physiologic processes of routine nuclear medicine radiopharmaceuticals than the strictly anatomic images of CT, x-ray, MRI, or even SPECT.
- Medicare/Medicaid coverage: Coverage was allowed on a conditional and temporary basis as of January 1, 1998.

Imaging

- Procedures vary greatly. Two examples of FDG imaging are as follows.

Jackson Memorial Hospital in Miami, FL

- Dual-head gamma camera with dedicated collimation.
- Patient NPO since midnight before examination.

- Blood glucose < 120 mg/dL.

- Inject ~6 mCi ^{18}F-FDG; 40 mg Lasix® may be injected to help clear radiotracer.

- Image in 1 hour; keep patient very relaxed and calm or radiotracer will uptake in muscle.

- Three consecutive SPECT-type studies performed, covering head to pelvis.

- If region of interest (ROI) is in pelvic area, patient is catheterized to keep bladder clear.

Halifax Medical Center, Daytona, FL

- Dual-head gamma camera with heavy collimation. Used in conjunction with CT.

- Patient NPO since midnight before examination.

- Inject 6–12 mCi ^{18}F-FDG depending on specific study.

- Whole-body scan, relatively fast sweep.

- If study concerns lungs, do transmission lung test (refer to manual).

- Do two SPECT-type studies of ROI consecutively. Add together.

- Catheterize bladder if ROI in pelvic area.

- For cardiac viability, serve two glucose-rich cola drinks with injection. Follow up with a thallium cardiac study for comparison.

- Especially good results experienced with tumor localization.

Isotope

- The isotope must be a pure β^+ emitter. If not, the detector is tied up sorting out single events, there is increased dead time, and there is markedly decreased resolution of the image.

- The isotopes of choice can be labeled with biologic and physiologic compounds used in the first step of metabolism of every cell.

Medical Importance

- Most medically significant compounds can be labeled with ^{11}C, ^{18}F, ^{13}N, or ^{15}O.

- These are physiologic, positron emitters and readily produced in "baby" cyclotrons.

- They produce high-resolution tomographic images.

- There are no gamma-emitting isotopes of carbon, nitrogen, or oxygen that can label these biologic compounds for SPECT, nor can ^{99m}Tc be labeled to most of these compounds at this time.

- Human disease is a biochemical process best diagnosed with a biochemical imaging modality.

Common Radiopharmaceuticals and Medical Applications

^{11}C-acetate	Myocardial metabolism
^{11}C-glucose	Cerebral glucose metabolism
^{11}C-1-butanol	Cerebral blood flow
^{11}C-N-methylspiperone	Dopamine receptor binding
^{11}C-palmitate	Myocardial metabolism

^{18}F-FDG	Cerebral glucose metabolism
	Myocardial glucose metabolism
	Tumor localization
^{18}F-16α-fluoro-17β-estradiol	Estrogen receptor binding
^{18}F-spiperone	Dopamine receptor binding
^{68}Ga-citrate/transferrin	Plasma volume
^{13}N-NH_3	Myocardial blood flow
^{15}O-CO	Cerebral blood volume
	Myocardial blood volume
^{15}O-H_2O	Cerebral blood flow
	Myocardial blood flow
^{15}O-O_2	Cerebral oxygen extraction and metabolism
^{82}Rb-Rb^+	Myocardial blood flow

Note
· · · · · ·

The Positron

Positrons are positive electrons emitted from the nucleus on decay of an unstable proton-rich isotope as it changes a proton into a neutron. Because of the abundance of electrons (negatively charged) in the electron cloud surrounding the nucleus of these large atoms, the escaping positron collides with an electron, resulting in annihilation of the positron and electron. The resulting annihilation radiation consists of two gamma photons, both of 511 keV and expelled from the atom at 180° of each other.

Technical Considerations

Considerations must be made regarding safety to compensate for the higher energies involved. Time, distance, and shielding are extremely important when using PET isotopes. Lead shielding must be thicker. For ^{99m}Tc, the lead half-value layer is 0.2 mm, whereas the half-value layer for 511 keV is 4.0 mm. This adds considerable thickness to shielding. Tungsten is more dense and is more suited to shielding the PET isotopes. Shipping and receiving the isotopes presents its own problems. They are packaged in routine lead-lined containers and centered in large boxes to keep the surface mR/h within Yellow Bar II shipping standards. It is imperative for the technologist who is receiving, calibrating doses, and handling these isotopes to do so expeditiously. The isotopes should be stored in well-shielded areas to reduce exposure to personnel and patients. Because the half-lives of these isotopes are relatively short, e.g., ^{18}F at 110 minutes, the 10-half-life rule for decay storage of spent syringes, tubing, stopcocks, saline flushes, wipes, etc., can be accomplished by 18–24 hours.

The imaging area needs special consideration as to room location, camera location, rest room facilities, and patient proximity to hospital staff and other patients and cameras. Walls may need thicker lead to reduce exposure to adjoining rooms. Dosing, waiting, and imaging areas should be isolated from other cameras and staff. These areas and rest room facilities should be planned to minimize patient movement within the department in an effort to reduce exposure to others and interference with other scans. The institution may have to amend its license to be authorized to receive and use the isotopes.

Detection

Several methods have been and are being developed to detect and use this phenomenon.

Special ring-shaped or doughnut-shaped cameras using arrays of photomultiplier tubes and surrounding the patient are currently in use to capture the gamma photons and pinpoint the location of the source. There are no collimators per se; rather, these devices use electronic collimation and special crystals to absorb the energy (bismuth germinate [BGO], barium fluoride [BaF$_2$], or cesium fluoride [CsF]). These cameras are extremely expensive, thus keeping them from most mainstream nuclear medicine departments.

Another method is to use the more common NaI crystals of a dual-head gamma camera with the addition of heavy collimation to accommodate the 511-keV photons and coincidence counting software in the computer. Modifications may also include changes to the electronics, a thicker crystal (5/8 inch as opposed to the standard 3/8 inch), and collimators changed out for scatter shields that contain a lining of lead around the perimeter to absorb oblique scattered radiation and horizontally aligned lead septa for absorbing low-energy photons. Improvements in hardware, software, and cost containment are making PET scanning more attractive and attainable to diagnostic departments. These can be used in planar, whole-body, and tomographic imaging.

Techniques are being developed to use single-head gamma cameras with heavy collimation and specialized software to allow many departments to take some advantage of the metabolic imaging that PET scanning affords without the use of coincidence counting. Processing is similar to SPECT and is usually included with the software to run the imaging programs.

SUGGESTED READINGS

Datz FL. Handbook of Nuclear Medicine. 2nd ed. St. Louis: Mosby, 1993.

Duncan K. Radiopharmaceuticals in PET imaging. J Nucl Med Technol 1998;26:228–234.

Early PJ, Sodee DB. Principles and Practice of Nuclear Medicine. 2nd ed. St. Louis: Mosby, 1995.

Murray IPC, Ell PJ, eds. Nuclear Medicine in Clinical Diagnosis and Treatment. Vols. 1 and 2. New York: Churchill Livingstone, 1994.

Wilson, MA. Textbook of Nuclear Medicine. Philadelphia: Lippincott-Raven, 1998.

Lasix® is a registered trademark of Hoechst-Roussel Pharmaceuticals, Inc., Somerville, NJ.

Notes

· · · · · · · ·

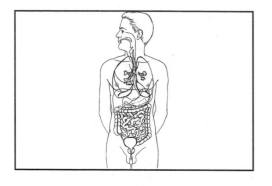

CHAPTER 38

ProstaScint® Scan

(Radioimmunoscintigraphy [RIS])

Radiopharmacy

Radionuclide

- ^{111}In $t_{1/2}$: 2.8 days

  Energies: 173, 247 keV

  Type: EC, γ, accelerator

Radiopharmaceutical

- ^{111}In-capromab pendetide, or ^{111}In-CYT-356, a whole murine monoclonal antibody, 7E11-C5.3 conjugated to the linker-chelator, glycyltyrosyl-(N,ϵ-diethylenetriaminepentaacetic acid)-lysine hydrochloride (GYK-DTPA-HCL).

Localization

- Chemical bonding to glycoprotein expressed by prostate epithelium known as prostate-specific membrane antigen (PSMA), more commonly known as prostate-specific antigen (PSA). PSA is located in the cytoplasmic domain and is not expressed on any other adenocarcinomas or transitional cell cancers.

Quality Control

- Produced by serum-free in vitro cultivation, purified by sequential protein isolation and chromatography. Chemical tag must be > 90%.

Adult Dose Range

- 5–17mCi (185–629 MBq)

Method of Administration

- IV using large-bore butterfly catheter and 10 mL of flush, slowly for 5 minutes. Vital signs monitored before injection and at 5, 15, 30, and 60 minutes after injection.

Indications

- Detection and localization of clinically suspected prostate cancer (via biopsy, x-ray, CT, MRI, ultrasonography (US), positive bone scan) with a high risk of metastasis. Metastatic growth occurs by both lymphatic and hematogenous routes.

- Evaluation of elevated PSA (8–10 times normal upper limit or Gleason score of 3–7, normals are 0–6.0 ng/mL in most cases); patients with a history of cancers, suspicious biopsy, or known cancers are candidates.

- Evaluation of patients with a high risk for lymph node metastasis, e.g., elevated prostatic acid phosphatase and PSAs ($\geq$ 8 times upper normal limits), corroborating CT, MRI, or US. Lymphatic metastasis first appears in areas of the obturator and internal and external iliac nodes.

- Evaluation of patients with a high clinical suggestion of occult recurrent or residual prostate cancer, elevated PSAs after radical prostatectomy, negative bone scan, and negative CT, MRI, or US, $\geq$ 0.8 ng/mL PSA levels and increasing.

- Evaluation of before and after surgical and therapy treatments.

Contraindications

- Patients who are sensitive to this or any other product of murine.
- Patients who are not at high risk for developing prostate cancer.
- Patients at risk of human anti-mouse antibody (HAMA) reaction.
- Not for screening for carcinomas.
- Female.

Patient History *(or use complete patient history in reference section)*

The patient should answer the following questions.

Do you have a history or family history of cancer?   Y   N

If so, what type and for how long?

Do you have any pain?   Y   N

If so, where and for how long?

Have you had any chemotherapy or radiation therapy?   Y   N

Have you had a recent ECG?	Y	N

Are there any recent or planned bone scans, other nuclear medicine, CT, MRI, US, x-ray, or biopsy?	Y	N

Are there any recent laboratory results
(e.g., PSA levels, electrolytes, glucose, blood
urea nitrogen [BUN], creatinine, calcium,
phosphorus, uric acid, total bilirubin, total
protein, albumin, aspartate aminotransferase
[AST], alanine aminotransferase [ALT], alkaline
phosphatase, acid phosphatase, urinalysis,
HAMA titer, complete blood cell count [CBC])?   Y   N

Other department-specific questions.

Patient Preparation

Before Day of Injection

- Physician to instruct patient to take a mild laxative (cathartic) evening before imaging. Also may be required to have a cleansing enema 1 hour before each imaging session.
- Instruct patient to increase fluid uptake for duration of examination.
- Obtain preinjection blood sample and baseline vital signs if protocol.

Day of Injection

- Identify the patient. Verify doctor's order. Explain the procedure and possible HAMA reaction.
- Obtain a written consent from patient.
- Administer injection to patient and wait according to protocol to image.
- Follow patient's vital signs after injection, 15–60 minutes as to protocol.
- Instruct patient to empty bladder completely (catheterize if necessary) before each imaging session.

Equipment

Camera

- Large field of view

Collimator

- Medium energy, general purpose

Computer Set-up

Statics

- Torso, 800,000 counts or 10 min/image; extremities and skull, 5 min/image

Whole Body

- 512 × 1024 matrix, 10 cm/min or longer (minimum 30 minutes) head to pelvis

Single Photon Emission Computed Tomography (SPECT)

- Noncircular 360°, 64 stops, 40–60 sec/stop, 64 × 64 word matrix, Weiner or Butterworth filter, cutoff 0.5, order 5.

Procedure *(time: ~1–2.5 hours each scan day)*

- Instruct patient to void before scan.

- Place patient in supine position on table; check for attenuating items.

- Instruct patient as to no movement during acquisition.

- Position camera as to images desired.

- Obtain images as to protocol: acquire 96-hour delays (most protocols and Cytogen Corporation opt for this time).

- Options
  - Immediates: inject and wait 30 minutes, then obtain statics, whole-body, or SPECT of pelvis to identify blood pool.
  - Delays: 48-, 72-, 96-, or 120-hour delays as to protocol. Include statics, whole-body, or SPECT. Check with nuclear physician or radiologist.
  - Planar: 800,000 counts or 10 minutes at 6–8 hours, and 24 hours after injection. Acquire marker planar image of bony prominences or other for reference.
  - Acquire anterior-posterior thorax, abdomen and pelvis, and tail-on-detector (TOD) for 10 min/image. Also images of proximal humeri, femurs, and skull for 5 min/image.
  - Whole-body sweep can be taken at each session.
  - SPECT: 6–8 hours and 24, 48, 72, 96, or 120 hours.

- Clinical trials used two sessions between 2 and 5 days after injection.

Normal Results

- Excretion is relatively slow: 10% after 72 hours is excreted in the urine.

- Uptake in immediates present blood pool, liver, spleen, bone marrow, kidneys, urinary bladder, and genitalia. Blood pool image differentiates blood vessels that can be confused with lymph node uptake in delayed images.

- Bowel activity changes between sessions.

- Blood pool, liver, spleen, kidney, and bone marrow diminish activity with time.

- Increased activity at the base of the penis serves as landmark for SPECT transaxial and sagittal images, identifying the inferior level of the prostatic fossa.

Abnormal Results

- Focal areas of uptake, particularly visible as time progresses and biologic activity diminishes background distribution.

- Focal areas of activity in the region of the prostatic fossa, distinct from activity in the bladder or rectum.

- Focal areas of uptake in bladder or seminal vesicles.

- Focal areas of activity may also show in bone, pelvic lymph node chains, extrapelvic or abdominal lymph nodes, and distant lesions throughout.

Artifacts

- There were high rates of false-positive and false-negative results in some clinical trials. This could result in the following:

  - Inappropriate surgical intervention to confirm results.

  - Inappropriate denial of curative therapy if results are not confirmed.

  - Inadequate surgical staging if only areas of uptake are sampled.

- ProstaScint® nonspecifically localizes to colostomy, degenerative joint disease, aneurysms, and inflammatory masses providing possible false-positive results.

- Staging pelvic lymphadenectomy, a sampling procedure that can miss metastatic spread, is still the standard for assessing the status of pelvic lymph nodes. Noninvasive modalities, e.g., US, CT, and MRI, are also used for evaluation. Correct staging is critical to the selection of patients and primary therapy.

- Bone scans are more sensitive to skeletal metastasis and should always be included.

SUGGESTED READINGS

Wilson, MA. Textbook of Nuclear Medicine. Philadelphia: Lippincott-Raven, 1998.

ProstaScint® is a registered trademark of Cytogen Corporation, Princeton, NJ.

Notes

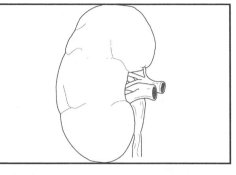

Renal: Cortical Imaging

(⁹⁹ᵐTc-DMSA)

Radiopharmacy

Radionuclide

- ⁹⁹ᵐTc $t_{1/2}$: 6 hours

  Energies: 140 keV

  Type: IT, γ, generator

Radiopharmaceutical

- ⁹⁹ᵐTc-DMSA (dimercaptosuccinic acid)

Localization

- Compartmental, blood stream; 90% binds to plasma proteins, preventing any significant glomerular filtration, hence slow clearance from renal cortex (proximal convoluted tubules).

Quality Control

- Chromatography, > 90%. Relatively unstable; a more stable form has been recently developed. Draw immediately after mixing into syringe. No O_2 introduction. Use within 30 minutes of preparation.

Adult Dose Range

- 1–6 mCi (37–222 MBq)

Method of Administration

- Direct IV injection or IV catheter with saline flush

Indications

- Evaluation of renal cortex.
- Evaluation and quantitation of regional relative function.

- Evaluation and quantitation of differential function.
- Detection and localization of renal mass.
- Detection and differentiation of acute and chronic pyelonephritis.
- Evaluation for renal blood supply obstruction and/or trauma.
- Evaluation of renal transplant.

Contraindications

- None

Patient History *(or use complete patient history in reference section)*

The patient should answer the following questions.

Do you have a history or family history of cancer?	Y	N
If so, what type and for how long?		
Do you have a history of kidney disease (e.g., stones, infections)?	Y	N
Do you have both kidneys?	Y	N
Are there any recent or planned operations?	Y	N
Have you had a kidney transplant?	Y	N
Do you have any pain?	Y	N
If so, where and for how long?		
Are you experiencing nausea or vomiting?	Y	N
Are you experiencing urinary frequency or urgency?	Y	N
Do you have any blood in your urine?	Y	N

Are you a diabetic?	Y	N
Do you have any cardiac diseases?	Y	N
Do you have high blood pressure?	Y	N
Do you have the results of any recent laboratory tests?	Y	N
Other department-specific questions.		

Patient Preparation

- Identify the patient. Verify doctor's order.
- Explain the procedure, especially the delay between injection and imaging.
- Patient is to be well hydrated and should void before test begins.
- Patient should discontinue angiotensin converting enzyme (ACE) inhibitors.

Equipment

Camera
- Large field of view

Collimator
- Low energy, all purpose, or low energy, high resolution

Computer Set-up
- Statics: 500,000–1,000,000 counts

Procedure *(varies greatly; time: injection ~15 minutes, images ~45 minutes)*

- DMSA is usually used for anatomic studies. Maintain patient hydration.
- Place patient in supine position, camera under table, except for kidney transplant patients for whom camera is placed above the abdomen.
- Position camera with upper abdomen centered in field of view.
- Obtain images: wide variation in protocols for pictures; 50% of injected dose is in kidneys within 1 hour. Here are some methods.
  - Some may require a flow study as in DTPA or MAG$_3$ (usually not).
  - Inject, take immediate statics (500,000–800,000 counts), then delays at 1 hour, using this 1-hour posterior view for processing. Also 4- to 6-hour delays, and 24-hour delays if requested.
  - Inject, take 2-hour delay(s), 24-hour delays if requested.
  - Inject, take 3-hour delay(s), 24-hour delays if requested.

- Inject, take 5-hour image(s), 24-hour delay if requested.
- Select image. Check with the radiologist.

- Images: 500,000–800,000 counts, posterior (at least). Some take RPOs and LPOs 30°, RLATs and LLATs, or anterior if horseshoe kidneys are suspected or kidney transplant. (May need to magnify views for pediatric patients.) RAOs and LAOs and PRPOs and PLPOs have also been suggested. Whole body and single photon emission computed tomography (SPECT) have been suggested as well. Check with radiologist for views.
- Generate percent uptake for each kidney. Select posterior static taken at least at 1 hour. Software differs: some have automatic programs, some will allow regions of interest to be drawn, giving counts within area. Add two counts together for total, divide each by total to give percent uptake for each kidney: combined percents should equal 100.
- Generate pictures of static images (and flow, whole body, and/or SPECT if taken).

Normal Results

- Assuming two kidneys, both kidneys visualizing about the same size and intensities if flow is performed.
- Static images should yield bilateral smooth renal contour.
- Hepatic uptake visualized, varies with degree of renal function.
- Because of extremely slow rate of clearance of DMSA, collecting system may not visualize.

Abnormal Results

- One or both kidneys are not visualized.
- One or both enlarged kidneys or decreased activity indicates pyelonephritis.
- Asymmetric activity indicates renal artery stenosis or hydroureteronephrosis.
- Gallbladder and gut are visualized in renal failure.

Artifacts

- Increased liver uptake with decreased renal uptake may be caused by chemical breakdown of radiotracer.
- Acidic urine may produce similar results as above.
- Some patients do not have both kidneys.
- Patient still on angiotensin-converting enzyme inhibitors before test.
- With dehydration, decreased kidney:liver ratio.
- Misalignment on positioning.

SUGGESTED READINGS

Datz FL. Handbook of Nuclear Medicine. 2nd ed. St. Louis: Mosby, 1993.

Early PJ, Sodee DB. Principles and Practice of Nuclear Medicine. 2nd ed. St. Louis: Mosby, 1995.

Murray IPC, Ell PJ, eds. Nuclear Medicine in Clinical Diagnosis and Treatment. Vols. 1 and 2. New York: Churchill Livingstone, 1994.

Wilson, MA. Textbook of Nuclear Medicine. Philadelphia: Lippincott-Raven, 1998.

Notes

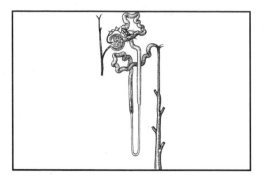

CHAPTER 40

Renal: Glomerular Filtration Rate

(GFR: ^{99m}Tc-DTPA)

Radiopharmacy

Radionuclide

- ^{99m}Tc $t_{1/2}$: 6 hours

  Energies: 140 keV

  Type: IT, γ, generator

Radiopharmaceutical

- ^{99m}Tc-DTPA (diethylenetriaminepentaacetic acid)

Localization

- Compartmental, blood (< 10% bound to protein, filtered by glomerulus)

Quality Control

- ^{99m}Tc-DTPA: chromatography, > 90%; use within 1 hour

Adult Dose Range

- 3 (for GFR) to 15 mCi (111–555 MBq)

Method of Administration

- Bolus IV (sometimes with furosemide [Lasix®] 40 mg given IV and/or captopril [Capoten®] 50 mg given PO)

Indications

- Evaluation of renal tubular function and perfusion (glomerular filtration).
- Evaluation of renal vascular flow.

- Evaluation of renal (renovascular) hypertension.
- Detection of acute tubular necrosis.
- Evaluation for renal tubular obstruction and/or trauma.
- Evaluation of renal transplant.

Contraindications

- Patient still on adrenal cortical extract (ACE, or angiotensin-converting enzyme) inhibitors (although some scans require the inclusion of their intake and function with the test).

Patient History *(or use complete patient history in reference section)*

The patient should answer the following questions.

Do you have a history or family history of cancer?	Y	N
If so, what type and for how long?		
Do you have a history of kidney disease (e.g., stones, infections)?	Y	N
Do you have both kidneys?	Y	N
Are there any recent or planned operations?	Y	N
Do you have any pain?	Y	N
If so, where and for how long?		
Are you experiencing nausea or vomiting?	Y	N
Are you experiencing urinary frequency or urgency?	Y	N
Do you have any blood in your urine?	Y	N

Are you a diabetic?	Y	N
Do you have any cardiac diseases?	Y	N
Do you have high blood pressure?	Y	N
Do you have the results of any recent laboratory tests?	Y	N

Other department-specific questions.

Patient Preparation

- Identify the patient. Verify doctor's order. Explain the procedure.
- Patient is to be well hydrated and should void before the test begins.
- Patient should discontinue any ACE inhibitors.

Equipment

Camera

- Large field of view

Collimator

- Low energy, all purpose, or low energy, high resolution

Computer Set-up
Flow

- 1–5 sec/frame for 1–2 minutes

Dynamic

- 20–60 sec/frame for 1800 seconds

Statics

- 500,000–800,000 counts at 1, 3, 5, 10, 15, 20, 25, and 30 minutes

Procedure *(varies greatly; time: ~30 [baseline] to 180 minutes [with captopril])*

Baseline

- DTPA is used for inexpensive and easy baselines, checking for normal renal function. If GFR is to be included, count the syringe before and after injection for 1 minute at 20–30 cm from camera face (use same distance both times).
- Place patient in supine position, camera posterior except for kidney transplant patients for whom camera is placed anterior covering the lower abdomen.

- Position camera by point source over xiphoid, umbilicus, pubic symphysis, and sides in field of view. Kidneys and bladder must be in view for processing.

- If study calls for Lasix® (furosemide), set IV up with butterfly, three-way stopcock, furosemide, flush, and bolus radiotracer.

- Inject bolus and start camera (and furosemide with flush, although some do not inject furosemide at this time but wait until later to see whether there is any obstruction). Note: some wait until they see activity blush in abdomen (the "umbrella" effect caused by the heart-liver-spleen and descending aorta) before starting camera. To be sure, set flow for 120 seconds, start camera just before injection.

- Acquire flow, then acquire dynamics or statics as to protocol.

- If furosemide is separate, acquire images for 5 minutes, inject for 2 minutes, and follow every 5 minutes for 30 minutes. Note time in study when Lasix® was given.

- Generate time–activity curve graph(s); renogram, and differential function.

- Generate percent uptake of each kidney. Select frame of dynamic study or static that has or appears to have the most counts. Software differs: some have automatic programs, some will allow regions of interest to be drawn, giving counts within the area. Add two counts together for the total, divide each by the total to give percent uptake for each kidney; combined percents should equal 100.

- Generate pictures of dynamic or static images.

Captopril

- Can be same day or separate day procedure. Captopril study can be performed first; if normal, it negates the need for a baseline study.

- Administer 50 mg Capoten® tablet PO with water (as much as 1 L).

- Patient is hooked to blood pressure cuff machine, arm level with machine and monitored (record blood pressures every 15 minutes) for 1 hour at which time patient should void.

- Patients may have reactions to the captopril.

  - Hypotension: small women or patient already on blood pressure medicines. Elevate legs, hydrate patient.

  - Allergic reaction: antihistamine (e.g., Benadryl® IV by nurse).

- Reposition patient and repeat baseline procedure from start.

- Take delays as per physician's order.

Normal Results

- Assuming two kidneys, both kidneys visualizing about the same size and intensities. Both graphs peaking with parallel upslope and within 3 seconds of aortic peak and dropping off (excretion) at about the same rate.

- Static images should yield a smooth renal contour.

- Furosemide suggested normals: $t_{1/2}$ washout time from injection is suggested at < 15 minutes; 15–20 minutes is indeterminate.

- GFR (glomerular filtration rate) = 125 mL/min.

- Normal renal uptakes are 4–9% for each kidney.

- ERPF (effective renal plasma flow) = 500–600 mL/min.

- Filtration fraction (GFR/ERPF) = 0.2

99mTc-DTPA With Captopril

- Captopril renal cortical activity (RCA) at 20 minutes < 30%.

- Captopril time to peak activity (t_{max}) is 3–6 minutes.

- Captopril renal function:tubular excretion rate (TER) ratio is 40:60.

Abnormal Results

- One or both kidneys not visualizing.

- One or both enlarged kidneys or decreased activity indicates pyelonephritis.

- Asymmetric activity indicates renal artery stenosis or hydroureteronephrosis.

- Graphs not having parallel input and excretion drop-off rates.

- Slow upslope and/or downslope in one or both kidneys. Corrected slopes after captopril would mean renal artery stenosis. Uncorrected slopes after captopril may mean obstruction or nephrosis of tissue, problems other than but perhaps as well as stenosis.

- Lasix® (furosemide) distinguishes benign dilated systems from mechanical obstruction.

- Furosemide: suggested abnormal $t_{1/2}$ washout time is > 20 minutes from injection.

- Increased spleen and liver activity indicates renal failure.

Grafts

- Acute rejection of transplanted kidney: delayed DTPA, diminished ¹³¹I-hippuran.

- ⁹⁹ᵐTc-sulfur colloid given to detect early graft rejection by increased uptake within kidney.

Artifacts

- Some patients do not have both kidneys.

- Patient still taking ACE inhibitors before test.

- With dehydration, curve may resemble obstruction.

- Misalignment on positioning.

- Injection problems for flow or bad start.

Note

Calculating the GFR: There are many methods. Some software has automatic programs; just punch in the information. The following is a simple method for the "do-it-yourselfers."

This is a rendition of the Gates Method. Using about 3 mCi (111 MBq), count syringe for 1 minute. Inject and obtain flow, then at least 5-minute dynamic or static images; choose the 2- to 3-minute picture for processing. If a renogram is also involved, let it run out. Either way, take a 1-minute postinjection count of syringe. Follow these easy steps:

- Net dose counts = preinjection syringe counts − postinjection syringe counts.

- Tonnesen method of kidney depth calculation:

Right kidney depth (cm) = [13.3 × weight/height] + 0.7

Left kidney depth (cm) = [13.2 × weight/height] + 0.7

where weight is the patient's weight in kilograms, and height is the patient's height in centimeters.

- Percent renal uptake of kidney (counts taken from ROIs of kidneys and backgrounds using 3-minute image).

$$\frac{\dfrac{\text{Right kidney counts} - \text{bkg counts}}{2.718 - (0.153 \times [\text{kidney depth}])} + \dfrac{\text{left kidney count} - \text{bkg counts}}{2.718 - (0.153 \times [\text{kidney depth}])}}{\text{preinjection counts} - \text{postinjection counts}} \times 100 = \text{percent uptake}$$

- GFR in mL/min = (percent renal uptake) × 9.81270 − 6.82519.

ACE inhibitors block the formation of angiotensin II. Angiotensin II is the potent vasoconstrictor that constricts the efferent glomerular arteriole. The normal renin–angiotensin II system helps maintain arterial blood pressure within normal limits, among other things. With renal artery stenosis, blood flow to the kidneys is reduced, stimulating the release of more than normal renin. This catalyzes the production of angiotensin I, which leads to angiotensin II. Angiotensin II then causes arterial constriction and sodium retention, resulting in increased systemic arterial pressure and blood flow to the stenotic kidney(s).

The following is a list of ACE inhibitors:

Altace®

Capoten®

Capozide®

Lotensin®

Monopril®

Prinivil®

Prinzide®

Vaseretic®

Vasotec®

Zestoretic®

Zestril®

SUGGESTED READINGS

Datz FL. Handbook of Nuclear Medicine. 2nd ed. St. Louis: Mosby, 1993.

Early PJ, Sodee DB. Principles and Practice of Nuclear Medicine. 2nd ed. St. Louis: Mosby, 1995.

Murray IPC, Ell PJ, eds. Nuclear Medicine in Clinical Diagnosis and Treatment. Vols. 1 and 2. New York: Churchill Livingstone, 1994.

Wilson, MA. Textbook of Nuclear Medicine. Philadelphia: Lippincott-Raven, 1998.

Notes

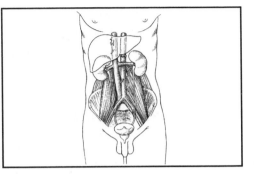

Renal: Tubular Function

(MAG$_3$®, ^{131}I-OIH)

Radiopharmacy

Radionuclide

- ^{99m}Tc t$_{1/2}$: 6 hours

  Energies: 140 keV

  Type: IT, γ, generator

- or: ^{131}I t$_{1/2}$: 8.1 days

  Energies: 364 keV

  Type: β$^-$, γ, fission product

Radiopharmaceutical

- ^{99m}Tc-MAG$_3$® (mercaptoacetyltriglycine)

- ^{131}I-OIH (orthoiodohippurate)

Localization

- Compartmental, blood flow

Quality Control

- ^{99m}Tc: chromatography, ^{99m}Tc-MAG$_3$®: > 95%

- ^{131}I: chemical purity test for ^{131}I iodide (< 1.5%), ^{131}I-OIH (orthoiodohippurate) > 97%, and ^{131}I orthoiodobenzoic acid; radionuclide purity for anything other than ^{131}I, spectrometer test for tracer tag.

Adult Dose Range

- ^{99m}Tc: 3–10 mCi (111–370 MBq)

- ^{131}I: 150–300 uCi (5.55–11.1 MBq)

Method of Administration

- Bolus IV (sometimes with furosemide [Lasix®] 40 mg and/or captopril [Capoten®] 50 mg given PO)

Indications

- Evaluation for renal artery stenosis.
- Evaluation for renal (renovascular) hypertension.
- Evaluation of renal tubular function.
- Evaluation of a kidney transplant.

Contraindications

- Patient still on adrenal cortical extract (ACE, or angiotensin-converting enzyme) inhibitors (although some scans require the inclusion of their intake and function with the test).
- Food intake too close to a captopril study will decrease the sensitivity of the test and slow the absorption of the ACE inhibitor.

Patient History *(or use complete patient history in reference section)*

The patient should answer the following questions.

Do you have a history or family history of cancer?	Y	N
If so, what type and for how long?		
Do you have a history of kidney disease (e.g., stones, infections)?	Y	N
Do you have both kidneys?	Y	N
Are there any recent or planned operations?	Y	N
Do you have any pain?	Y	N
If so, where and for how long?		
Are you experiencing nausea or vomiting?	Y	N

Are you experiencing urinary frequency or urgency?	Y	N
Do you have any blood in your urine?	Y	N
Are you a diabetic?	Y	N
Do you have any cardiac diseases?	Y	N
Do you have high blood pressure?	Y	N
Do you have the results of any recent laboratory tests?	Y	N
Other department-specific questions.		

Patient Preparation

- Identify the patient. Verify doctor's order. Explain the procedure.
- Instruct patient to hydrate well (up to 10 mL/kg) and void just before test.
- Physician is to instruct patient to discontinue ACE inhibitors for several days before examination. They may also be asked to discontinue diuretics and β-blockers.
- Instruct patient to be NPO for morning before captopril study.

Equipment

Camera

- Large field of view

Collimator

- ^{131}I: medium to high energy
- ^{99m}Tc: low energy, all purpose, or low energy, high resolution

Computer Set-up
Flow

- 2–4 sec/frame for 1 minute.

Dynamic

- 20–60 sec/frame for 1800 seconds.

Statics

- 500,000–1,000,000 counts at 1, 3, 5, 10, 15, 20, 25, and 30 minutes.

Procedure *(varies greatly; time: ~30 [baseline] to 180 minutes [with captopril])*

Baseline

- Place patient in supine position, camera under table, except for kidney replacement patients for whom camera is placed anterior over the abdomen.

- Position camera by point source over xiphoid, umbilicus, pubic symphysis, and sides in field of view. Some inject 100–200 μCi of ^{99m}Tc-MAG$_3$® before starting camera to visualize kidney placement.

- Bolus IV push, start camera. Note: some wait until they see activity blush in abdomen (the "umbrella" effect caused by the heart-liver-spleen and descending aorta) before starting camera. To be sure, set flow for 120 seconds; start camera just before injection.

- If using furosemide then:

    - Set IV up with butterfly, three-way stopcock, furosemide, flush, and bolus radiotracer.

    - For 1-minute flow: inject bolus, start camera, inject furosemide, and flush. (Some do not inject furosemide at this time but wait until later [at 10–15 minutes] to see whether there is any obstruction.)

    - Acquire statics at 2- to 5-minute intervals for 30 minutes or serial 1-minute images for 30 minutes. (Most systems have a preset for renogram, renal qualitative, or renal perfusion.)

- If furosemide is separate, take images for 5 minutes, inject for 2 minutes, and follow every 5 minutes for 30 minutes.

- Calculate effective renal plasma flow (ERPF). Generate graphs.

Captopril

- Can be same day or separate day procedure. Captopril study can be performed first; if normal, it negates the need for a baseline study.

- Administer 50 mg Capoten® tablet PO with water (as much as 1 L).

- Patient is connected to blood pressure cuff machine, arm level with machine, and monitored closely (record blood pressures every 15 minutes, watch for reactions) for 1 hour at which time patient is to void.

- Reposition patient and repeat baseline procedure from start.

- Take delays as per physician's order.

Normal Results

- Assuming two kidneys, both kidneys visualizing about the same size and intensities. Both graphs peaking with parallel upslope and within 3 seconds of aortic peak and dropping off (excretion) at the same rate.

- Static images should yield a smooth renal contour.

- Furosemide suggested normals: $t_{1/2}$ washout time from injection is suggested at < 15 minutes; 15–20 minutes is indeterminate.

- A normal captopril or enalaprilat renogram obviates the need for a baseline study.

- ERPF 500–600 mL/min.

^{99m}Tc-MAG$_3$® With Captopril

- Captopril renal cortical activity (RCA) at 20 minutes $< 30\%$.
- Captopril time to peak activity (t_{max}) is 3–6 minutes.
- Captopril renal function:tubular excretion rate (TER) ratio is 40:60.

Abnormal Results

- One or both kidneys not visualizing.
- Graphs not having parallel input and excretion drop-off rates.
- Furosemide: Suggested abnormal $t_{1/2}$ washout time is > 20 minutes from injection.
- Slow upslope or downslope in one or both kidneys. Corrected slopes after captopril would mean renal artery stenosis. Uncorrected slopes after captopril may mean obstruction or nephrosis of tissue, problems other than but perhaps as well as stenosis.
- Increased spleen and liver activity indicates renal failure.

Artifacts

- Some patients do not have both kidneys.
- Patient still taking ACE inhibitors before test.
- Misalignment on positioning.
- Injection problems for flow or bad start.

Note

Baseline and captopril studies are routinely performed on a 1- or 2-day protocol. If a 1-day protocol is desired, usually a baseline renogram is performed, captopril is given (or enalaprilat; 40 µg/kg IV for 3–5 minutes) with the patient monitored closely for 1 hour (peak activity for captopril), then a second injection and renogram are performed.

Patients may have reactions to the captopril.

- Hypotension: small women or patient already on blood pressure medicines. Elevate legs, hydrate patient.
- Allergic reaction: antihistamine (e.g., Benadryl® IV by nurse).

There are many methods to calculate ERPF: here are two.

$$\text{ERPF} = -51.1 + (8.21X) - (0.019X^2) \text{ in mL/min}$$

where X = dose injected (counts/s) ÷ counts/s per liter of plasma from blood specimen taken 45 minutes after injection.

Schegel Method for ^{131}I-OIH

- Take 1-minute counts of preinjection and postinjection syringe at 20–30 cm from camera face (same distance for both).
- Preinjection counts − postinjection counts = net injected counts.
- From the 2-minute image regions of interest:

$$ERPF = \frac{(\text{kidney counts} - \text{bkg counts} \times Y^2 \times 100}{\text{net injected counts}}$$

where Y = kidney depth.

Tonnesen Method of Kidney Depth Calculation

Right kidney depth (cm) = [13.3 × weight/height] + 0.7

Left kidney depth (cm) = [13.2 × weight/height] + 0.7

where weight is the patient's weight in kilograms, and height is the patient's height in centimeters.

ACE inhibitors block the formation of angiotensin II. Angiotensin II is the potent vasoconstrictor that constricts the efferent glomerular arteriole. The normal renin–angiotensin II system helps maintain arterial blood pressure within normal limits, among other things. With renal artery stenosis, blood flow to the kidneys is reduced, stimulating the release of more than normal renin. This catalyzes the production of angiotensin I, which leads to angiotensin II. Angiotensin II then causes arterial constriction and sodium retention, resulting in increased systemic arterial pressure and blood flow to the stenotic kidney(s).

The following is a list of ACE inhibitors

Altace®

Capoten®

Capozide®

Lotensin®

Monopril®

Prinivil®

Prinzide®

Vaseretic®

Vasotec®

Zestoretic®

Zestril®

SUGGESTED READINGS

Datz FL. Handbook of Nuclear Medicine. 2nd ed. St. Louis: Mosby, 1993.

Early PJ, Sodee DB. Principles and Practice of Nuclear Medicine. 2nd ed. St. Louis: Mosby, 1995.

Murray IPC, Ell PJ, eds. Nuclear Medicine in Clinical Diagnosis and Treatment. Vols. 1 and 2. New York: Churchill Livingstone, 1994.

Wilson, MA. Textbook of Nuclear Medicine. Philadelphia: Lippincott-Raven, 1998.

Altace® is a registered trademark of Hoechst-Roussel Pharmaceuticals, Inc., Somerville, NJ.
Benadryl® is a registered trademark of Parke-Davis, Morris Plains, NJ.
Capoten® is a registered trademark of ER Squibb & Sons, Inc., Princeton, NJ.
Capozide® is a registered trademark of ER Squibb & Sons, Inc., Princeton, NJ.
Lasix® is a registered trademark of Hoechst-Roussel Pharmaceuticals, Inc., Somerville, NJ.
Lotensin® is a registered trademark of CIBA Consumer Pharmaceuticals, Edison, NJ.
MAG$_3$® is a registered trademark of Mallinckrodt Medical, Inc., St. Louis, MO.
Monopril® is a registered trademark of Mead Johnson Pharmaceuticals, Evansville, IN.

Prinivil® is a registered trademark of Merck, Sharp, & Dohme, West Point, PA.
Prinzide® is a registered trademark of Merck, Sharp, & Dohme, West Point, PA.
Vaseretic® is a registered trademark of Merck, Sharp, & Dohme, West Point, PA.
Vasotec® is a registered trademark of Merck, Sharp, & Dohme, West Point, PA.
Zestoretic® is a registered trademark of Stuart Pharmaceuticals, Wilmington, DE.
Zestril® is a registered trademark of Stuart Pharmaceuticals, Wilmington, DE.

Notes

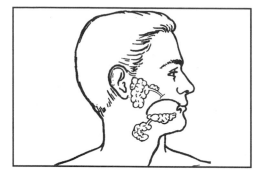

Salivary Gland Imaging

Radiopharmacy

Radionuclide

- ^{99m}Tc $t_{1/2}$: 6 hours

  Energies: 140 keV

  Type: IT, γ, generator

Radiopharmaceutical

- Na ^{99m}TcO$_4^-$ (pertechnetate)

Localization

- Compartmental to blood supply. ^{99m}TcO$_4^-$ is taken up by the parenchyma cells of the parotid and salivary glands.

Quality Control

- Moly-Al breakthrough, chromatography > 90%

Adult Dose Range

- 8–12 mCi (296–444 MBq)

Method of Administration

- IV injection, good bolus for flow

Indications

- Differentiation of Warthin's tumor from other malignant or benign salivary tumors.
- Evaluation of function of palpable masses in parotid or salivary tissue.
- Evaluation of salivary gland function, especially after head and neck irradiation.
- Evaluation of anatomic size and position of salivary glands.
- Evaluation and assessment of salivary glands for preexternal or interstitial radiotherapy candidates.

Contraindications

- None

Patient History

The patient should answer the following questions.

Do you have a history or family history of cancer?	Y	N
If so, what type and for how long?		

Do you have a history or family history of salivary dysfunction?	Y	N
Do you have "dry mouth"?	Y	N
Do you have any palpable lumps in or under your jaw?	Y	N
Do you have any pain in or under your jaw?	Y	N
Have you had a labial biopsy (minor salivary gland tissue)?	Y	N

Other department-specific questions.

Patient Preparation

- Identify the patient. Verify doctor's order. Explain the procedure.
- Withhold thyroid-blocking agents (e.g., iodide or perchlorate) for 48 hours before examination.
- Administer gum to stimulate salivary glands.

Equipment

Camera

- Large field of view

Collimator

- Low energy, all purpose, or low energy, high resolution

Computer Set-up

- 128 × 128 matrix, some magnify at ×2–×4

Flow

- 1 sec/image for 60 seconds

Dynamic

- 1- to 3-minute images for 30–60 minutes

Statics

- 300,000 counts or 180 seconds per view

Procedure *(time: 60–90 minutes)*

- Place patient in supine position on table, pillow under shoulders, neck extended, camera as close as possible.
- Administer injection to patient; start camera.
- Obtain one of the following:
  - Flow and dynamics for 30–60 minutes. Then, obtain anterior marker, left and right laterals.
  - Flow with statics at 15 minutes after injection, 3 minutes per view. Obtain anterior marker, anterior, left and right laterals.
  - Statics only at least at 15 minutes after injection, 3 minutes per view. Some obtain images at 2, 5, 10, 15, 20, and 30 minutes. Obtain anterior marker, anterior, left and right laterals.
- Lemon phase:
  - Place lemon extract or lemon juice-soaked gauze on both sides of patient's mouth. (Or patient can suck lemon juice through straw and hold in mouth to stimulate salivaries.)
  - Some do this during dynamics at 40 minutes or after dynamics and statics. Use 2 mL of lemon juice through straw (intraorally).
  - Remove gauze after 5 minutes, allow patient to expectorate excess saliva and rinse with water.
  - Repeat static anterior, left, and right lateral images at 15 and 30 minutes after lemon administration.
- Salivary function evaluation:
  - Draw regions of interest around thyroid, submandibular, parotid glands, and backgrounds on appropriate lateral or anterior view.
  - Record counts and repeat for all sequential timed images.

Normal Results

- Symmetric uptake in the parotid and submandibular glands.
- Uptake in sublingual and thyroid glands and nasal cavity.
- Significant reduction of activity in salivary glands after lemon administration.

Abnormal Results

- Increased uptake nonsymmetrically on one side or both sides of face, different from the bilateral uptake of the salivary glands.

- Activity remains local after lemon administration.

- Malignant (Warthin's) tumor presents with increased concentration of radiotracer and will retain tracer within the mass.

- Space-occupying lesions or filling defects: 1.5–2 cm in diameter, patchy decreases in activity in Sjögren's syndrome (autoimmune disease affecting the salivary and lacrimal glands, occurs in postmenopausal women; presents with rheumatoid arthritis, xerostomia [dryness of mouth caused by malfunctioning salivary glands], and keratoconjunctivitis sicca [dryness in eyes]).

- Mixed tumors of the parotid: patchy decrease in activity in area of lesion; lesion may have normal or even increased count rate.

- Lymphomatous infiltration: patchy areas of decreased concentration and may have normal count rates; with increasing infiltration, count rate decreases.

- Metastatic lesions: space-occupying and slightly ragged with no activity.

- Abscesses: smooth and round with no activity, tender to palpation.

- Cysts: smooth and round, no activity, not tender to palpation.

- Bacterial or viral acute sialadenitis (inflammation of the salivary glands): marked increase in uptake of affected gland(s).

Artifacts

- Patient movement will blur images.

SUGGESTED READINGS

Early PJ, Sodee DB. Principles and Practice of Nuclear Medicine. 2nd ed. St. Louis: Mosby, 1995.

Murray IPC, Ell PJ, eds. Nuclear Medicine in Clinical Diagnosis and Treatment. Vols. 1 and 2. New York: Churchill Livingstone, 1994.

Wilson, MA. Textbook of Nuclear Medicine. Philadelphia: Lippincott-Raven, 1998.

Notes

CHAPTER 43

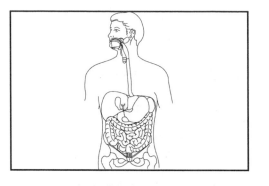

Schilling Test

Radiopharmacy

Radionuclide

- ^{57}Co $t_{1/2}$: 270 days

  Energies: 122 keV

  Type: EC, γ, accelerator

Radiopharmaceutical

- ^{57}Co-cyanocobalamin (vitamin B-12)

Localization

- Bound to plasma proteins. Combined to intrinsic factor in the gastric mucosa, absorbed into the bloodstream in the terminal ileum, and stored in the liver.

Quality Control

- Capsule(s) come with kit. Calibrated by dose.

Adult Dose Range

- 0.3–1 μCi (11.1–37 kBq)

Method of Administration

- PO; intrinsic factor given IM

Indications

- Diagnosis of pernicious anemia (decreased red blood cells, muscular weakness, gastrointestinal and neural disturbances).
- Diagnosis of macrocytic (megaloblastic) anemia (degenerative disease of spinal cord).
- Evaluation of low B-12.
- Evaluation of small intestinal malabsorption.
- Evaluation of thrombocytopenia or leucopenia.

Contraindications

- Pregnant women or nursing mothers.

Patient History

The patient should answer the following questions.

Do you have a history or family history of cancer?   Y   N

If so, what type and for how long?

When was your last meal?

Do you have a history or family history of
  low B-12?   Y   N

Do you have a history of intestinal disease?   Y   N

Have you had any recent abdominal trauma?   Y   N

Have you had any stomach disease or surgery
  (e.g., ulcers, tapeworm, gastrectomy)?   Y   N

Are you a strict vegetarian?   Y   N

Are you taking vitamins?   Y   N

Do you feel that you are tired?   Y   N

Are you on any drug therapy?   Y   N

What medications are you taking?

Have you received any vitamin B-12 recently?   Y   N

Have you had any recent nuclear medicine
  or related tests?   Y   N

Do you have the results of any recent laboratory tests (especially serum creatinine)?   Y   N

Other department-specific questions.

Patient Preparation

- Identify the patient. Verify doctor's order. Explain the procedure.
- Instruct patient to be NPO from midnight before test (NPO at least 4 hours before test) and continue to do so for 2 hours after ingestion of radiotracer.
- Instruct patient to discontinue parenteral B-12 for 3 or more days before test.
- Complete all patient paperwork.
- Instruct patient to collect *all* urine in container during the 24-hour period after ingestion of radiotracer.
- Instruct patient to drink only water for liquid.
- Instruct patient to have no other tests, enemas, or laxatives for the duration of this test.

Equipment

Detector

- Well counter

Collimator

- N/A

Computer Set-up

- Energy window set at 114–144 keV. Count for 5–10 minutes per sample (count all the same way).

Procedure *(time: ~30 minutes)*

Before Dosing Patient

- Obtain kit supplied by radiopharmacy.
- Calibrate patient dose; record.
- Calibrate standard dose (if separate); record.
- Label paperwork, collection container, and doses.
- Collect a predose urine sample from patient if background test tube is indicated. Label and store for 24-hour count. Also needed if patient has had recent nuclear scan.

Stage 1: Without Intrinsic Factor

- Instruct patient to empty bladder. Collect some urine for testing for radioactivity if previous nuclear medicine tests have been performed.

- Instruct patient to ingest capsule containing ^{57}Co-labeled B-12. Note time on paperwork.
- Patient is given 24-hour urine collection container to begin collection, still fasting.
- Instruct patient to return in 1–2 hours for IM "flushing dose" of 1000 μg of cold B-12, which saturates the remaining B-12 binding sites in body so whatever labeled (hot) B-12 was absorbed from intestine is excreted in the urine.
- Instruct patient to return in 24 hours with collection container(s). Some collect for 48 hours if serum creatinine levels are more than 2.5 mg/dL. Record total amount of urine brought in.

Stage 2: With Intrinsic Factor

- Instruct patient to return in 5 days.
- Same test is repeated with patient receiving a capsule containing intrinsic factor (30 mg) along with the ^{57}Co-labeled B-12 capsule.

Stage 3: After Antibiotic Treatment

- Physician prescribes antibiotic therapy to patient.
- Instruct patient to return in 5 days.
- Same test as in Stage 2.

Stage 4: Dual-Isotope Study

- Use ^{58}Co with study.
    - ^{58}Co $t_{1/2}$: 72 d
    - Energies: 810 keV
    - Type: EC, β^+, γ, accelerator
- Administer ^{57}Co-labeled B-12 and ^{58}Co-labeled B-12 and intrinsic factor at the same time (kit form).
- Count using two standards and two windows.
- Counting, procedure, and results are same as above, just performed in one step.

Process Information

- Check lot numbers for correctness.
- Record total amount of urine in sample.
- Pipet two patient samples, 4 mL each, into test tubes.
- Place standard into test tube, or pour into test tube to make 4 mL (typically 0.5 mL of labeled B-12 and 3.5 mL of water, check kit insert).
- Count samples using program provided by probe. Usually something similar to counting background sample (or room background) for 5 minutes, count two patient 24-hour samples for 5 minutes each, count reference standard for 5 minutes. Some go 10 minutes for each.
- Manual calculations (all in cpm):
    - Net standard counts (net std cts) = standard − background (bkg)
    - Corrected patient (pt) sample counts 1 = pt sample 1 − bkg
    - Corrected patient sample counts 2 = pt sample 2 − bkg

- Net corrected patient sample counts (net corr pt sample cts) = (corrected 1 + corrected 2)/2

$$\% \text{ excreted in urine} = \frac{\text{net corr pt sample cts} \times \text{total urine vol (mL)}}{\text{net std cts} \times 4} \times 100$$

- or (using counts per milliliter [divide counts by 4]):

$$\frac{\text{pt urine cts/mL} \times \text{total urine vol} \times 100}{\text{diluted standard cts/mL} \times \text{dilution factor}} = \% \text{ excreted labeled B-12}$$

where dilution factor is calculated as follows: if 4 mL of dilute standard contains 1% of the standard (check kit insert), 1 mL will contain 0.25%. The dilution factor will then be 400.

Normal Results

- Greater than or equal to 7% of dose excreted in urine at 24 hours. Some use > 10% with 6–10% indeterminate. Less than 7% is abnormal, indicating failure to absorb B-12.

- Others: > 10% excreted at 24 hours is normal; 5–9.9% indeterminate. Less than 5% is abnormal, indicating failure to absorb B-12.

Abnormal Results

- Stage 1: < 7% of dose excreted in urine at 24 hours. Deficient absorption because of either intrinsic factor or intestinal deficiency.

- Stage 2: Greater than or equal to 7% of dose excreted in urine at 24 hours indicates malabsorption due to intrinsic factor deficiency (ulcers, cancer, etc.).

- Less than 7% indicates malabsorption caused by intestinal illness (bacterial, viral, etc.).

Artifacts

- It is extremely important that the patient collects all urine into the collection container. Missing any will cause falsely low results.

- Medications and vitamin supplements, recent food intake, etc., are all important to the outcome of the test. Patient history is a must.

- Impaired renal function makes test inappropriate. Physical problems with renal system, e.g., benign prostatic hypertrophy that results in urinary retention can affect the 24-hour collection. Elderly patients with slowed renal function will similarly affect the 24-hour collection. In these and other situations, a second 24-hour collection is indicated.

Note

Vitamin B-12 and folic acid (B-complex vitamins) are involved with the production of red blood cells. B-12 is naturally absorbed from meats and dairy products, is bound to intrinsic factor by gastric mucosa, and is a coenzyme needed, along with folic acid from vegetables, for DNA synthesis and cell division in all tissues, especially bone marrow. Normal nutritional requirements are 1 μg/d. Normal diets usually provide 2–30 μg/d. B-12 is stored for up to 800 days. Neurologic changes are often associated with severe B-12 and folate deficiencies. These may not be reversible. Deficiencies (malabsorption) of B-12 can be caused by lack of intrinsic factor from pernicious anemia or gastrectomy, dietary lack of the vitamin, bacterial overgrowths within the bowel that consume the vitamin, or inability to absorb the intrinsic factor–B-12 complex in the terminal ileum because of resection or disease states, e.g., Crohn's disease.

SUGGESTED READINGS

Datz FL. Handbook of Nuclear Medicine. 2nd ed. St. Louis: Mosby, 1993.

Early PJ, Sodee DB. Principles and Practice of Nuclear Medicine. 2nd ed. St. Louis: Mosby, 1995.

Murray IPC, Ell PJ, eds. Nuclear Medicine in Clinical Diagnosis and Treatment. Vols. 1 and 2. New York: Churchill Livingstone, 1994.

Wilson, MA. Textbook of Nuclear Medicine. Philadelphia: Lippincott-Raven, 1998.

Notes

CHAPTER 44

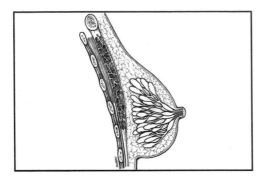

Scintimammography

Radiopharmacy

Radionuclide

- ^{99m}Tc $t_{\frac{1}{2}}$: 6 hours

  Energies: 140 keV

  Type: IT, γ, generator

Radiopharmaceutical

- ^{99m}Tc-sestamibi (hexakis[2-methoxyisobutylisonitril]),
  ^{99m}Tc-1,2-bis(bis[2-ethoxyethyl]phosphino)ethane

Localization

- Passive transport through cell membranes in proportion to blood flow, active transport into myocardial mitochondria. High affinity to myocytes and carcinoma cells.

Quality Control

- Chromatography > 90%

Adult Dose Range

- 20–30 mCi (740–1110 MBq)

Method of Administration

- IV injection in foot or hand contralateral to breast with suspected lesion.

- If bilateral lesions suspected or postmastectomy, inject in foot vein.

- For hand or arm injections, use IV catheter or butterfly and stopcock to avoid infiltration (very important), which may appear as false-positive axillary node uptake.

- Flush with at least 10 mL of saline.

Indications

- Detection and localization of breast carcinoma, particularly in women with palpable breast mass. Usually done in conjunction with and to help improve the sensitivity and specificity of mammography, and aid in decisions about biopsy.
- Evaluation of women with mammographically dense breasts, palpable mass, and negative fine needle aspiration (FNA).
- Detection and localization of metastases in the axillary lymph nodes. Test helps breast cancer patients decide between lumpectomy or mastectomy: for high-risk patients with prior history or family history of premenopausal breast cancer, patients with palpable lumps or abnormal lesions on mammography, and patients with dense, as opposed to fatty, breast tissue.
- Evaluation of known but nonpalpable breast lesions.
- Evaluation of elevated tumor markers.
- Differentiation between true-positives (e.g., invasive ductal carcinoma, ductal carcinoma in situ, colloid carcinoma, medullary carcinoma, and infiltrating lobular carcinoma) and true negatives (e.g., fibrocystic changes, fibroadenoma, atypical ductal hyperplasia, florid epithelial hyperplasia, stromal sclerosis, complex sclerosing lesion, cysts, and combinations thereof).
- Evaluation of therapy.
- Evaluation of breast implants.

Contraindications

- None.

Patient History *(or use complete patient history in reference section)*

The patient should answer the following questions.

**Do you have a history or family history
of cancer?**   Y   N

If so, what type and for how long?

Do you have any palpable nodules?   Y   N

If so, since when?

Do you have any tenderness in your breasts?   Y   N

Have you had any discharge from your breasts?	Y	N
Have you had any recent trauma to your chest area?	Y	N
Have you had any recent surgery or mastectomy?	Y	N
Have you had any implants?	Y	N
Have you received any chemotherapy or radiation therapy?	Y	N
Have you had any recent mammograms, CT, MRI, NM, biopsy, x-rays, or laboratory work?	Y	N
Other department-specific questions.		

Patient Preparation

- Identify the patient. Verify doctor's order.
- Explain the procedure; mid-menstrual cycle is best time for exam.
- Patient dressed in hospital gown open to the front, no bra or jewelry.
- Obtain recent mammogram or other relevant scans and results for lesion correlation.

Equipment

Camera

- Large field-of-view or dedicated scintimammographic camera (SPEM: single photon emission mammograph)

Collimator

- Low energy, high resolution

Computer Set-up

- 10% window (to reduce scatter from table, which appears as a vertical line during processing), centered on 140 keV, 128 × 128 matrix, zoom as allowed to include large breasts and anterior chest wall in field of view. Acquisition on "time" (600 seconds).

Procedure *(time: ~90 minutes)*

Prone Dependent-Breast Position

- Patient is injected; imaging begins 5 minutes after injection. Consider dorsal foot injection to minimize extravasation and false-positive lymph node presentation.

- Images: All pictures are 10-minute (600 seconds) views.

  - Place patient in prone position on imaging bed, sternum on edge of bed, arms comfortably over head, shoulder flat on bed, head to one side.

  - On dual-pendant table, include an attachment for a lead shield to be placed between the breasts to eliminate shine-through from opposite breast.

  - Maintain collimator face as close to the patient's side and breast as possible to improve image resolution and patient safety.

  - Reposition patient and camera as needed for the acquisitions.

- or Images: All pictures are 10-minute (600 seconds) views.

  - Place patient in sitting position or standing upright with camera positioned for anterior chest image, arms up (around detector) for evaluation of axillae (ipsilateral). This can also be done supine, arms up with breasts taped up and away from interfering liver-spleen-gut-cardiac activity.

  - Obtain 180-second marker image (nipples and known lesions, with or without ^{57}Co transmission image).

  - Obtain left and right laterals with patient prone (if both breasts are pendant, a lead shield is placed between to eliminate shine-through).

  - Optional view: position camera under table, patient prone, to take the "anterior" picture.

  - Obtain 30° posterior obliques, arms up, for better separation if deep lesion is visualized close to chest wall.

Single Photon Emission Computed Tomography (SPECT) Scintimammography (usually 20–30 minutes after injection)

- Place patient in prone position, with breast dependent.

- 180° acquisition; 32 30-second frames.

- 45° anterior oblique to 45° posterior oblique.

- 64 × 64 matrix with zoom as permitted.

- Reconstruct using Hamming/Hanning or Butterworth filter. Transverse, coronal, and sagittal images in gray scale, masking chest and abdominal organs.

- SPECT is said not to improve sensitivity of test because of the high counts in heart and gut.

Normal Results

- Diffuse, mild, or no uptake of sestamibi (Miraluma™) or tetrofosmin (Myoview®) in normal breast tissue.

Abnormal Results

- Focal area(s) of increased uptake in either or both breast tissue and axillary lymph nodes.
- Localization in tumors in thorax, neck, or abdomen.

Artifacts

- Imaging of prone dual dependent breasts (dual- or single-head camera) without lead shield between allows for shine-through.
- Supine anterior views require taping of breasts up and away from interfering liver-spleen-gut-cardiac activity.
- Be aware of possible thyroid shine-through on laterals.
- Extreme kyphosis can result in poor images. Supporting the patient's lower extremities with pillows will allow chest wall to be as close to the imaging table as possible.
- Cannot detect lesions smaller than 5–8 mm; hence, those with malignant calcifications may be missed. However, at present, very accurate with lesions of 1 cm or greater.
- Artifacts caused by perspiration, table, clothing, jewelry, heart monitors, movement, and shine-through from background organs.
- Implants may mask possible sites.
- Care must be taken with positioning of pendent breast, patient, and camera. Stay with patient throughout study.

Biopsy Table

- Surgeons may use gamma probe to localize uptake and remove site.

Role of Technologist in Operating Room (OR)

- Many institutions are using these studies to localize and resect suspected lesions. The role of the technologist differs with the institution, but they generally perform the following tasks.
- Inject patient as per protocol of institution.
- Images taken as suggested above; patient and images are brought to preoperative area to prepare for surgery.
- In OR
  - Technologist uses gamma probe to locate "hot" lesion(s). (Only in some institutions, others hire a company to manipulate the probe.)
  - Technologist takes resected material to pathology for inspection.
  - Technologist assays material for storage (10 half-lives) if > 0.05 mR at 1 m or disposal if background ≤ 0.05 mR at 1 m.
  - Technologist assays pathology room and equipment for contamination.
  - Technologist assays OR for contamination after removal of patient.

Note

Mammograms will find normal tissue, fibroglandular breast pattern, architectural distortion, mass, fatty tissue, dense tissue, calcification, and combinations thereof, along with a lesion of a centimeter in size or larger if present. Other helpful tracers are ^{99m}Tc-MDP, ^{111}In-octreotide, ^{18}F- fluorodeoxyglucose, various monoclonal antibodies, ^{99m}Tc-sulfur colloid, ^{99m}Tc-dextran, ^{99m}Tc-O$_4$$^-$, ^{67}Ga-citrate, ^{201}Tl, and estrogen and progesterone receptor markers. Cardiolite® and Miraluma™ are the same sestamibi DuPont agent. Tests are being conducted with tetrofosmin (Myoview® from Amersham). There are companies manufacturing dedicated scintimammography tables or cushions that accommodate the patient very well.

SUGGESTED READINGS

Early PJ, Sodee DB. Principles and Practice of Nuclear Medicine. 2nd ed. St. Louis: Mosby, 1995.

Murray IPC, Ell PJ, eds. Nuclear Medicine in Clinical Diagnosis and Treatment. Vols. 1 and 2. New York: Churchill Livingstone, 1994.

Wilson, MA. Textbook of Nuclear Medicine. Philadelphia: Lippincott-Raven, 1998.

Cardiolite® is a registered trademark of DuPont Merck, Wilmington, DE.
Miraluma™ is a trademark of DuPont Merck, Wilmington, DE.
Myoview® is a registered trademark of Amersham International Plc, Amersham, UK.

Notes

CHAPTER 45

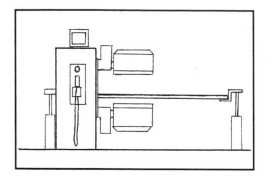

SPECT Imaging

(Single Photon Emission Computed Tomography): An Overview

Radiopharmacy

Radionuclide and radiopharmaceutical

- SPECT imaging can be performed with any in vivo nuclear medicine radiotracer given the proper collimation for the chosen isotope and software for collection and processing of data.

Localization

- Same as in planar imaging

Quality Control for the SPECT Camera

- ^{99m}Tc source, ^{57}Co flood disc, cylindrical phantom.

- Daily floods: 2–4 million counts for camera uniformity.

- Gantry index search or alignment: daily to maintain gantry positioning.

- Table-camera alignment: daily, axis of rotation must be absolutely parallel to table.

- Weekly bar phantoms: for linearity and spatial resolution (ability to resolve fine lines in bar phantoms).

- Center of rotation (COR): weekly, 500 μCi line source on end of table, 1 mm in diameter. SPECT performed. Center should not vary more than 0.5 pixel (2 mm).

- Uniformity correction: 30 million counts (64 × 64 matrix) or 100 million counts (128 × 128 matrix) every 3 months to make matrix uniform.

- Overall performance: every 3 months, SPECT performed on cylindrical phantom containing radioisotope of choice. Examine images for artifacts, adjustments made to table leveling, reconstruction, display, or components.

- Extrinsic floods: every 3 months, bar phantom floods with collimators on for system resolution.

Adult Dose Range

- Microcuries to many millicuries (same for megabecquerels). On the low end, the dosage must provide adequate photon flux from the region of interest (ROI) for the collection of data for processing into an image within the amount of time given to each step. On the high end, the amount should not be so much as to create dead time in which the camera is locked up and not taking counts. There remains a considerable range.

Method of Administration

- Radiotracer administration is the same for SPECT as it is for planar imaging. Camera(s) positioned as close as possible to body surface without brushing. Patient comfort is a consideration.

Indications

- SPECT is often performed if planar images turn up negative when a lesion or abnormality is highly suspected.
- Visualization of "buried" or blocked lesions within an organ or hidden by other structures.
- Additional information to planar (20% benefit from adding SPECT study).
- Gated SPECT for cardiac studies.

Advantages

- Three-dimensional processing.
- Better target to nontarget ratio than planar.
- Improved resolution in any given plane.
- Better definition of lesion shape.
- Accurate quantification.
- Wide selection of radiotracers.

Contraindications

- Patient unable to cooperate physically or psychologically for scan.
- Radiographic examinations under way or recent, using contrast that would hamper acquisition in the ROI.

Patient History

The patient should answer the following questions.

Are you physically or psychologically challenged in any way that would impede this study?   Y   N

Can you lie flat on your back and remain motionless for about 20 minutes?   Y   N

Are you claustrophobic?	Y	N
Do you have any monitors, pumps, pacemakers, or surgically implanted devices?	Y	N
Do you have any attenuating articles on or in clothing?	Y	N
Have you had any recent diagnostic examinations with contrast?	Y	N
Other scan-specific questions.		
Other department-specific questions.		

Patient Preparation

- Identify the patient. Verify doctor's order. Explain the procedure.
- Instruct patient to void before exam.
- Instruct patient to remain motionless for duration of imaging.

Equipment

Camera

- Single-, dual-, triple-, or quadruple-head large field-of-view gamma camera

Collimator

- Matched to radioisotope. Make sure a COR has been performed for the collimators of choice and flood tables loaded for the radioisotope.

Computer Set-up

- Circular, noncircular (elliptic), peanut-shaped, helical (whole body), or mapped orbit.
- Gated SPECT: three or five leads on patient, pictures triggered by R wave of electrocardiogram.
- Matrix is 64×64, 128×128, or larger. The larger the matrix, the higher the resolution of the image, and more computer memory is used.
- Rotation usually covers 360°, although cardiac studies cover 180° (right anterior oblique to left posterior oblique except for those with dextrocardia). Some use double or triple orbits, others use a helix orbit to cover the whole body.
- Projections usually 32 or 64 steps for step-and-shoot. Can also do continuous.
- Acquisition time usually 20–40 seconds per step. Depends on study (usually preset) and patient (size and cooperation).
- Reconstruction filters, attenuation correction, and slice thickness are usually preset although most software has opportunities to change these during processing.

Procedure *(time: ~20-40 minutes [depending on number of camera heads])*

- Place patient in supine position. No attenuating items in field of view. Make note of any surgically implanted devices.
- Position arm(s) over head if ROI requires it.
- Secure head to table with Ace bandage for cranial studies to minimize movement.
- Verify the existence of the raw data on computer before the patient leaves.

Processing: *(General)*

- Processing is very camera and software specific and department specific as to what the radiologists or nuclear physicians wish to see. Basically, though, the following must always be performed.

General SPECT

- Pick SPECT reconstruction, pick patient, select raw data.
- Select image or series of images for reconstruction.
- Select a filter(s). Most have defaults already set. You may be able to pick prefilters (affect the two-dimensional raw data) and reconstruction filters. There are many. A simple ramp is usual although a Butterworth works well. Choose one that is not too smooth nor too grainy. Also, adjustments can be made as to the strength of the filter. Postprocessing filters can be applied and usually only affect or smooth the three-dimensional image.
- Transverse (transaxial) slices: move parameter lines to cover ROI. Software differs greatly but usually gives instructions on screen. Set slice thickness, attenuation correction, working color, and intensity. When parameters are set, there is usually a "complete reconstruction" or "exit and save" or the like.
- Some now complete sagittal and coronal slices automatically whereas others ask you to click reconstruct, reformat, or continue, etc.
- At the end, always save your work. Some will automatically annotate the slices. If not (usually but not always, software differs) do the following:
  - Transverse slices: if superior to inferior, then images usually marked top is anterior, right is right side of patient, bottom is posterior, left is left side of patient.
  - Sagittal slices: if right side to left side of patient, then images usually marked left is posterior, top is superior, right is anterior.
  - Coronal slices: if anterior to posterior, then images usually marked left is right side of patient, top is superior, right is left side of patient.
- If there is a three-dimensional command, complete this and save to create a three-dimensional rotational or cine picture for review.

To Display Images

- Usually there is a SPECT display or dynamic display command.
- Select patient, select proper data set (there should be at least four: raw, transverse, sagittal, and coronal, maybe more).
- You may still be able to sum images for slice numbers, magnify images if needed, and adjust intensity.

- Annotate (type of slices, direction, dose, hospital, etc.).
- Usually one page each for transverse, sagittal, and coronal slices.
- May want one page (e.g., four on one) for positive study of frame or frames best depicting affected area.
- Display three-dimensional by choosing cine or three-dimensional cine or similar for physicians. Select three-dimensional data set. Select create cine data. Adjust intensity, speed, and color (usually gray).

Cardiac SPECT

- Because of the orientation of the heart within the body, names of slices are unique. Most systems have dedicated software for heart processing that allows the stress and rest or stress and redistribution data sets of the patient to be processed in the same session. A correlation of general to cardiac SPECT planes is as follows:
    - Transverse (transaxial) = horizontal long axis (slices: superior to inferior; image, left is septal wall, top is apex, right is lateral wall).
    - Sagittal = vertical long axis (slices: right side of heart to left; image, top is anterior wall, right is apex, bottom is inferior wall).
    - Coronal = short axis (slices: apex to base; image, top is anterior wall, right is lateral wall, bottom is inferior wall, left is septal wall).
- Software differs greatly but, again, certain things must be accomplished. Many have auto-SPECT programs and most have instructions on screen.
- Select cardiac SPECT processing, select patient, select raw data group(s).
- For each set, select working color, intensity, orientation, and parameters for processing.
- Adjust filter(s) and set line(s) for masking (to remove background), slice thickness, and magnification.
- Proceed, complete, or save and exit, etc.
- Bull's eye images may also be processed from data.

To Display Images

- Refer to cardiologist's preferences.
- Select image display type (full-page three-axes stress/rest slices, single-page single-axis stress/rest slices), select patient, select appropriate data set(s).
- Align stress/rest images, adjust intensities, annotate.
- Film up slices and bull's eye as well if requested. Some software supplies an ejection fraction program. Physician may want to view cine of gated study for wall motion.

Artifacts

- "Star" artifact: caused by overlap of projections, removed by ramp filter.
- Concentric rings indicate nonuniform flood source.
- Image blurring indicates camera not leveled.
- Mottled image indicates insufficient count density.
- "Starburst" effect indicates injection site in slice.
- Arm shadows indicates attenuation from extremities, patient not positioned correctly.
- Blurring indicates wrong COR.

- Loss of resolution indicates improper use of filters.
- Ring around the edge indicates little or no attenuation correction because of uniformity problems.

SUGGESTED READINGS

Datz FL. Handbook of Nuclear Medicine. 2nd ed. St. Louis: Mosby, 1993.

Early PJ, Sodee DB. Principles and Practice of Nuclear Medicine. 2nd ed. St. Louis: Mosby, 1995.

Murray IPC, Ell PJ, eds. Nuclear Medicine in Clinical Diagnosis and Treatment. Vols. 1 and 2. New York: Churchill Livingstone, 1994.

Wilson, MA. Textbook of Nuclear Medicine. Philadelphia: Lippincott-Raven, 1998.

Notes

CHAPTER 46

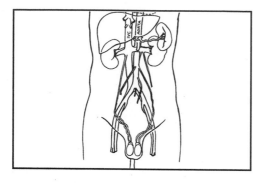

Testicular Scan

Radiopharmacy

Radionuclide

- ^{99m}Tc $t_{1/2}$: 6 hours

  Energies: 140 keV

  Type: IT, γ, generator

Radiopharmaceutical

- Na ^{99m}TcO$_4^-$ (pertechnetate)

Localization

- Compartmental to blood supply

Quality Control

- Moly-Al breakthrough, chromatography > 90%

Adult Dose Range

- 8–20 mCi (296–740 MBq)

Method of Administration

- IV injection, good bolus for flow

Indications

- Evaluation of groin pain.
- Evaluation of patency of blood supply to testes.
- Evaluation of increased perfusion caused by inflammatory disease.
- Differentiation between torsion (twisting and lack of blood supply to one or both testes), acute epididymitis (infection or trauma to epididymis or scrotum), and orchitis (infection of testes).
- Evaluation of scrotal mass.

Contraindications

- None

Patient History

The patient should answer the following questions.

Do you have a history or family history
   of cancer?   Y   N

If so, what type and for how long?

Are you in pain now?   Y   N

How long since pain started?

Where exactly is the pain?

What was the activity at the onset of pain
   (e.g., fighting, lifting, exercising, walking,
   sexual calisthenics)?

Do you have a history of this type of pain?   Y   N

Have you had any recent trauma to that
   region?   Y   N

Have you had any prostate problems?   Y   N

Other department-specific questions.

Patient Preparation

- Identify the patient. Verify doctor's order. Explain the procedure.
- Instruct the patient to empty bladder if possible.
- Use discretion as patient is usually experiencing some degree of pain; modesty will
  be compromised.

Equipment

Camera

- Small field of view (FOV) is best; if large FOV, use magnification

Collimator

- Low energy, high sensitivity, or low energy, all purpose (flow) and low energy, high resolution (statics); pinhole for pediatric statics

Computer Set-up

Flow

- 2–6 sec/frame for 1 minute

Statics

- Collect 500,000–700,000 counts at immediate, 5, 10, 15, 20, 25, and 30 minutes as per protocol. Magnification, 1.5 to 2 times.

Procedure *(time: ~30 minutes)*

- Place patient in supine position on table, legs abducted or frogleg.
- Secure penis to abdomen (or chest in some cases) with tape.
- Position towel or tape sling under testicles for support while imaging.
- Drape privacy cloth after set-up. Ensure tape cannot stick to legs, scrotum, or penis.
- Insure testes are separated.
- Position camera anterior, as close as possible, with scrotum centered in FOV.
- Position lead shielding over thighs and abdomen or under scrotum to reduce background vascularity.
- Inject and wait a few seconds to start flow study.
- Image immediate blood pool, then statics every 5 minutes for 30 minutes or as per protocol.
- Optional imaging includes right and left anterior obliques, magnified views, and placement of a thin marker on raphe of scrotum in one static.

Normal Results

- Flow: medial border of iliac artery is smooth.
- No significant activity is seen in area of testicular, deferential, or pudendal artery.
- Scrotal perfusion, if present, is seen only as poorly marginated, minimally intense area of activity.
- Tissue phase: scrotum and contents with homogeneous activity.

Abnormal Results

- Torsion
  - Flow (perfusion) scan will be missing perfusion to affected side. Tissue phase

(statics) will show photopenic area with activity less than opposite testicle and less than that of thigh. Increased activity may be seen high in cord.

- Infarcted tissue: Flow (perfusion) scan will show increased blood flow through pudendal vessels. Tissue phase will have halo sign on affected side.

- Spontaneous detorsion: Flow and tissue phase will have increased perfusion.

- Epididymitis (acute): Flow and tissue phase will show increased activity.

- Orchitis: Similar but more medial testicular involvement.

- Trauma: Diffuse increase with decreased areas (hematoma, hematocele, hydrocele).

- Tumor: Diffuse increase with decreased areas.

- Vascular tumor: Increased flow, increased tissue phase.

Artifacts

- Lead shielding can be used to block out background vascularity from torso and legs.

- Testicles not separated for imaging.

- Sticky side of tape on scrotum or penis.

- $^{99m}TcO_4^-$ in a filled bladder could interfere with interpretation.

- Patient movement will blur images.

- Female or previously castrated patients make visualization a long and tedious process.

SUGGESTED READINGS

Datz FL. Handbook of Nuclear Medicine. 2nd ed. St. Louis: Mosby, 1993.

Early PJ, Sodee DB. Principles and Practice of Nuclear Medicine. 2nd ed. St. Louis: Mosby, 1995.

Murray IPC, Ell PJ, eds. Nuclear Medicine in Clinical Diagnosis and Treatment. Vols. 1 and 2. New York: Churchill Livingstone, 1994.

Wilson, MA. Textbook of Nuclear Medicine. Philadelphia: Lippincott-Raven, 1998.

Notes

CHAPTER 47

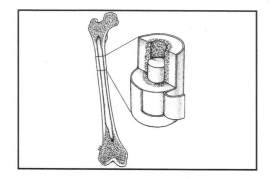

Therapy: Bone Pain

(Palliation)

Radiopharmacy

Radionuclide

- ^{89}Sr $t_{1/2}$: 50.5 days

    Energies: 1463 keV (max), 583.3 keV (mean)

    Type: β^-, fission product

- ^{153}Sm $t_{1/2}$: 46.7 hours

    Energies: β^- 632, 702, 805 keV (max), 198, 224, 263 keV (mean), γ 103 keV

    Type: β^-, γ, fission product (neutron irradiation of ^{152}Sm)

Radiopharmaceutical

- ^{89}Sr-chloride

- ^{153}Sm-lexidronam (ethylenediamine-tetramethylene phosphonate [EDTMP])

Localization

- ^{89}Sr: Uptake of strontium at sites of osteoblastic skeletal metastases remaining in the same concentration for 100 days after injection. Metastron® (^{89}Sr-chloride) behaves like calcium analogs, preferentially localizing in areas of active osteogenesis.

- ^{153}Sm: Phosphonate compounds concentrate in bone mineral. Metallic ions are chelated with phosphonate complexes, with the resulting compound used to deliver metallic radioactive ions to bone mineral turnover in association with hydroxyapatite. Quadramet® (^{153}Sm-lexidronam) accumulates in osteoblastic lesions at a 5:1 ratio compared with normal bone.

Quality Control

- Radiochemical purity must be $\geq$ 90%

Adult Dose Range

- ^{89}Sr: 4 mCi (148 MBq) or 40–60 µCi (1.48–2.22 MBq) per kg

- ^{153}Sm: 1 mCi (37MBq) per kg

Method of Administration

- It is suggested that the syringe be shielded with a lead syringe shield rather than plastic even though Sr-89 is a pure β-emitter.

- Existing IV catheter or 21-gauge butterfly.

- Three-way stopcock.

- Ten milliliters of flush or more. It is suggested to flush the radiopharmaceutical syringe several times to ensure the entire dose is administered.

- Performed by authorized user: nuclear physician, radiologist, or ordering physician.

Indications

- Palliation of intractable bone pain for patients with two or more osseous metastases (osteoblastic metastatic bone lesions) documented by bone scan from primary cancer. Candidates should have multiple bone metastases sites, bone pain, white blood cell (WBC) count of > 2400, and a platelet count of $> 60,000$. Other candidates are those who have failed hormonal therapy for prostate cancer management.

- Assessment of painful bone metastases for the use of palliation in conjunction with, or instead of, radiotherapy.

Contraindications

- Patients with no bone pain, multiple sites of metastases, WBC counts of < 2400, platelet counts of $< 60,000$, or doing well with other methods of pain palliation.

- A solitary metastatic site.

- Patients with evidence of seriously compromised bone marrow from previous therapy or disease infiltration.

- Quadramet®: patients who have a known hypersensitivity to EDTMP or similar phosphonate compounds.

- *No* contraindications are indicated for the following:

  - Previous heavy external beam irradiation.

  - Previous failure of ^{89}Sr therapy.

  - Anemia; can be corrected by infusion.

  - Conventional methods of pain palliation (e.g., analgesics, nonsteroidal anti-inflammatory drugs, hormonal therapy, and radiotherapy) that have not yet been used or are being used and have not yet failed.

Patient History

The patient should answer the following questions.

Do you have a history or family history of cancer?   Y   N

If so, what type and for how long?

When was your last chemotherapy?

_____

When was your last radiotherapy?

_____

Are you on any other type of therapy for pain?   Y   N

_____

Have you had a recent chest radiograph?   Y   N

_____

When was your last bone scan?

_____

Do you have a copy of the images or results
   with you?   Y   N

_____

Do you have recent laboratory results with
   you (hemoglobin, WBC [> 2,500], platelets
   [> 60,000])?   Y   N

_____

Do you have bone pain at present?   Y   N

   If so, where and for how long?

_____

Do you have the results of any related
   examinations with you?   Y   N

_____

Are you taking any pain medication?   Y   N

   Please list.

_____

Have you received and read your
   information sheet?   Y   N

_____

Other department-specific questions.

_____

Patient Preparation

- Identify the patient. Verify doctor's order. Explain the procedure.
- Ensure patient has and reads package insert information.
- Obtain a signed, informed consent from patient.
- Patient to bring results of latest laboratory tests.
- Patient to bring images and results of latest bone scan (within the last 6 weeks).

- Instruct patients with incontinence as to toilet instructions and if necessary, catheterize 2 days before injection.
- Instruct patient to ingest 500 mL of fluid before injection and to void often before and after injection.

Equipment

Camera

- Large field of view

Collimator

- Low energy, all purpose, or low energy, high resolution

Computer Set-up

- ^{153}Sm; peak for 103 keV, 20% window

Statics

- 500,000–750,000 counts

Whole Body

- 10 cm/min, head to toe

Procedure *(time: injection, 20 minutes; images, ~30–50 minutes)*

- Place patient in supine position on table or sitting upright in chair.
- The following is in preparation for the injection:
  - Place a butterfly needle in (preferably) the antecubital fossa, secure with tape, or use indwelling catheter.
  - Attach a three-way stopcock to the line.
  - Attach a syringe containing 10 mL (or more) of saline to the straight port.
  - Ensure that the needle is properly in the vein by withdrawing and reinjecting small amounts of blood; the blood should flow freely.
  - Cover area with absorbent material in case of spill or leak.
- The injection is performed by an authorized user (e.g., nuclear physician):
  - Attach the syringe containing the radiopharmaceutical to the side port.
  - Turn the stopcock to connect the radiopharmaceutical syringe to the patient and inject the radiopharmaceutical for 30–60 seconds.
  - Turn the stopcock to connect the saline syringe to the patient and flush the radiopharmaceutical syringe three times to ensure the entire dose has been injected into the patient.
  - Observe injection site for extravasation; apply warm compresses to area if detected to encourage venous and lymphatic absorption.
  - The IV catheter (once removed), the saline syringe, tubing, and radiopharmaceutical syringe can be counted before proper disposal to ensure that there is not an abundance of residue.
- Samarium-153: Optional imaging:
  - Obtain whole-body scan or statics of areas of bone pain at 3–48 hours after

injection, if desired, to confirm success of skeletal uptake and lesion affinity. These have been shown to be very comparable to routine bone imaging agents.

- Compare results with most recent bone scan.

Normal Results

- Decreased bone pain lasting 10–16 weeks or more.
- Increased quality of life.
- Patients can be treated again as early as 10 weeks if symptoms reappear.

Abnormal Results

- No change or short-term change in pain levels or deteriorating conditions.
- Platelet count should be monitored as 80% of patients experience a 20–30% decrease by 6 weeks.

The Role of the Nuclear Medicine Technologist in Therapy

- Order and receive the radiopharmaceutical from the radiopharmacy into the department.
- Properly prepare patient and paperwork for physician and therapy.
- Some institutions have other personnel to start IV catheter. If not, the nuclear medicine technologist must start and test the IV catheter and tubing for patency.
- Provide a sterile area and proper equipment for the injection.
- Calibrate the therapy dose and confirm the amount of activity with the injecting physician.
- Record the time, dose, patient, doctor, and any pertinent information about the therapy.

Artifacts

- Nonpatent IV site leading to leakage or extravasation of radiopharmaceutical and hence less than or no therapeutic amount delivered to patient.
- Myelosuppression (bone marrow toxicity) is one of the major concerns with therapy, and the patient should be monitored for any signs during this and other types of therapy.

Note

The carcinomas that account for most of the metastatic bone disease are breast, prostate, bronchial, renal, lung, and thyroid. Research is presently under way to develop therapeutic administrations to use in conjunction with pain palliation. Typical strategies include nonnarcotic analgesics, narcotic analgesics, nonsteroidal anti-inflammatory drugs, hormone therapy, chemotherapy, local-field external beam radiotherapy, and wide-field external beam radiotherapy. Although palliation has been the intention of using these agents, there is serious attention now being paid to the use of these agents as tumor-controlling therapeutic drugs.

Other bone palliation agents include the following:

^{32}P-orthophosphate; t$_{1/2}$ 14.3 days, 1.710 MeV (max), 0.695 MeV (mean).

^{186}Re-etidronate (hydroxyethylidene diphosphonate [HEDP]), chelate; t$_{1/2}$ 3.8 days, 1.077 MeV (max), 0.362 MeV (mean), γ, 137 keV.

^{188}Re-phosphonate, chelate; t$_{1/2}$ 16.98 hours, 2.120 MeV (max), 0.795 MeV (mean), γ, 155 keV.

^{131}I-diphosphonate; t$_{1/2}$ 8.0 days, 0.606 MeV (max), 0.191 MeV (mean), γ, 365 keV.

^{90}Y-citrate; t$_{1/2}$ 2.7 days, 2.284 MeV (max), 0.935 MeV (mean).

^{117m}Sn-chelate; t$_{1/2}$ 13.6 days, isomeric transition, γ, 159 keV.

SUGGESTED READINGS

Early PJ, Sodee DB. Principles and Practice of Nuclear Medicine. 2nd ed. St. Louis: Mosby, 1995.

Klingensmith W, Eshima D, Goddard J. Nuclear Medicine Procedure Manual 1997–98. Englewood, CO: Wick, 1998.

Murray IPC, Ell PJ, eds. Nuclear Medicine in Clinical Diagnosis and Treatment. Vols. 1 and 2. New York: Churchill Livingstone, 1994.

Wilson, MA. Textbook of Nuclear Medicine. Philadelphia: Lippincott-Raven, 1998.

Metastron® is a registered trademark of Amersham International Plc, Amersham, UK.
Quadramet® is a registered trademark of Cytogen Corporation, Princeton, NJ.

Notes

CHAPTER 48

. . . .

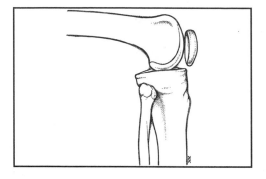

Therapy: Intra-articular (Joint); Synovectomy

Radiopharmacy

Radionuclide

- ^{32}P $t_{1/2}$: 14.26 days

  Energies: 1710 keV (max), 694.9 keV (mean)

  Type: β^-, fission product

- ^{99m}Tc $t_{1/2}$: 6 hours

  Energies: 140 keV

  Type: IT, γ, generator

Radiopharmaceutical

- ^{32}P-chromic phosphate as a colloid, 0.6–2.0 μm
- ^{99m}Tc-sulfur colloid (SC)

Localization

- Compartmental to synovial cavity

Quality Control

- ^{32}P-chromic phosphate: > 95% radiochemical purity
- ^{99m}Tc-SC: > 92% radiochemical purity

Adult Dose Range (weight based)

- ^{32}P-chromic phosphate:
  - 10–25 kg: knee, 0.500 mCi (18.5 MBq); elbow/ankle, 0.250 mCi (9.25 MBq)
  - 25–40 kg: knee, 0.750 mCi (27.75 MBq); elbow/ankle, 0.375 mCi (13.875 MBq)
  - > 40 kg: knee, 1.000 mCi (37.0 MBq); elbow/ankle, 0.500 mCi (18.5 MBq)
- ^{99m}Tc-SC: 1 mCi (37 MBq)

Method of Administration
- Injection through needle placement into a joint (synovial) cavity.

Indications

- Palliation of joint pain caused by rheumatoid arthritis.
- Palliation of joint pain caused by hemophilic arthropathy (hemorrhage into synovial space because of hemophilia).
- Palliation of joint pain caused by villonodular synovitis (nodular projections of the synovial membrane into the synovial cavity).

Contraindications

- None

Patient History

The patient should answer the following questions.

Do you have a history or family history of cancer?	Y	N
If so, what type and for how long?		
Do you have a history of rheumatoid arthritis?	Y	N
Do you have a history of joint disease?	Y	N
Are you experiencing pain at present?	Y	N
Do you have the results of recent laboratory tests and recent x-ray films with you?	Y	N

What other means of therapy are currently or recently under way (e.g., aspirin, nonsteroidal anti-inflammatory agents, steroids, remission-inducing agents [gold or D-penicillamine], intra-articular corticosteroid injections, osmic acid, alkylating agents [thiotepa-T])?

Have you had any recent operations?	Y	N

Other department-specific questions.

Patient Preparation

- Identify the patient. Verify doctor's order. Explain the procedure.
- The written directive must be signed by an authorized user.
- Obtain a signed consent from the patient.
- Patients with hemophilia are usually given factor VIII before therapy (50 U/kg) and at 24 and 72 hours after therapy (20 U/kg). This is also required in known cases of factor IX deficiency.
- Patient must bring laboratory results and recent x-ray films of area of interest.

Equipment

Camera

- Large field of view

Collimator

- Low energy, all purpose, or low energy, high resolution

Computer Set-up

- ^{99m}Tc-SC: 140 keV, 20% window
  Statics: 250,000 counts or 180-second images

Procedure *(with optional ^{99m}Tc-SC imaging; time: injection, ~30 minutes; imaging, ~15 min/session)*

- Place patient in supine position on table or in a suitable position for proper placement of injection needle.
- Procedure is performed by authorized user (physician) under fluoroscopy guidance.
  - Wipe area to be injected with povidone-iodine solution (Betadine®).
  - Anesthetize the skin in area to be injected using 1% lidocaine.
  - Enter the synovial (joint) space with needle. For the knee, the needle is placed beneath the lateral side of the patella.
  - Connect tubing and three-way stopcock to the needle.
  - Attach a 50-mL syringe to the stopcock and aspirate the synovial fluid. Optional: instill iothalamate (Conray®) through needle to ensure needle is in the joint space using fluoroscopy.
  - Attach the syringe containing the ^{32}P-chromic phosphate, or, optionally, ^{99m}Tc-SC if imaging is desired, to the stopcock.
  - Optional: inject 1 mCi (37MBq) ^{99m}Tc-SC into synovial space for imaging. (This ensures therapeutic agent will not loculate, but disperse throughout joint space.) Obtain static images: anterior, posterior, and laterals both before therapy dose and after therapy dose.

- Inject the ^{32}P-chromic phosphate and (optionally) any remaining ^{99m}Tc-SC. Again optional: image area again to ensure thorough dispersal within the joint.
- Flex the joint to ensure thorough distribution of therapy dose. Optional: image area of interest as before.
- Attach the syringe containing 1% lidocaine and dexamethasone.
- Inject 3–5 mL of 1% lidocaine/dexamethasone along the needle track while withdrawing the needle from the joint to prevent inflammation and leakage of the therapy dose.
- Immobilize joint in a protective splint for 2 days (helps to minimize leakage into lymphatics and blood vessels).
- Optional:
  - At 24 and 72 hours and optionally at 7 days, patient may be counted by Geiger-Müller (GM) counter to assess nodal uptake of therapeutic colloid in draining lymphatic nodes and liver.
  - Imaging using bremsstrahlung radiation from ^{32}P can be performed to document distribution within the synovial cavity. Use a high-energy collimator and energy window of 150–450 keV.
  - Blood and urine samples may be obtained every few hours after injection and counted for radioactivity to document presence or absence of leakage.

Normal Results

- Reduction of pain associated with the affected joint.
- Reduction of inflammation within the affected joint.
- Reduction of degradation of cartilage and bone within the affected joint.
- Improvement of function of the affected joint.
- With the use of ^{99m}Tc-SC imaging, joint space presents as thoroughly and evenly perfused with radiotracer.

Abnormal Results

- Little or no palliative effect felt in affected joint.
- Images may have clumping or subspaces with more activity than others (inhomogeneous mixture within the synovial cavity).

The Role of the Nuclear Medicine Technologist in Therapy

- Order and receive the radiopharmaceutical from the radiopharmacy into the department.
- Properly prepare patient and paperwork for physician and therapy.
- Provide a sterile area and proper equipment for the injection.
- Be prepared to take pretherapy dose images of area of interest if that avenue is being pursued.
- Calibrate the therapy dose and confirm the amount of activity with the injecting physician. Pure beta emitters do not dose calibrate well. Low-energy bremsstrahlung

radiation can be used to assay the dose. The radiopharmacist can be contacted for verification.

- Record the time, dose, patient, doctor, and any pertinent information about the therapy.

- Be prepared to take posttherapy dose images of area of interest if that avenue is being pursued.

Artifacts

- Extravasation of therapy dose or misplacement of needle will, depending on extent, negatively affect the usefulness of the therapy.

- Do not use as IV injection. Radiotherapy colloid will localize in liver. The preparation should be a cloudy, brownish-green colloidal suspension, not the clear ^{32}P solution used for IV injection for polycythemia vera.

Note

Other radiopharmaceuticals used in synovectomy include the following:

^{165}Dy-FHMA (ferric hydroxide macroaggregates): $t_{1/2}$, 2.3 hours; energies, 1285, 1190 keV (max), 453, 414 keV (mean).

^{90}Y-calcium oxalate or FHMA: $t_{1/2}$, 64.1 hours; energies, 2284 keV (max), 935 keV (mean).

^{198}Au: $t_{1/2}$, 2.7 days; energies, 961 keV (max), 315 keV (mean), 412 keV.

SUGGESTED READINGS

Early PJ, Sodee DB. Principles and Practice of Nuclear Medicine. 2nd ed. St. Louis: Mosby, 1995.

Klingensmith W, Eshima D, Goddard J. Nuclear Medicine Procedure Manual 1997–98. Englewood, CO: Wick, 1998.

Murray IPC, Ell PJ, eds. Nuclear Medicine in Clinical Diagnosis and Treatment. Vols. 1 and 2. New York: Churchill Livingstone, 1994.

Wilson, MA. Textbook of Nuclear Medicine. Philadelphia: Lippincott-Raven, 1998.

Betadine® is a registered trademark of Purdue Fredrick Co., Norwalk, CT.
Conray® is a registered trademark of Mallinckrodt Medical, Inc., St. Louis, MO.

Notes

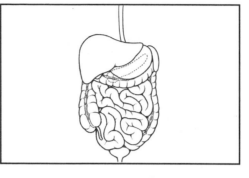

Therapy: Intracavitary

(Serosal)

Radiopharmacy

Radionuclide

- ^{32}P t$_{1/2}$: 14.26 days

    Energies: 1710 keV (max), 694.9 keV (mean)

    Type: β^+, fission product

- ^{99m}Tc t$_{1/2}$: 6 hours

    Energies: 140 keV

    Type: IT, γ, generator

Radiopharmaceutical

- ^{32}P-chromic phosphate as a colloid, 0.1–0.3 μm in size
- ^{99m}Tc-sulfur colloid (SC)

Localization

- Compartmental to serosal cavity. Macrophages consume colloid particles and become fixed on serosal compartment lining. Confined to lining, beta emitters deliver ablation energy to serosal and lymphatic deposits. Some reach the local lymph nodes and are deposited there.

Quality Control

- ^{32}P-chromic phosphate: > 95% radiochemical purity
- ^{99m}Tc-SC: > 92% radiochemical purity

Adult Dose Range

- ^{99m}Tc-SC: 2–3 mCi (74–111 MBq)
- ^{32}P-chromic phosphate:
    - Pleura: 10–15 mCi (370–555 MBq)

- Pericardium: 5–10 mCi (185–370 MBq)
- Peritoneum: 15–20 mCi (555–740 MBq)

Method of Administration

- IV catheter into cavity of concern. This may be a patent access left from surgical treatments or a new installation.

Indications

- Palliation by reduction of recurrent effusions in serosal cavities (e.g., peritoneal, pericardial, and pleural) secondary to malignant disease, especially those not successfully treated with sclerosing agents such as tetracycline.
- Prevention of recurrence of malignant disease on serosal surfaces.
- Treatment of cystic neoplasms.
- Treatment of malignant ascites (especially ovarian source).
- Treatment, in limited role, of ovarian cancer. Patients with stage I or II ovarian carcinoma are treated with 15 mCi (555 MBq) of ^{32}P-chromic phosphate colloid premixed with 250 mL of normal saline.

Contraindications

- Patients with intraperitoneal infection.
- Patients with longer than 6 months' life expectancy.
- Detection of the presence of loculated fluid (through the use of ^{99m}Tc-SC).

Patient History

The patient should answer the following questions.

**Do you have a history or family history
of cancer?**   **Y**   **N**

If so, what type and for how long?

Are you presently experiencing pain?   **Y**   **N**

If so, where and for how long?

Do you feel you have fluid build-up?	Y	N

If so, where and for how long?

_____

Do you have the results of any other related examinations?   Y   N
_____

Do you have the results of any recent laboratory tests?   Y   N
_____

Have you had any other therapy?   Y   N

If so, what type and when?

_____

Other department-specific questions.
_____

Patient Preparation

- Identify the patient. Verify doctor's order. Explain the procedure.
- The written directive must be signed by an authorized user.
- Obtain a signed consent from the patient.
- Patients receiving intrapleural administration must have a thoracentesis to remove the effusion.

Equipment

Camera

- Large field of view

Collimator

- Low energy, all purpose, or low energy, high resolution

Computer Set-up

- ^{99m}Tc-SC: 140 keV, 20% window

Statics

- 250,000 counts or 180-second images

Procedure *(with optional ^{99m}Tc-SC imaging; time: injection, ~30 minutes; imaging, ~15 min/session)*

- Place patient in supine position on table or in a suitable position for proper placement of injection needle.
- Injection:
  - Using aseptic technique and 1% lidocaine to anesthetize the skin, place the intracatheter into the cavity and secure with tape. (Ultrasound imaging may be helpful in documenting the location of ascites.)
  - Attach a connecting tube to the intracatheter.
  - Attach a three-way stopcock to the connecting tube.
  - Attach the second connecting tube to the three-way stopcock.
  - Attach the collecting bag to the free end of the connecting tube.
  - Attach the 50-mL syringe to the stopcock and withdraw the bulk of the fluid, but not all of it.
  - Document free flow of injected fluid within the cavity by injecting iodinated contrast material and obtaining a radiograph or by injecting ^{99m}Tc-SC or ^{99m}Tc-macroaggregated albumin (MAA) and acquiring a gamma camera image.
    - Attach the syringe containing the ^{99m}Tc-SC, if imaging is desired, to the stopcock.
    - Optional: inject 1 mCi (37MBq) ^{99m}Tc-SC into serosal cavity for imaging. (This ensures therapeutic agent will not loculate, but disperse throughout serosal cavity.) Obtain static images: anterior, posterior, and laterals both before and after therapy dose.
    - Some attach up to 500-mL (for peritoneum) bag of saline to tubing leading into cavity.
    - Inject the ^{32}P-chromic phosphate (into saline bag if used) and (optionally) any remaining ^{99m}Tc-SC. Again optional: Image area again to ensure thorough dispersal within the cavity.
- Peritoneum or pleural cavity: have the patient roll from side to side and lie prone to ensure adequate distribution of the radiotherapy throughout the cavity. Heart motion ensures adequate distribution in the pericardial cavity.
- Confirmation that fluid will disperse can be obtained by injecting a water-soluble radiopaque agent and taking a KUB (kidneys, ureter, and bladder x-ray).
- Optional: image peritoneum or pleural cavity using bremsstrahlung radiation from ^{32}P to confirm dispersal. Use a high-energy collimator and energy window of 150–450 keV.
- Cystic volume measurement in brain neoplasms can be obtained with computed tomography (CT).
- After injection, patient is repositioned repeatedly in first hour, then several times each hour for the next 24 hours.

Normal Results

- Palliation of the pain caused by excess fluid within affected cavity. Maximum effect occurs at 3 months. Dose may need repeating.
- Temporary therapeutic treatment (remission) of cancer causing the production of excess fluid within the affected cavity.

- With the use of ^{99m}Tc-SC imaging, serosal cavity presents as thoroughly and evenly perfused with radiotracer.

Abnormal Results

- Little or no palliative relief of pain or cancer causing the production of excess fluid within the affected cavity.

- Images may have clumping or subspaces with more activity than others (inhomogeneous mixture within the serosal cavity).

The Role of the Nuclear Medicine Technologist in Therapy

- Order and receive the radiopharmaceutical from the radiopharmacy into the department.

- Properly prepare patient and paperwork for physician and therapy.

- Provide a sterile area and proper equipment for the injection.

- Calibrate the therapy dose and confirm the amount of activity with the injecting physician. Pure beta emitters do not dose calibrate well. Low-energy bremsstrahlung radiation can be used to assay the dose. The radiopharmacist can be contacted for verification.

- Record the time, dose, patient, doctor, and any pertinent information about the therapy.

- Be prepared to take posttherapy dose images of area of interest if that avenue is being pursued.

Artifacts

- Do not use as IV injection. Radiotherapy colloid will localize in liver. The preparation should be a cloudy, brownish-green colloidal suspension, not the clear ^{32}P solution used for IV injection for polycythemia vera.

- Any leakage from the therapy site must be treated as a radioactive spill and cleaned in accordance with precautions pertaining to beta emitters.

Note

Tumors in the peritoneal or pleural cavity cause serosal irritation, resulting in excess cavity transudate. This excess fluid can be a source of extreme discomfort to the patient. The beta emitter ^{32}P-chromic phosphate is used as a palliative treatment, irradiating the surfaces of cavity and reducing the amount of fluid production. Macrophages within the system engulf the colloid particles and settle on the surfaces. Little systemic colloid absorption occurs.

SUGGESTED READINGS

Early PJ, Sodee DB. Principles and Practice of Nuclear Medicine. 2nd ed. St. Louis: Mosby, 1995.

Klingensmith W, Eshima D, Goddard J. Nuclear Medicine Procedure Manual 1997–98. Englewood, CO: Wick, 1998.

Murray IPC, Ell PJ, eds. Nuclear Medicine in Clinical Diagnosis and Treatment. Vols. 1 and 2. New York: Churchill Livingstone, 1994.

Wilson, MA. Textbook of Nuclear Medicine. Philadelphia: Lippincott-Raven, 1998.

Notes

. . . .

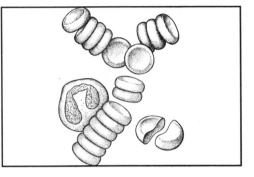

CHAPTER 50

Therapy: Polycythemia Vera

Radiopharmacy

Radionuclide

- ^{32}P $t_{1/2}$: 14.26 days

  Energies: 1710 keV (max), 694.9 keV (mean)

  Type: β^-, fission product

Radiopharmaceutical

- ^{32}P-sodium phosphate (clear, injectable solution)

Localization

- Approximately 85% of administered dose metabolically localizes in bone tissue (bone marrow and trabecular bone) because of its high inorganic phosphorous content. Incorporates into DNA with subsequent damage from beta particles and decays to ^{32}S, altering nucleic acid structure.

Quality Control

- No other radiochemical forms are present. Administered dose must be within 10% of requested dose.

Adult Dose Range

- 2.3 mCi (85.1 MBq) per square meter body surface.

- 3–5 mCi (111–185 MBq), dosage not to exceed 7 mCi (259 MBq) during any 6-month period.

- If no response within 3 months, repeat dose at 25% of original dose.

- If no response in subsequent 3 months, repeat dose at 25% of previous dose (dose not to exceed 7 mCi [259 MBq]).

Method of Administration
- IV injection through butterfly or indwelling catheter with a 10-mL saline flush.

Indications

- Palliation of erythrocytosis not controllable by phlebotomy alone.
- Treatment of thrombocytosis with platelet counts approaching 1 million.
- Treatment of extramedullary hematopoiesis with painful spleen, hypersplenism, abdominal pain, or splenic infarct.
- Palliation of pruritus or hyperuricemia not controlled by phlebotomy, allopurinol, or antihistamines.
- Treatment of cardiovascular problems contraindicating frequent phlebotomies.
- Treatment of patients with a risk of thrombosis.
- Treatment is reserved for the elderly ($>$ 75 years old) to minimize concerns of possible subsequent development of acute leukemia.
- Treatment of patients who cannot tolerate or be relied on to take hydroxyurea according to instructions.

Contraindications

- Treatment should not be used if
    - platelet count is $<$ 15,000.
    - reticulocyte count is $<$ 0.2%.
    - white blood cell count is $<$ 3,000.

Patient History

The patient should answer the following questions.

Do you have a history or family history of cancer?	**Y**	**N**
If so, what type and for how long?		
Do you have documentation of a bone disorder?	**Y**	**N**
Do you have the results of any related examinations?	**Y**	**N**
Do you have the results of recent laboratory tests?	**Y**	**N**

Have you received any recent therapy?   Y   N

If so, what type and when?

_____

Other department-specific questions.

_____

Patient Preparation

- Identify the patient. Verify doctor's order. Explain the procedure.
- The written directive must be signed by an authorized user.
- Obtain a signed consent from the patient.

Equipment

Camera
- N/A

Collimator
- N/A

Computer Set-up
- N/A

Procedure (time: ~20 minutes)

- Place patient in supine position on table or sitting upright in chair.
- The following is in preparation for the injection:
  - Place a butterfly needle in (preferably) the antecubital fossa and secure with tape, or use indwelling catheter.
  - Attach a three-way stopcock to the line.
  - Attach a syringe containing 10 mL (or more) of saline to the straight port.
  - Ensure that the needle is properly in the vein by withdrawing and reinjecting small amounts of blood; the blood should flow freely.
  - Cover area with absorbent material in case of spill or leak.
- The injection is performed by an authorized user (e.g., nuclear physician):
  - Attach the syringe containing the radiopharmaceutical to the side port.
  - Turn the stopcock to connect the radiopharmaceutical syringe to the patient and inject the radiopharmaceutical for 30–60 seconds.
  - Turn the stopcock to connect the saline syringe to the patient and flush the radiopharmaceutical syringe three times to ensure the entire dose has been injected into the patient.
  - Observe injection site for extravasation; apply warm compresses to area if detected to encourage venous and lymphatic absorption.

- The IV catheter (once removed), the saline syringe, tubing, and radiopharmaceutical syringe can be counted before proper disposal to ensure that there is not an abundance of residue.
- Extravasation can be checked with a Geiger-Müller counter moving up the arm. The count rate should remain pretty much the same all the way.

Normal Results

- Patient's blood chemistry returns to normal levels within 4–6 weeks. It may stay in remission for 2 years or more.

Abnormal Results

- No reduction of production of red blood cells even after repeated doses of the therapy.

The Role of the Nuclear Medicine Technologist in Therapy

- Order and receive the radiopharmaceutical from the radiopharmacy into the department.
- Properly prepare patient and paperwork for physician and therapy.
- Some institutions have other personnel to start IV catheter. If not, the nuclear medicine technologist must start and test the IV catheter and tubing for patency.
- Provide a sterile area and proper equipment for the injection.
- Calibrate the therapy dose and confirm the amount of activity with the injecting physician. Pure beta emitters do not dose calibrate well. Low-energy bremsstrahlung radiation can be used to assay the dose. The radiopharmacist can be contacted for verification.
- Record the time, dose, patient, doctor, and any pertinent information about the therapy.

Artifacts

- Extravasation of the therapy dose may cause collateral tissue damage and lessen the desired therapeutic affect. This can occur up to 2 weeks after injection.
- 10–20% of ^{32}P patients contracted acute leukemia as opposed to 1% with phlebotomy alone.
- Median survival of patients treated with ^{32}P is 10–16 years, 7–8 years with phlebotomy only, and 1.5 years without any therapy.
- Myelofibrosis with myeloid metaplasia occurs in 10–20% of polycythemia patients and is considered a natural outcome, unrelated to therapy.

Note

Other treatment plans include phlebotomy and chemotherapy with chlorambucil.

Polycythemia rubra vera is a chronic hematologic disease characterized by increased proliferative activity of erythroid, myeloid, megakaryocytic, and fibroblastic cells. The early phase often progresses to the myelofibrosis phase with myeloid metaplasia (spent phase). This entails anemia, a leukoerythroblastic blood condition, and hepatosplenomegaly. This evolves into an accelerated malignant phase closely resembling acute myeloblastic leukemia.

SUGGESTED READINGS

Early PJ, Sodee DB. Principles and Practice of Nuclear Medicine. 2nd ed. St. Louis: Mosby, 1995.

Klingensmith W, Eshima D, Goddard J. Nuclear Medicine Procedure Manual 1997–98. Englewood, CO: Wick, 1998.

Murray IPC, Ell PJ, eds. Nuclear Medicine in Clinical Diagnosis and Treatment. Vols. 1 and 2. New York: Churchill Livingstone, 1994.

Wilson, MA. Textbook of Nuclear Medicine. Philadelphia: Lippincott-Raven, 1998.

Notes

CHAPTER 51

· · · · · · · ·

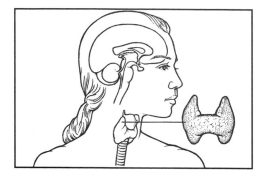

Thyroid: Ablation

Radiopharmacy

Radionuclide

- ^{131}I $t_{1/2}$: 8.1 days

  Energies: 364 keV (γ), 606 keV (β^-)

  Type: β^-, γ, fission product

Radiopharmaceutical

- ^{131}I as sodium iodide capsule or liquid

Localization

- Active transport. Organified by thyroid and held in cells or follicular lumen. T_e = 3-5 days.

Quality Control

- Dose calibrate capsule or vial to confirm amount of radioactivity

Adult Dose Range

- 30-300 mCi (1,110-11,100 MBq)

Method of Administration

- PO, usually with radiation safety officer (RSO), nuclear physician, or resident nuclear physicist present

Indications

- Ablation of residual functioning thyroid carcinoma.
- Ablation of residual functioning normal thyroid tissue after total or partial thyroidectomy.

Contraindications

- Pregnancy or nursing.
- Allergy to iodine.
- Iodinated studies under way or done recently.
- Patient taking thyroid medications or vitamins, or not on low-iodine diet.
- Patient extremely likely to regurgitate dose.

Patient History

The patient should answer the following questions.

Do you have a history of adenocarcinoma?	Y	N
Do you have a history or family history of any cancer?	Y	N
If so, what type and for how long?		
Have you recently had thyroid surgery?	Y	N
Do you feel that there is a possibility of nausea or vomiting?	Y	N
Do you have the results of recent laboratory tests?	Y	N
Have you had any recent iodinated radiographic studies?	Y	N
Are you presently taking any thyroid medications?	Y	N
Do you have any questions about the stay in the hospital, procedure, or possible side effects?		
Female patients:		
Are you pregnant or nursing?	Y	N

When was your last menstrual period?

Have you experienced amenorrhea
(suppression of menstruation)?   Y   N

Other department-specific questions.

Patient Preparation

- Identify the patient. Verify doctor's order. Explain the procedure.
- Low-iodine diet 1 week before therapy.
- Patient should discontinue thyroid medication for 2–4 weeks before therapy.
- No iodinated radiographic studies 3 weeks before therapy.
- Female patients cannot be pregnant or nursing nor should they have plans to be until the therapy and follow-up studies are completed.
- Additional preparation is considerable with this therapy. Examples are given below.

Equipment

Camera
- N/A

Collimator
- N/A

Computer Set-up
- N/A

Procedure *(time: dosing, ~15 minutes; hospital stay, ~3–5 days)*

- Obtain initial room clearance from hospital admitting (see Note).
- Prepare patient's room (see Note).
- In-service the nurses involved with that patient (see Note).
- Admit patient into room.
- Explain therapy and answer all questions (see Note).
- Obtain signed consent from patient and signature in log book.
- Calibrate dose and bring to room (see Note).
- Remove family and friends from patient's room.
- Administer Reglan® to patient as anti-vomitus if deemed necessary.
- Obtain the written directive (prescription) from physician.
- Administer dose to patient quickly (in the presence of RSO or physician). Watch for signs of vomiting.
- Obtain an initial assay of patient, room, doorway, adjoining wall, record results.
- Monitor and record assays of patient and room b.i.d. until readings fall below limits

(usually 5–7 mR at 1 m from patient's chest and/or < 30 mCi remaining in body. As of 1998, the Nuclear Regulatory Commission has made changes to the rules for handling ^{131}I about the need for patient hospitalization and release. Not all of the agreement states have instituted these changes. (Check the hospital protocol). Have patient void before taking the reading.

- Release patient when appropriate, clean and assay room for residual contamination (see Note).

Normal Results

- Residual thyroid tissue and thyroid carcinoma tissue ablated. Patient is treated with thyroid medication.
- No naturally occurring elevated levels of thyroid hormones.
- No residual thyroid tissue or carcinoma is found on follow-up whole-body scan.
- Upon reevaluation, patient is naturally hypothyroid, but with medication, can be adjusted to proper levels of hormones.

Abnormal Results

- On reevaluation, elevated levels of thyroid hormones in laboratory tests.
- Whole-body scan reveals areas of uptake in neck and/or thorax, perhaps other places as well, suggesting insufficient ablation, metastasis, or recurrence.

Artifacts

- Patient may vomit dose immediately or some time soon after dosing. Prepare for that type of radioactive spill (gloves, absorbent cloths, some type of containment).
- Distances from patient must be consistent when recording readings.
- Patient must force hydration and empty bladder often.

Note

Scheduling patient: Something similar to the following must occur to admit the patient into the hospital for the therapy.

- Get a signed prescription from the authorized user along with written order from physician.
- Call ordering physician to confirm order.
- Call the chief radiologist to confirm dose ordered.
- Call admitting office and/or floor to confirm room availability (usually a corner room).
- Call patient to confirm date and time for dosing.
- Confirm that patient has completed all laboratory and other tests before being admitted to the hospital or before dosing.
- Call pharmacy to order dose.
- Call ordering doctor's office to have them confirm admitting orders by calling admitting office.
- Prepare the room (next section).

Room preparation: Some form of the following is needed for room preparation.

- Bring radiation signs, therapy patient log book, dosimeter(s), tape measure, several packs of "chucks," masking tape, 3 mL of stable iodine, two waste containers double lined with signs for linen and trash, small and large plastic bags.
- Use small plastic bags to cover phone and call button or other small items likely to be held and used, e.g., TV controller.
- Cover floor by bed, bathroom floor, back of toilet bowl, table tops, the chair of use. If the patient is incontinent or unstable, it is not out of the question to cover the floor and walls with chucks and plastic.
- Place chucks on bed under sheets.
- Wrap pillows in plastic bag under pillow case.
- Squirt 3 mL of stable iodine into toilet and sink (this takes up possible iodine sites).
- Store plenty of linen in room.
- Mark a tape line on the floor behind which visitors must remain (usually 10 feet from where patient will usually be).
- Some hospitals supply a cooler stocked with patient's choice of soft drinks and juices.
- Set a small table outside room for charting dosimeter and Geiger counter readings.

Nursing in-service: Check specific hospital rules for nursing status.

- No pregnant nurses.
- These patients are not sick unless they are already inpatients for something else, hence no daily care or vital signs are needed. They will be there for about 3 days on average.
- No housekeeping personnel are permitted.
- Explain dosimeter, how to read, and how to log with each visit.
- Explain time, distance, and shielding for radiation safety.
- Explain what the ^{131}I does to the patient and that 95% of the dose will be excreted in bodily fluids and urine.
- Always glove up and discard just before leaving room.
- Chart all orders, medications, and visual assessments. Document each visit.
- Nurse is usually allowed 2 mR/day, or about 1 min/visit at 3 feet.
- Make sure patient remains completely hydrated and encourage using the bathroom frequently.
- Food trays should contain only disposable utensils, all must stay in room.
- Everything must remain in the room, either placed in the waste cans or flushed (three times) down the toilet.
- Try to do whatever needs to be done quickly, then leave and chart.
- Any problems, call nuclear medicine department, the RSO, or a nuclear physician.

Patient explanation:

- Most institutions have forms explaining their specific protocols for the therapy.
- Patient may experience a dry mouth or soreness in the salivary glands and throat.
- Patient may experience nausea and vomiting and neck swelling and pain. These symptoms should be reported immediately and are treatable.

- Whatever the patient brings into the room must remain in the room until checked out by Geiger counter after patient leaves. If articles are found to be "hot," they must remain in storage until decayed to background.
- Once dosed, the patient is restricted to the room until released.
- Stay hydrated and use the facilities often. Flush three times after each use.
- After eating, rinse out milk and juice containers before throwing into waste cans, rinse off disposable plates and utensils. Flush sink or toilet well after each use. Nothing leaves the room.
- Report any sickness immediately.
- Visitors may only stay for 20 minutes per day and at a distance of (usually) 10 feet or at the door.
- No pregnant visitors or those younger than 18 years old.
- Have patient sign the informed consent and allow for any questions.
- Call the RSO or physician, get the dose.

Dosing Patient: Bring these items:

- Dose calibrate the dose, replace into lead container; therapy log book; Geiger counter; dosimeter(s); tape measure; masking tape and signs; cup for water if capsule; straw and 12-mL or more syringe for water to rinse vial if liquid; gloves and booties; absorbent cloths for possible accident; stable iodine for toilet and sink; dose of Reglan® (anti-vomitus) if required.
- With RSO or physician present and signed consent, administer dose to patient as quickly as possible. Watch for any signs of regurgitation. Take initial readings of patient, 1 m, 2 m, doorway, adjacent walls (follow hospital protocols). Make sure signs are posted. Inform nursing staff that patient is dosed.

Room decontamination:

- When readings at 1 m from patient fall < 5 mR/hr, the patient may be discharged with the blessing of the RSO or physician.
- Nothing is to leave the room except the patient (hopefully in a new set of clothes brought for that purpose).
- Glove up; put booties on.
- With a Geiger counter, survey the room and its contents. Articles in drawers, phone, buttons, books, linen, chairs, tables, closet, bed, etc. Anything that registers > 5 mR/hr at 1 m must be stored for decay.
- All chucks must be surveyed and disposed of properly and according to activity.
- The bathroom must be surveyed and scrubbed until levels are < 5 mR/hr at 1 m.
- Check the sink and plumbing below for activity; it may have to be dismantled and stored.
- Check the waste cans for activity and store or discard.
- Mark for storage and decay any containers and bags that remain contaminated.
- Mark separate bag(s) for personal items left by patient that need storage.
- When room is below levels of contamination, let the floor know that the room is ready and that housekeeping can go in.
- Call admitting to let them know the room is now available.

Most of the destruction is caused by the 606 keV of the β^- particles causing ionization and chromosomal damage. Cells cannot replicate. Delay in effect is caused by remaining thyroid tissue that is still functional, although not replicating, until natural cell death. Built-up hormone produced from before therapy must be metabolized.

Some physicians, for postsurgery and posttherapy follow-up, opt for a regular thyroid uptake and scan, prescribe < 30 mCi therapy if something is found, then follow laboratory results before they attempt an ablation. Some say this sensitizes the remaining tissue, which becomes more resistant, making it more difficult to eradicate.

SUGGESTED READINGS

Datz FL. Handbook of Nuclear Medicine. 2nd ed. St. Louis: Mosby, 1993.

Early PJ, Sodee DB. Principles and Practice of Nuclear Medicine. 2nd ed. St. Louis: Mosby, 1995.

Murray IPC, Ell PJ, eds. Nuclear Medicine in Clinical Diagnosis and Treatment. Vols. 1 and 2. New York: Churchill Livingstone, 1994.

Wilson, MA. Textbook of Nuclear Medicine. Philadelphia: Lippincott-Raven, 1998.

Reglan® is a registered trademark of AH Robbins Company, Richmond, VA.

Notes
. . . .

Patient Information for > 30 mCi Thyroid Therapy

1. You are not here because you are sick. The nursing staff will not be coming in to take daily vital signs like blood pressure and temperature.

2. This room is to keep you isolated during your therapy. Please confine yourself to the room.

3. The usual stay is about 3 days depending on how much of the iodine is excreted as measured by a Geiger counter.

4. No visitors under the age of 18 or pregnant persons are allowed.

5. Visiting time permitted is no more than 20 minutes per visitor per day. The time increases slightly as the days progress.

6. Visitors must remain at the doorway (at least 10 feet from patient).

7. Iodine is released from the body in perspiration as well as waste so everything brought into the room and touched stays in the room. The clothes you wear and possessions handled will be bagged and stored for 3 months. Games and other items can be wrapped in plastic before being handled, then released once checked by the Geiger counter.

8. You will be given disposable plates and utensils. These must be stored for 3 months, then opened and surveyed with the Geiger counter. Please thoroughly rinse off dishes; rinse out cans and milk cartons before placing them in the storage bag.

9. Flush what you do not finish down the toilet (except for larger items like chicken bones, etc.). If you do not touch a meal at all, it can be surveyed and removed from the room.

10. When using the toilet, be careful not to contaminate the surrounding area, and, when done, flush three times to ensure dilution within the plumbing system. Wash hands often.

11. Questions: call the nuclear medicine department.

CHAPTER 52

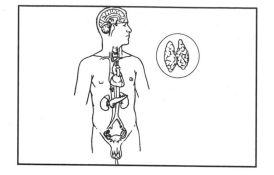

Thyroid: Ectopic Tissue Scan

(Substernal)

Radiopharmacy

Radionuclide

- ^{131}I $t_{1/2}$: 8.1 days

  Energies: 364 keV (γ), 606 keV(β^-)

  Type: β^-, γ, fission product

- or ^{123}I $t_{1/2}$: 13.1 hours

  Energies: 159 keV

  Type: EC, γ, accelerator

- or ^{99m}Tc $t_{1/2}$: 6 hours

  Energies: 140 keV

  Type: IT, γ, generator

Radiopharmaceutical

- ^{123}I and ^{131}I: sodium iodide as capsules

- $^{99m}TcO_4^-$: (pertechnetate)

Localization

- Active transport

- ^{131}I and ^{123}I organified by thyroid and held in cells or follicular lumen. T_e = 3-5 days.

- $^{99m}TcO_4^-$ trapped but not organified.

Quality Control

- ^{99m}Tc: chromatography, moly and Al breakthrough

- ^{123}I and ^{131}I: dose calibrate capsules to confirm amount of radioactivity

Adult Dose Range

- ^{131}I: 10–100 uCi (0.37–03.7 MBq)
- ^{123}I: 200–400 uCi (7.4–14.8 MBq)
- $^{99m}TcO_4^-$: 10–20 mCi (370–740 MBq)

Method of Administration

- ^{131}I, ^{123}I: capsules PO
- $^{99m}TcO_4^-$: IV

Indications

- Detection and localization of substernal and other ectopic thyroid tissue.
- Differentiation of anterior mediastinal mass from substernal thyroid tissue.
- Evaluation of suspected autonomously functional ectopic thyroid tissue in hyperthyroidism.
- Evaluation of normally positioned thyroid gland.
- Evaluation of ectopic thyroid tissue in hypothyroidism.

Contraindications

- Allergy to iodine if that is being used.
- Patient still taking thyroid medication.
- Contrast studies under way.

Patient History

The patient should answer the following questions.

Do you have a history or family history
   of cancer?   Y   N

  If so, what type and for how long?

Why does the physician suspect ectopic tissue?

Do you have a history of thyroid disease?   Y   N

Are you presently taking any iodine-containing
   medications, thyroid hormones, or
   antithyroid drugs?   Y   N

Have you had any surgery?   Y   N

   If so, what type and when?

_____

Do you have difficulty swallowing?   Y   N

_____

Do you have any swelling or tenderness
   in the neck?   Y   N

_____

Have you had any recent weight loss or gain?   Y   N

_____

Have you had any recent change in your
   appetite?   Y   N

_____

Have you recently experienced fevers?   Y   N

_____

Have you had any recent change in your
   overall energy levels?   Y   N

_____

Have you had any thyroid therapy,
   chemotherapy, or radiation therapy?   Y   N

_____

How does cold or heat affect you?

_____

Are you taking vitamins?   Y   N

_____

Have you had any tests using iodine or
   radiographic contrast?   Y   N

_____

Have you had (or do you have planned) any
   recent related US, CT, x-ray, or nuclear
   medicine examinations?   Y   N

_____

Do you have any recent laboratory work
   results?   Y   N

_____

Are you pregnant or nursing?   Y   N

_____

Other department-specific questions.

_____

Patient Preparation

- Identify the patient. Verify doctor's order. Explain the procedure.
- Obtain a prescription signed by physician for iodine studies.

Equipment

Camera

- Large field of view

Collimator

- High energy, parallel hole for ^{131}I
- Low energy, high resolution, or low energy, all purpose, and pinhole for ^{99m}Tc and ^{123}I

Computer Set-up

- ^{131}I: 30% window at 364 keV
- ^{123}I: 20% window at 159 keV
- ^{99m}Tc: 20% window at 140 keV

Statics

- ^{131}I: 10-minute images (600 seconds)
- ^{123}I, $^{99m}TcO_4^-$: 50,000–100,000 counts

Procedure *(time: ~45–60 minutes)*

^{131}I

- Images taken at 24 hours after ingestion.
- Place patient in supine position, chin hyperextended (very important when looking for ectopic tissue), camera anterior.
- Obtain all images, taking one with and one without markers.
- Obtain anterior view, centered over thyroid, markers on chin, thyroid cartilage, and suprasternal notch (SSN).
- Position camera centered over thorax, markers on SSN and xiphoid process.
- Position camera over lower abdomen. If ectopic tissue is suspected in ovaries (struma ovarii), markers on xiphoid, umbilicus, and pubic symphysis.

^{123}I Capsule

- Images taken at 4–6 hours after ingestion.
- Same procedure as above. Be sure camera is peaked for radiotracer.
- Counts or time to get good images (10 minutes or 50,000–100,000 counts).

$^{99m}TcO_4^-$

- Images taken at 15–30 minutes after injection

- Administer injection to patient; give patient; water (some use lemon water to decrease uptake in salivary glands).
- Place patient in supine position with pillow under shoulders and chin up (Water's position).
- Utilizing LEHR collimator, obtain images (300 seconds or 100,000 counts) with and without markers as above.
- Optional study: Any of these can be performed in conjunction with a routine thyroid uptake and scan.

Normal Results

- Increased activity within normal thyroid gland tissue around the trachea between the thyroid cartilage and the SSN.
- Some have left lobe smaller than right lobe or a pyramidal lobe.

Abnormal Results

- Increased activity higher or lower on the trachea, usually separated from the normal thyroid gland tissue (not to be confused with salivary gland uptake if $^{99m}TcO_4^-$ is being used).
- Increased activity beneath and shining through the sternum.
- Increased activity around one or both ovaries is not unlikely in cases of struma ovarii.
- The thyroid gland embryonically migrates from the base of the tongue caudally into the neck. Remnants are possible anywhere along this path (usually hypofunctioning lingual thyroid tissue at the midline base of the tongue, thyroglossal duct cyst superior to thyroid and slightly off midline, and, occasionally, further caudally beneath sternum to the diaphragm and perhaps the abdomen).

Artifacts

- ^{123}I and $^{99m}TcO_4^-$ will allow imaging although they are easily attenuated by the sternum.
- $^{99m}TcO_4^-$ lingers in many places, making visualization of ectopic tissue an uncertainty or obscured by uptake in other systems.
- ^{131}I is the best for substernal, although there is the consideration of β^- and 364 keV gamma radiation to the tissue.

SUGGESTED READINGS

Datz FL. Handbook of Nuclear Medicine. 2nd ed. St. Louis: Mosby, 1993.

Early PJ, Sodee DB. Principles and Practice of Nuclear Medicine. 2nd ed. St. Louis: Mosby, 1995.

Murray IPC, Ell PJ, eds. Nuclear Medicine in Clinical Diagnosis and Treatment. Vols. 1 and 2. New York: Churchill Livingstone, 1994.

Wilson, MA. Textbook of Nuclear Medicine. Philadelphia: Lippincott-Raven, 1998.

Notes
. . . .

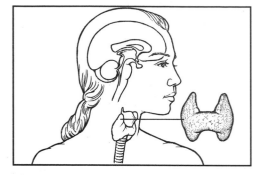

Thyroid: Hyperthyroid Therapy

(< 30 mCi)

Radiopharmacy

Radionuclide

- ^{131}I $t_{1/2}$: 8.1 days

  Energies: 364 keV (γ), 606 keV(β^-)

  Type: β^-, γ, fission product

Radiopharmaceutical

- ^{131}I as sodium iodide capsule or liquid

Localization

- Active transport. Organified by thyroid and held in cells or follicular lumen.
  T_e = 3-5 days.

Quality Control

- Dose calibrate capsule or vial to confirm amount of radioactivity

Adult Dose Range

- 1 to < 30 mCi (37 to < 1110 MBq). Diffuse goiter (Graves' disease) 5-10 mCi,
  nodular (Plummer's disease) usually 10-29 mCi. All < 30 mCi according to patient
  gland size and to avoid Nuclear Regulatory Commission mandatory hospitalization
  for doses > 30 mCi.

Method of Administration

- PO administered by physician

Indications

- Detection of hyperthyroidism.
- Evaluation for treatment of Graves' disease (thyrotoxicosis, diffuse toxic goiter).
- Detection and localization of toxic (multiple) nodular goiter.
- Evaluation for Plummer's disease (true autonomous toxic nodular goiter).
- Detection and localization of toxic nodule (toxic adenoma).

Contraindications

- Pregnancy.
- Allergy to iodine.

Patient History

The patient should answer the following questions.

Do you have a history or family history of cancer? Y N

If so, what type and for how long?

Have you had any of the following (Graves' disease): exophthalmos, lid lag, goiter, fine tremor in extremities, tachycardia, high metabolism, vomiting, diarrhea, nervousness, anxiety, perspiration, hot feeling, brittle thinning hair, heat intolerance, weight loss, pretibial myxedema (swelling of legs), acropachy (clubbing of fingers and toes)? Y N

What medications are you currently taking?

Are you taking any thyroid medications? Y N

If not, how long have you been off them?

What were the results of your nuclear medicine uptake and scan?		
Have you had any previous treatments?	Y	N
Do you have the results of any recent laboratory tests (elevated thyroid function tests)?	Y	N
Female patients:		
Are you pregnant or nursing?	Y	N
When was your last menstrual period?		
Have you experienced amenorrhea (suppression of menstruation)?	Y	N
Other department-specific questions.		

Patient Preparation

Before Ingestion

- Identify the patient. Verify doctor's order. Explain the procedure.
- Physician to instruct patient to discontinue all thyroid medication for at least 2 days.
- Ensure there has been no iodinated radiographic studies for 3 weeks before test.
- Instruct patient to consume no food or vitamins containing large amounts of iodine.

After Ingestion

- Instruct patient not to have close contact with anyone for 48 hours after ingestion.
- Instruct the patient not to share food or utensils.
- Instruct the patient to flush toilet twice (some suggest 3 mL of normal iodine into toilet to take up possible iodine sites).
- Instruct the patient to wash clothes and linen thoroughly.
- Inform the patient that they may feel a scratchy throat.
- Inform the patient that there is no immediate benefit, it is a week or more to feel effect.
- Instruct the patient to contact department immediately if dose is vomited.

Equipment

Camera

- N/A

Collimator

- N/A

Computer Set-up

- N/A

Procedure *(time: ~20 minutes)*

- Ensure procedure is preceded by uptake and scan procedures within 2 weeks.
- Calibrate the dose (the amount is decided by ordering physician and ordered through pharmacy).
- Obtain a signed informed consent (some have a booklet to read) from patient.
- Obtain a prescription prepared and signed by physician.
- Obtain a signature from physician on requisition and appropriate paperwork.
- Ensure that the physician explains benefits and disadvantages.
- Provide a glass of water to the patient.
- Ensure that the dose is administered by physician (or technologist in presence of physician).
- Inform the patient that they will be reevaluated in 2–3 months.
- Instruct the patient to exit the department (immediately, after making sure patient does not vomit dose).

Normal Results

- Goiter shrinks and symptoms decrease with earliest effect 2–6 weeks after ingestion.
- Patient becomes euthyroid after 2–6 months (follow-up laboratory tests and/or uptake and scan to confirm).

Abnormal Results

- In 3 months to a year, patient does not become euthyroid as confirmed by follow-up tests; retreatment may be ordered.
- Hypothyroidism that must be rectified by thyroid medications.
- Possible errors:
  - Make sure patient has signed form for treatment.
  - Patient may be reluctant to inform of loss of dose.
  - Paperwork a must for Nuclear Regulatory Commission regulations for radioiodine.

Artifacts

- Patient regurgitates dose shortly after dosing.

- Patient does not discontinue thyroid medications.

Note

Most of the destruction is caused by the 606 keV (89%) of the β^- particles causing ionization and chromosomal damage. Cells cannot replicate. Delay in effect is caused by remaining thyroid tissue that is still functional until cell death although not replicating. Built-up hormone produced before therapy must be metabolized.

Graves' disease (exophthalmic goiter): autoimmune disease usually of middle age and women. Antibodies attach to thyroid-stimulating hormone (TSH) receptors of thyroid cells, causing glandular hypertrophy and increased production of thyroid hormone (T_4 and T_3). Toxic diffuse goiter, elevated T_3 and T_4, and low TSH produces LATS (long-acting thyroid stimulator, an autoantibody). Signs of Graves' disease are caused by excessive deposits of mucopolysaccharides.

Toxic nodular goiter: higher doses used as there is little uptake in nodules. Estimation of gland size is difficult because of irregularity and retrotracheal and substernal extensions. Relapse occurs more frequently with this disease.

Plummer's disease: toxic nodular goiter, solitary or multiple autonomous nodules, elevated T_3 and T_4, low TSH, no LATS, normal suppressed gland receives little radiation.

SUGGESTED READINGS

Datz FL. Handbook of Nuclear Medicine. 2nd ed. St. Louis: Mosby, 1993.

Early PJ, Sodee DB. Principles and Practice of Nuclear Medicine. 2nd ed. St. Louis: Mosby, 1995.

Murray IPC, Ell PJ, eds. Nuclear Medicine in Clinical Diagnosis and Treatment. Vols. 1 and 2. New York: Churchill Livingstone, 1994.

Wilson, MA. Textbook of Nuclear Medicine. Philadelphia: Lippincott-Raven, 1998.

Notes

Patient Information for (< 30 mCi) Hyperthyroid Therapy

1. For at least 2 days, keep a distance of 3 feet or more between you and any persons.

2. Do not hug or hold children close for 2 days.

3. Do not share utensils at home with anyone. Wash the ones you use thoroughly.

4. Keep your clothes and linen separate and wash them thoroughly. The iodine exits your body over time by bowel movements, urine, saliva, and perspiration.

5. Sleep alone for the first 2 nights.

6. When using the toilet, be careful not to contaminate the surrounding area, and, when done, flush two times to ensure dilution within the plumbing system. Wash hands often.

7. You may feel a scratchy throat within a few days but that will subside.

8. It may take a couple of weeks to feel any benefit related to your condition from the capsules.

9. If you get sick and throw up the capsule(s), try to do so in a toilet, sink, or, at last resort, on the pavement. Call the nuclear medicine department so that they will know you no longer have the capsule(s) inside you. This is extremely rare and is usually caused by food or sickness unrelated to the iodine capsules.

10. Although any allergic reaction to the iodine capsules is extremely rare, if you feel you are having one, contact your doctor's office.

11. You have taken a capsule that contains radioactive iodine that emits beta and gamma rays. It is designed to do its therapeutic work on your thyroid and does not present a danger to anyone. These steps are taken only to reduce unnecessary exposure to people with whom you may come in contact.

12. Questions: call the nuclear medicine department.

CHAPTER 54

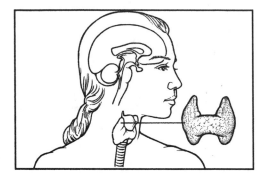

Thyroid Scan

Radiopharmacy

Radionuclide

- ^{123}I $t_{\frac{1}{2}}$: 13.1 hours

  Energies: 159 keV

  Type: EC, γ, accelerator

- or ^{131}I $t_{\frac{1}{2}}$: 8.1 days

  Energies: 364 (γ), 606 keV (β^-) keV

  Type: β^-, γ, fission product

- or ^{99m}Tc $t_{\frac{1}{2}}$: 6 hours

  Energies: 140 keV

  Type: IT, γ, generator

Radiopharmaceutical

- ^{123}I and ^{131}I as capsules

- $^{99m}TcO_4^-$ (pertechnetate)

Localization

- Active transport. $^{99m}TcO_4^-$ trapped but not organified. Iodine organified by thyroid and held in cells or follicular lumen. T_e = 3–5 days.

Quality Control

- ^{99m}Tc: chromatography, moly and Al breakthrough

- ^{123}I and ^{131}I: dose calibrate capsules to confirm amount of radioactivity

Adult Dose Range

- ^{131}I: 1–10 μCi (0.037–0.37 MBq)

- ^{123}I: 100–300 μCi (3.7–11.1 MBq)

- $^{99m}TcO_4^-$: 2–10 mCi (74–370 MBq)

Method of Administration

- ^{123}I and ^{131}I capsule PO
- ^{99m}Tc by IV injection

Indications

- The test is usually performed in conjunction with the thyroid uptake test.
- Detection and evaluation of hyperthyroidism and hypothyroidism.
- Detection and localization of metastases from thyroid cancer.
- Differentiation of benign from malignant nodules.
- Detection, localization, and evaluation of independent functioning nodule(s).
- Evaluation of heterogeneity of function within a hyperthyroid gland.
- Detection and localization of benign ectopic thyroid tissue.

Contraindications

- Allergy to iodine if that is being used.
- Patient has not discontinued thyroid medication.

Patient History *(or use complete patient history in reference section)*

The patient should answer the following questions.

Do you have a history or family history of cancer?	Y	N
If so, what type and for how long?		
Do you have a history of thyroid disease?	Y	N
Are you presently taking any iodine-containing medications, thyroid hormones, or antithyroid drugs?	Y	N
Have you had any surgery?	Y	N
If so, what type and when?		

Do you have difficulty swallowing?	Y	N
Do you have any swelling or tenderness in the neck?	Y	N
Have you had any recent weight loss or gain?	Y	N
Have you had any recent change in your appetite?	Y	N
Have you recently experienced fevers?	Y	N
Have you had any recent change in your overall energy levels?	Y	N
Have you had any thyroid therapy, chemotherapy, or radiation therapy?	Y	N
How does cold or heat affect you?		
Are you taking vitamins?	Y	N
Have you had any tests using iodine or radiographic contrast?	Y	N
Have you had (or do you have planned) any recent related US, CT, x-ray, or nuclear medicine examinations?	Y	N
Do you have any recent laboratory work results?	Y	N
Are you pregnant or nursing?	Y	N
Other department-specific questions.		

Patient Preparation

- Identify the patient. Verify doctor's order. Explain the procedure.
- Patient to discontinue thyroid medications and avoid contrast material, Betadine®, or amiodarone.

- Refrain from eating foods containing iodine such as cabbage, turnips, greens, seafood, kelp, or large amounts of table salt.
- ^{123}I: Patient will be returning at 4–6 hours and 24 hours for scan.

Equipment

Camera

- Large field of view

Collimator

- Low energy, high resolution, or low energy, all purpose and pinhole for ^{99m}Tc and ^{123}I

- High energy, parallel hole for ^{131}I

Computer Set-up

- ^{131}I: 30% window at 364 keV
- ^{123}I: 20% window at 159 keV
- ^{99m}Tc: 20% window at 140 keV; 50,000–100,000 counts

Procedure *(usually two parts; time: ~40 minutes)*

$^{99m}TcO_4{}^-$

- Administer injection to patient; wait 15–20 minutes before imaging. Give patient water (optional lemon to clear salivary glands).

- Place patient in supine position with pillow under shoulders and chin up (Water's position).

- Using the LEHR collimator, obtain anterior views (300 seconds or 100,000 depending on protocol) with and without markers as per protocol (thyroid cartilage and suprasternal, marker strip, right side, etc). RAO and LAO and perhaps a "pull-back" image (more distant) for ectopic thyroid tissue are optional images if a pinhole collimator is not available.

- Using a pinhole collimator if available, obtain anterior views with and without markers as per protocol, then RAO and LAO and perhaps a "pull-back" image (more distant) for ectopic thyroid tissue.

^{123}I Capsule

- Same procedure as above without injection. Be sure camera is peaked for radiotracer.

^{131}I Capsule

- Same procedure as above without injection. Usually used to locate residual and recurrent cancers. 24-, 48-, and 72-hour pictures may be the most useful. Collect 100,000 counts over thyroid and whole body if cancer is suspected. Check peak and collimator(s).

Normal Results

- Euthyroid: homogeneous uptake of radiotracer.
- Left lobe smaller than right lobe or having pyramidal lobe.
- Straight or convex outer margins.
- Uptake equal to or greater than that of salivary glands (water or lemon given to reduce salivary uptake).

Abnormal Results

- Plummer's disease: autonomous multinodular goiter; nodules, solitary or multiple: cold or hot (solitary: adenoma, thyroiditis; multiple: goiter).
- Nonvisualization of thyroid gland caused by, e.g., subacute thyroiditis.
- Graves' disease: enlarged gland, high uptake (LATS [long-acting thyroid stimulator, an autoantibody]).
- Hashimoto's thyroiditis: enlarged gland, mottled (checkerboard) areas.
- Thyroid carcinoma: usually solitary cold nodule (4% show high uptake).

Artifacts

- Compton scatter and downscatter from contaminates may contribute to ^{123}I spectrum.
- ^{99m}TcO$_4^-$ not as accurate because of low absolute uptake, high neck background, changing biodistribution, concentrations in extrathyroid tissues, and trapping without organification.
- High collar metal buttons or medallions may interfere with pictures.
- Improper collimator and computer changes.
- Careless marker placement.
- Patient movement (particularly with pinhole collimator).

Note

Definitions

T$_3$ = triiodothyronine = Cytomel® (most metabolically active).

T$_4$ = thyroxine (highest concentration in blood).

TSH = thyrotropin, anterior pituitary hormone stimulates thyroid to release T$_3$ and T$_4$.

TRH = thyrotropin-releasing hormone from hypothalamus, stimulates release of TSH from anterior pituitary.

Calcitonin = from the C cells or parafollicular cells; regulates calcium or bone building.

Parathormone = parathyroid hormone; breaks down calcium in bone (resorption).

Hypothyroidism

Hypothyroidism may be the result of iodine deficiency (large, endemic goiter), inherited enzyme deficiency, postradioiodine ablation (iatrogenic), end-stage toxic goiter, metastatic cancer, chronic thyroiditis, iodine excess, or pituitary or hypothalamic injury. Hypothyroidism is characterized by myxedema (end-stage hypothyroidism, puffy face, fluid retention, and lethargy) or cretinism in infants (lethargy, pot belly, enlarged tongue, stunted growth, and mental retardation). Hashimoto's thyroiditis is characterized by inflammation, chronic lymphocytic thyroiditis, lymphoid goiter, and struma lymphomatosa; autoimmune thyroiditis is diffuse lymphocytic infiltration.

Hyperthyroidism

Plummer's disease (toxic nodular goiter) is characterized by solitary or multiple autonomous nodules (goiter), elevated T_3 and T_4, low TSH, and no LATS. Graves' disease (exophthalmos, pretibial myxedema, and acropachy) results in hyperthyroidism, thyrotoxicosis, toxic diffuse goiter, elevated T_3 and T_4, and low TSH, and produces LATS. Subacute thyroiditis is the absence of uptake illustrating shutdown of the thyroidal iodine extraction and hormonal synthesis pathway. Patient presents sporadically with (among other things) sore neck, difficulty in swallowing, fever, dehydration, and slightly elevated white blood cell count. Serum thyroid hormone levels may present as normal or elevated to the point of hyperthyroidism or even "thyroid storm."

SUGGESTED READINGS

Datz FL. Handbook of Nuclear Medicine. 2nd ed. St. Louis: Mosby, 1993.

Early PJ, Sodee DB. Principles and Practice of Nuclear Medicine. 2nd ed. St. Louis: Mosby, 1995.

Murray IPC, Ell PJ, eds. Nuclear Medicine in Clinical Diagnosis and Treatment. Vols. 1 and 2. New York: Churchill Livingstone, 1994.

Wilson, MA. Textbook of Nuclear Medicine. Philadelphia: Lippincott-Raven, 1998.

Betadine® is a registered trademark of Purdue Fredrick Co., Norwalk, CT.
Cytomel® is a registered trademark of SmithKline Beecham Pharmaceuticals, Philadelphia, PA.

Notes

CHAPTER 55

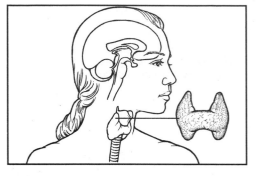

Thyroid Uptake

(usually in conjunction with thyroid scan)

Radiopharmacy

Radionuclide

- ^{123}I $t_{1/2}$: 13.1 hours

  Energies: 159 keV

  Type: EC, γ, accelerator

- or ^{131}I $t_{1/2}$: 8.1 days

  Energies: 364 (γ), 606 keV (β^-) keV

  Type: β^-, γ, fission product

- or ^{99m}Tc $t_{1/2}$: 6 hours

  Energies: 140 keV

  Type: IT, γ, generator

Radiopharmaceutical

- ^{123}I and ^{131}I as capsules

- $^{99m}TcO_4^-$ (pertechnetate)

Localization

- Active transport. $^{99m}TcO_4^-$ trapped but not organified. Iodine organified by thyroid and held in cells or follicular lumen. T_e = 3–5 days.

Quality Control

- ^{99m}Tc: chromatography, moly and Al breakthrough

- ^{123}I and ^{131}I: dose calibrate capsules to confirm amount of radioactivity

Adult Dose Range

- ^{131}I: 1–10 μCi (0.037–0.37 MBq)

- ^{123}I: 100–300 μCi (3.7–11.1 MBq)

- $^{99m}TcO_4^-$: 2–10 mCi (74–370 MBq)

Method of Administration

- ^{123}I and ^{131}I capsule PO
- ^{99m}Tc by IV injection

Indications

- The test is usually performed in conjunction with the thyroid scan.
- Evaluation of thyroidal radioactive iodine uptake (RAIU). This provides an index of thyroid trapping and organification of iodide measured as a percentage of radiotracer actively transported into thyroid tissue during a period of time. It is dependent on thyroid function and the body's iodine pool.
- Evaluation of hyperthyroidism and hypothyroidism.
- Detection and localization of metastases from thyroid cancer.
- Differentiation of benign from malignant nodules.
- Detection, localization, and evaluation of independent functioning nodule(s).
- Evaluation of heterogeneity of function within a hyperthyroid gland.
- Detection and localization of benign ectopic thyroid tissue.

Contraindications

- Allergy to iodine if that is being used.
- Patient has not discontinued thyroid medication or other interfering medications.
- Patient discontinued thyroid medication too long.

Patient History *(or use complete patient history in reference section)*

The patient should answer the following questions.

Do you have a history or family history of cancer?   Y   N

If so, what type and for how long?

Do you have a history of thyroid disease?   Y   N

Are you presently taking any iodine-containing medications, thyroid hormones, antithyroid drugs, or antiarrhythmics?   Y   N

Have you had any surgery?   Y   N

If so, what type and when?

_____

Do you have difficulty swallowing?	Y	N
Do you have any swelling or tenderness in the neck?	Y	N
Have you had any recent weight loss or gain?	Y	N
Have you had any recent change in your appetite?	Y	N
Have you recently experienced fevers?	Y	N
Have you had any recent change in your overall energy levels?	Y	N
Have you had any thyroid therapy, chemotherapy, or radiation therapy?	Y	N

How does cold or heat affect you?

Are you taking vitamins?	Y	N
Do you have a list of all medications presently being taken?	Y	N
Have you had any tests using iodine or radiographic contrast?	Y	N
Have you had (or do you have planned) any recent related US, CT, x-ray, or nuclear medicine examinations?	Y	N
Do you have any recent laboratory work results?	Y	N
Are you pregnant or nursing?	Y	N

Other department-specific questions.

_____

Patient Preparation

- Identify the patient. Verify doctor's order. Explain the procedure.
- Physician to instruct patient to discontinue thyroid medications, contrast material, Betadine®, or amiodarone (antiarrhythmics).
- Instruct patient to refrain from eating iodine-containing foods such as cabbage, turnips, greens, seafood, kelp, or large amounts of table salt.
- Instruct patients taking ^{123}I to return at 4–6 hours and 24 hours for scan and uptake.

Equipment

Camera

- Thyroid probe or small or large field of view

Collimator

- Flat-field scintillation probe with pulse-height analyzer or low energy, all purpose, or low energy, high resolution

Computer Set-up

- ^{131}I: 30% window at 364 keV
- ^{123}I: 20% window at 159 keV
- ^{99m}Tc: 20% window at 140 keV

Procedure *(time: ~15 minutes)*

- Dose calibrate radiotracer of choice.
- Count capsule in neck phantom with thyroid probe or gamma camera; record count(s) (this can also serve as the "standard" or count standard capsule if separate). Count room background; record count(s).
- Ensure that the patient has discontinued all interfering medications (e.g., thyroid medications, antiarrhythmics) for the appropriate amount of time.
- Administer the capsule with water (or inject the ^{99m}TcO$_4{}^-$). Instruct patient to return in 4–6 hours and 24 hours (for capsules) or counted under camera in 20 minutes (for ^{99m}TcO$_4{}^-$). If performed in conjunction with scan, take images along with the 4- to 6-hour uptake. Peak camera for use with iodine.
- Probe: facing thyroid gland (usually 25–30 cm from patient's neck), 1-minute counts, usually twice, then averaged. Record counts.

  Camera: place patient in supine position, pillow under shoulders to extend neck with camera anterior and close (record position to use for 24-hour uptake), thyroid centered; start count or camera (1-minute counts, usually two, then averaged); record count(s).
- Probe: position as per protocol for patient background, usually facing thigh, 25–30 cm, start count, 1-minute counts, usually twice, then averaged. Record count(s). (This applies to 24-hour uptake as well.)

  Camera: count standard in neck phantom at same distance as patient as per protocol. (This applies to 24-hour uptake as well.)
- Calculate uptake (two examples of the many methods):

Probe (most new probes automatically calculate after thyroid and thigh counts): Using this manual method:

- the patient is given one capsule and one standard capsule is retained.
- or two capsules are given to the patient and two are retained as standard.
- or two capsules are given to the patient and one is retained as standard and counted twice.
- or one or two capsules are counted first, then given to the patient, then mathematically decayed using the decay factors.

$$\% \text{ uptake} = \frac{[\text{patient thyroid CPM} - \text{patient background (thigh) CPM}]}{(\text{standard count or original capsule CPM} \times \text{decay factor}) - \text{original background (room)}} \times 100$$

Camera: Using this manual method:

- two capsules are given to the patient and one standard capsule is retained.
- or count one or two capsules first, then give them to patient, then mathematically decay the original count as the standard as in the example above.

$$\% \text{ uptake} = \frac{\text{Two 60-sec patient counts/2}}{\text{Two 60-sec standard counts added together}} \times 100$$

- Whichever method is used, one must end up using the same number of standard capsules (real, counted twice, or mathematically derived) as is given to the patient.
- Repeat count procedure at 24 hours and calculate uptake.
- Decay factors: these are for decaying the counts, not the activity.

  4 hours: 0.810548

  6 hours: 0.72974

  24 hours: 0.283578

Normal Results *(percents vary greatly between hospitals according to local populations)*

- 4-6 hours = 5-20%
- 24 hours = 7-35%
- $^{99m}TcO_4^-$: 20 minutes = ~4%

Abnormal Results

- At 24 hours, less than ~7% indicates hypothyroidism, especially with concordant history.
- More than ~35% indicates hyperthyroidism with concordant history.

Artifacts

- Capsule not dose calibrated for activity or counted before administration.
- Compton scatter and downscatter from contaminates may contribute to ^{123}I spectrum.

- $^{99m}TcO_4^-$ not as accurate because of low absolute uptake, high neck background, changing biodistribution, concentrations in extrathyroid tissues and trapping without organification.
- High collar metal buttons or medallions may interfere with counts.
- Placement of probe must be consistent with department protocol or readings can be false-positive or false-negative.
- Patient on interfering food or medications, e.g., thyroid or antiarrhythmic agents.

Additional Interventions

- Thyrotropin-releasing hormone (TRH) and thyrotropin (thyroid-stimulating hormone, TSH) stimulating tests can be performed to indicate suppressed tissue, functioning metastasis, and functional reserve.
- Perchlorate washout test to diagnose organification defects such as Hashimoto's thyroiditis or congenital enzyme deficiencies.
- Triiodothyronine (T_3, Cytomel®) suppression test to diagnose borderline hyperthyroidism.

Note

Definitions

T_3 = triiodothyronine = Cytomel® (most metabolically active).

T_4 = thyroxine (highest concentration in blood).

TSH = thyrotropin, anterior pituitary hormone stimulates thyroid to release T_3 and T_4.

TRH = thyrotropin-releasing hormone from hypothalamus, stimulates release of TSH from anterior pituitary.

Calcitonin = from the C cells or parafollicular cells; regulates calcium or bone building.

Parathormone = parathyroid hormone; breaks down calcium in bone (resorption).

Hypothyroidism

Hypothyroidism may be the result of iodine deficiency (large, endemic goiter), inherited enzyme deficiency, postradioiodine ablation (iatrogenic), end-stage toxic goiter, metastatic cancer, chronic thyroiditis, iodine excess, or pituitary or hypothalamic injury. Hypothyroidism is characterized by myxedema (end-stage hypothyroidism, puffy face, fluid retention, and lethargy) or cretinism in infants (lethargy, pot belly, enlarged tongue, stunted growth, and mental retardation). Hashimoto's thyroiditis is characterized by inflammation, chronic lymphocytic thyroiditis, lymphoid goiter, and struma lymphomatosa; autoimmune thyroiditis is diffuse lymphocytic infiltration.

Hyperthyroidism

Plummer's disease (toxic nodular goiter) is characterized by solitary or multiple autonomous nodules (goiter), elevated T_3 and T_4, low TSH, and no LATS (long-acting thyroid stimulator, an autoantibody). Graves' disease (exophthalmos, pretibial myxedema, and acropachy) results in hyperthyroidism, thyrotoxicosis, toxic diffuse goiter, elevated T_3 and T_4, and low TSH, and produces LATS. Subacute thyroiditis is the absence of uptake illustrating shutdown of the thyroidal iodine extraction and hormonal synthesis pathway. Patient presents sporadically with (among other things) sore neck, difficulty in swallowing, fever, dehydration, and slightly elevated white blood cell count. Serum thyroid hormone levels may present as normal or elevated to the point of hyperthyroidism or even "thyroid storm."

SUGGESTED READINGS

Datz FL. Handbook of Nuclear Medicine. 2nd ed. St. Louis: Mosby, 1993.

Early PJ, Sodee DB. Principles and Practice of Nuclear Medicine. 2nd ed. St. Louis: Mosby, 1995.

Murray IPC, Ell PJ, eds. Nuclear Medicine in Clinical Diagnosis and Treatment. Vols. 1 and 2. New York: Churchill Livingstone, 1994.

Nuclear Medicine Handbook. Princeton, NJ: ER Squibb & Sons, 1990.

Wilson, MA. Textbook of Nuclear Medicine. Philadelphia: Lippincott-Raven, 1998.

Betadine® is a registered trademark of Purdue Fredrick Co., Norwalk, CT.
Cytomel® is a registered trademark of SmithKline Beecham Pharmaceuticals, Philadelphia, PA.

Notes:

CHAPTER 56

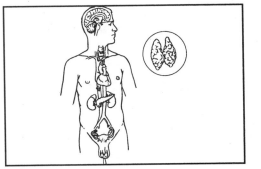

Thyroid: Whole-Body ^{131}I Cancer Study and rTSH Augmentation

Radiopharmacy

Radionuclide

- ^{131}I $t_{1/2}$: 8.1 days

  Energies: 364 keV (γ), 606 keV(β^-)

  Type: β^-, γ, fission product

Radiopharmaceutical

- ^{131}I as sodium iodide capsule or liquid

Localization

- Active transport. Organified by thyroid and held in cells or follicular lumen. T_e = 3-5 days.

Quality Control

- Calibrate capsule or vial to confirm amount of radioactivity

Adult Dose Range

- 1-5 mCi (37-185 MBq)

Method of Administration

- PO

Indications

- Localization and evaluation for metastasizing or recurrent thyroid carcinoma.
- Localization and evaluation for residual functioning thyroid tissue after total thyroidectomy.

Contraindications

- Allergy to iodine.
- Iodinated radiographic studies recently or under way.
- High-iodine diet or taking thyroid medications.

Patient History

The patient should answer the following questions.

Do you have a history or family history of cancer?	Y	N
If so, what type and for how long?		

Do you have a history of adenocarcinoma?	Y	N
Do you have a history of thyroid problems?	Y	N
Have you had any recent pain or problems in neck or throat area?	Y	N
Have you had any thyroid surgery?	Y	N
If so, when?		

Have you had any thyroid therapy, chemotherapy, or radiation therapy?	Y	N
If so, when and what type?		

Do you have any recent laboratory results?	Y	N

If rTSH (recombinant thyroid-stimulating hormone) study, do you have Tg (thyroglobulin) results?	Y	N

When was your last injection of Thyrogen®?

Have you had any recent iodinated radiographic studies (IV pyelogram, CT with contrast, x-ray with contrast, myelogram, angiogram, nuclear medicine)?	Y	N

Other department-specific questions.

Patient Preparation

- Identify the patient. Verify doctor's order. Explain the procedure.
- Physician to instruct patient to be on low-iodine diet.
- Physician is to discontinue thyroid medication (hormone supplements or antithyroid medication). Patient should be clinically hypothyroid with elevated TSH levels at time of study unless it is an rTSH study.
- Instruct patient to be NPO for at least 4 hours before ingestion of dose and remain so for 1 hour after ingestion of dose.
- Instruct patient to bring results of recent laboratory tests.
- For rTSH augmentation study, ^{131}I injection: 24 hours after the final Thyrogen® injection. Patient need not discontinue medication.

Equipment

Camera
- Large field of view, single or dual head

Collimator
- Medium- or high-energy parallel hole

Computer Set-up
Statics
- [131]I peaks, 15–20% windows, 128×128 or 256×256 matrix, 600 seconds or more per view ($> 1,000,000$ counts). Anterior–posterior, head, thorax, abdomen, and pelvis.

Whole Body (usually head to thigh)
- 10 cm/min or slower

Procedure *(time: dosing, ~15 minutes; imaging, ~30–60 minutes)*

- Procedure is usually performed 6 months to 1 year after surgery or therapy (see Note).

- Ensure patient has discontinued medications and is following physician's orders as to diet.

- Administer dose to patient as to protocol, by physician or technologist.

- Instruct patient to return at appropriate time for images, according to protocol.

- Place patient in supine position, remove attenuating articles from clothing.

- Instruct patient to remain motionless during acquisition.

- Obtain images at 48 and 72 hours. These present with better target to background ratios.

- Optional: obtain images at 24 hours after ingestion of dose if protocol.

- Obtain whole-body statics (5–10 min/image) or whole-body sweep, anterior–posterior from head to thigh.

- Obtain optional statics with markers if suspicious areas are found (see Note).

Normal Results

- No focal areas of iodine uptake.

- Salivary glands may present dim to bright.

- Mouth, stomach (may extend into intestine), and bladder present well.

Abnormal Results

- Focal areas of uptake, especially in thyroid bed, although other places (lymph metastases, etc.) are not unlikely.

- Areas of lungs and breasts may have uptake, suggesting pulmonary or breast metastases, etc. Lateral images may better define area.

- False-positive focal uptake in liver indicating metastatic lesion may be caused by retention in intrahepatic duct dilation, particularly in patients with history of biliary tract disease.

Whole-Body Scans With rTSH Augmentation

This test is based on serum thyroglobulin levels and stimulation of thyroid tissue with a recombinant form of TSH to detect recurring thyroid cancer or residual functioning thyroid tissue in patients without necessitating the discontinuation of thyroid hormone medications (e.g., Synthroid®).

Description

- Thyrogen® (thyrotropin alfa for injection) is a highly purified, heterodimeric glycoprotein, recombinant form of human pituitary TSH. It is synthesized using a genetically modified Chinese hamster ovary cell line.

Localization

- Thyrotropin alfa binds to TSH receptors on normal thyroid epithelial cells or on well-differentiated thyroid cancer tissue, stimulating iodine uptake and organification, and synthesis and secretion of thyroglobulin (Tg), triiodothyronine (T_3), and thyroxine (T_4).

Adult Dose Range

- $\geq$ 4 mCi (148 MBq) ^{131}I-sodium iodide. Clearance of radioiodine is 50% greater when euthyroid (posttreatment patient taking thyroid medications) as opposed to hypothyroid (posttreatment patient not taking thyroid medications). This may be a consideration when selecting the activity for imaging.

Procedure

- Thyrogen® injections: 0.9 mg IM into buttock every 24 hours for two injections, every 72 hours for three injections.
- ^{131}I injection: 24 hours after the final Thyrogen® injection.
- Scanning: whole-body images are obtained at 48 hours after ^{131}I injection (72 hours after final Thyrogen® injection).
- Parameters:
  - Whole body: $\geq$ 30 minutes or minimum of 140,000 counts.
  - Statics: 10–15 minutes each or 60,000 counts for large field-of-view cameras or 35,000 counts for small field-of-view cameras.
- For a serum Tg test: a blood sample is obtained at 72 hours after final Thyrogen® injection (at time of imaging).

Artifacts

- Patient has not discontinued medications or not on low-iodine diet.
- Patient not clinically hypothyroid or with elevated TSH levels. This may preclude the test because there must be autonomous tissue producing hormone.

Note

The whole body cancer study can also be performed with ^{201}Tl (~4 mCi IV, image 20 minutes after injection), alleviating the need to discontinue thyroid medication. Also with ^{131}I-*meta*-iodobenzylguanidine (^{131}I-mIBG, same as pheochromocytoma study with emphasis on neck and chest).

Some physicians, for after surgery or therapy follow-up, opt for a regular thyroid uptake and scan, a < 30 mCi therapy if something is found, then monitor laboratory results before they attempt an ablation. Some say this sensitizes the remaining tissue, which becomes more resistant, making it more difficult to eradicate.

One way for markers, if a ^{131}I marker is not available, is to make up a ^{99m}Tc marker (a drop on a cotton-tipped swab stuffed into a needle cap works well) and take a quick marker image on ^{99m}Tc peak, then switch to ^{131}I peak and take image. Do this for all views, put ^{99m}Tc images on one film and ^{131}I images in same order on one film to allow direct overlay.

SUGGESTED READINGS

Datz FL. Handbook of Nuclear Medicine. 2nd ed. St. Louis: Mosby, 1993.

Early PJ, Sodee DB. Principles and Practice of Nuclear Medicine. 2nd ed. St. Louis: Mosby, 1995.

Genzyme Therapeutics. Thyrogen®, thyrotropin alfa for injection. Pamphlet. Cambridge, MA: Genzyme and Knoll, 1999.

Murray IPC, Ell PJ, eds. Nuclear Medicine in Clinical Diagnosis and Treatment. Vols. 1 and 2. New York: Churchill Livingstone, 1994.

Wilson, MA. Textbook of Nuclear Medicine. Philadelphia: Lippincott-Raven, 1998.

Notes

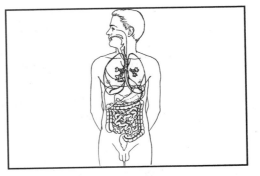

CHAPTER 57

Verluma™-Scan: Small Cell Lung Cancer

(Radioimmunoscintigraphy: RIS)

Radiopharmacy

Radionuclide

- ^{99m}Tc $t_{1/2}$: 6 hours

  Energies: 140 keV

  Type: IT, γ, generator

Radiopharmaceutical

- ^{99m}Tc-nofetumomab merpentan (murine monoclonal antibody [Moab] fragments [Fabs]). Generated from NR-LU-10, a murine IgG$_2$b; binds to an approximately 40-kd glycoprotein (carcinoma-associated) antigen that is expressed in a number of cancers and some normal tissue. Fabs minimize the induction of human anti-mouse antibody (HAMA) reaction. (DuPont has temporarily removed this product from the market.)

Localization

- Compartmental, blood flow; dose-dependent, antibody binding

Quality Control

- If made from kit, chromatography > 85% radiochemical purity

Adult Dose Range

- 15–30 mCi (550–1110 MBq) in a final volume of 15–20 mL

Method of Administration

- IV butterfly (large-bore, 18–22 gauge) for 5 minutes. The recommended volume of 20 mL may require a special syringe shield.
- 10 mL of saline flush.
- Make available a physician or nurse to observe patient for possible allergic reaction (1 mg of epinephrine available).
- Monitor vital signs: baseline, 5, 15, 30, 45, and 60 minutes after injection (some only observe patient for 15–30 minutes looking for redness at injection site or signs of nausea and vomiting).

Indications

- Used in conjunction with standard diagnostic evaluations and after histologic diagnosis is established.
- Detection, localization, and staging (as limited or extensive) of primary or metastatic small cell lung carcinoma.
- Detection and localization of non–small cell lung cancer and adenocarcinomas of the breast, ovary, colorectum, and prostate. The antigen expresses in a variety of cancers and some normal tissue.
- Evaluation of elevated or rising serum CEA (carcinoembryonic antigen) or other tumor markers.
- Evaluation and detection of extent of regional lesions and occult metastases by clarifying equivocal diagnostic modality findings.
- Localization of recurrent disease in surgical candidate patients (biopsy, exploratory laparotomy, and surgical resection).

Contraindications

- Should not be administered to patients who are hypersensitive to murine products.
- Not intended for differential diagnosis of suspected lung cancer or suspected metastases.
- Not intended for single use before treatment or assessment of response or evaluation after chemotherapy or radiation therapy.
- Should not be used in patients with impaired renal or hepatobiliary function because those systems are the main routes of radiotracer excretion.

Patient History *(or use complete patient history in reference section)*

The patient should answer the following questions.

Do you have a history or a family history
of cancer?   Y   N

If so, what type and since when?

Do you have any pain?   Y   N

    If so, where and since when?

Do you have a history of allergies?   Y   N

Have you had any recent surgery?   Y   N

Have you had any recent radiation therapy
    or chemotherapy?   Y   N

Have you had any murine-based examinations?   Y   N

    If so, what type, when, and where?

Have you had any recent or planned nuclear
    medicine, CT, MRI, x-ray, or US examinations?   Y   N

Have you had any recent abnormal laboratory
    test results?   Y   N

    If so, please list (CEA, CA-19–9, HAMA, other).

Other department-specific questions.

Patient Preparation

- Identify the patient. Verify doctor's order. Explain the procedure.
- Obtain a signed consent form from patient.
- Obtain a history of allergies and prior examinations.
- Instruct patient to hydrate and void often for 12–14 hours after injection.
- Physician to order a mild cathartic between injection and imaging if timed so that cleansing is completed before imaging time (cathartic at about 4 hours after injection).

Equipment

Camera

- Large field of view

Collimator

- Low energy, all purpose, or low energy, high resolution

Computer Set-up
Statics

- Initial image for 500,000 counts. Time noted; subsequent statics taken for that amount of time. 256 × 256 byte mode.

Whole Body

Statics

- 10-minute (600-second) images, at least head to midthigh, anterior and posterior

Sweep

- 10 cm/min or slower (30 minutes [1800 seconds] or greater) anterior–posterior; check patient length

Single Photon Emission Computed Tomography (SPECT)

- Rotation, 360° step and shoot; projections, 60; 30 sec/frame (single head), 45–60 sec/frame (dual head); matrix, 64 × 64 or 128 × 128 word mode; axis/center of rotation, < 2 mm or 0.5 pixels; uniformity correction, yes (± 1%).

Procedure *(images 14–17 hours after injection; time: ~1–2 hours)*

- Instruct patient to void; check clothing for possible artifacts.
- Place patient in supine position on imaging table.
- Instruct patient to remain motionless during acquisition.
- Acquire whole-body statics or sweep: 14–17 hours after injection.
- Acquire statics: 500,000 counts or 10 minutes (600 seconds) per view (whichever comes first, then use that time for subsequent images); anterior-posterior, obliques, laterals, thorax, abdomen, pelvis. Spot views often provide the best diagnostic pictures. Arms up for obese patients to help eliminate skinfolds.
- Acquire SPECT of thorax or suspected area of interest.
- Optional images: 24-hour or more delays (advisable because of reduced target to background ratios, especially for questionable areas or suggested normal bowel activity).

Normal Results

- Activity in gallbladder, intestines, kidneys, and urinary bladder because of excretion.
- Activity in testes, midline nasal area, liver, and spleen because of nonspecific vascularization.

- Bowel activity may be present because of radiolabel in stool (ask patient if they cleansed bowel between injection time and imaging).
- Specific reactivity found in pituitary gland, salivary gland, and thyroid.
- Background tissue and vascularity should be diminished and diffuse.

Abnormal Results

- Focal areas of increased uptake in lesions, especially of the lungs; also hilar, mediastinal, supraclavicular, bone, bone marrow, lymphatic, brain, cervical, hepatic, abdominal, or renal areas indicating adenopathies and/or metastases.
- Focal areas of increased activity that remain persistent and stationary over time with delayed images, particularly over lymph nodes and/or organ of interest.
- There may be accumulation of activity in nontumor areas such as regions of inflammation, increased vascular pool, or recent surgical sites (possible false-positive results, making detection of small lesions in these areas difficult). Patient history is vital, along with confirmation of areas using other modalities.
- Skinfolds in areas of axillas, breasts, and abdomen, especially in obese patients, may result in false-positive results.
- Large lesions may present as cold spots and remain cold because of poor vascularization or central necrosis.

Processing

- Slice thickness to 2 mm. Using a low-pass filter, e.g., Butterworth, with a 0.4 Nyquist cutoff and seventh-order (or 0.5 and fifth-order) has produced acceptable images.

Artifacts

- Watch patient for allergic reaction, e.g., anaphylactic shock, nausea, redness or rash at injection site, transient eosinophilia, bursitis, headache, itching, upset stomach, and fever.
- Patient motion blurs possible areas of interest.
- A negative scan should not alter the patient-care management.
- Small lesions may not present (< 2 cm).

Note

Nofetumomab has been shown not to visualize in some sites of known involvement by small cell lung cancer. Localization that suggests limited staging does not exclude the possibility of extensive stage disease. This test should always be used in conjunction with other diagnostic modalities.

- Patient treatment can begin within 1–5 days after MoAb imaging; composed of chemotherapy consisting of cyclophosphamide, doxorubicin, vincristine (or etoposide), or cisplatin; etoposide; and/or radiation therapy.

SUGGESTED READINGS

Wilson, MA. Textbook of Nuclear Medicine. Philadelphia: Lippincott-Raven, 1998.

Verluma™ is a trademark of DuPont Merck, Wilmington, DE.

Notes

CHAPTER 58

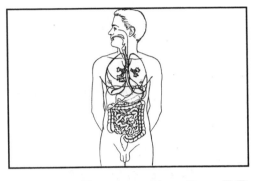

White Blood Cell

(^{111}In-oxime and ^{99m}Tc-Ceretec™)

Radiopharmacy

Radionuclide

- ^{111}In t$_{1/2}$: 2.8 d

  Energies: 173, 247 keV

  Type: EC, γ, accelerator

- or ^{99m}Tc t$_{1/2}$: 6 hours

  Energies: 140 keV

  Type: IT, γ, generator

Radiopharmaceutical

- ^{111}In-oxine (oxyquinoline)
- ^{99m}Tc-HMPAO (D,L-hexamethylpropyleneamine oxime or Ceretec™)

Localization

- White blood cell (WBC) migration through chemotaxis

Quality Control

- ^{111}In-oxine: > 90%
- ^{99m}Tc-HMPAO: > 95% radiochemical purity

Adult Dose Range

- ^{111}In-oxine: 500 μCi (18.5 MBq)
- ^{99m}Tc-HMPAO: 10–24 mCi (370–888 MBq)

Method of Administration

- Slow IV straight stick or IV catheter with flush

Indications

- Detection and localization of acute and chronic osteomyelitis (especially acute).
- Detection and localization of acute abscesses (e.g., liver, renal, intra-abdominal sepsis).
- Detection and localization of infection (especially in fever of unknown origin [FUO]).
- Detection of acute inflammatory disease (e.g., bowel, cellulitis, genitourinary).
- Evaluation for prosthesis rejection.
- Differentiation of pulmonary infiltrates (infarct versus pneumonia).

Contraindications

- Antibiotics decrease leukocyte chemotaxis and have negative effect on leukocytes.
- Not particularly effective on spinal cord infections.
- Patient should not be leukopenic.

Patient History *(or use complete patient history in reference section)*

The patient should answer the following questions.

**Do you have a history or family history
of cancer?**   Y   N

If so, what type and for how long?

Do you have a history of bowel disease?   Y   N

If so, what type and for how long?

Have you had any recent surgery?   Y   N

Have you had any recent infections?   Y   N

Do you have any blood-borne infections?   Y   N

Do you have any pain?   Y   N

If so, where and for how long?

Are you taking antibiotic therapy?	Y	N
Have you had recent fevers?	Y	N
Have you had any recent trauma?	Y	N
Are you a diabetic?	Y	N
Are there any recent or planned related studies (e.g., US, CT, MRI, nuclear medicine, x-ray, biopsy)?	Y	N
Discern discreetly whether the study is AIDS-related.		
Other department-specific questions.		

Patient Preparation

- Identify the patient. Verify doctor's order. Explain the procedure (especially blood draw, reinjection, then delay for pictures).
- Document name, date, and time for procedure to begin.

Equipment

Camera

- Large field of view

Collimator

- ^{111}In: medium energy; general purpose, or medium energy, high resolution
- ^{99m}Tc: low energy, all purpose, or low energy, high resolution

Computer Set-up

- Set energies for radiotracer if not automatic

Statics (spots)

- 800,000–2,000,000 counts or 15–20 min/image (cover head to pelvis, extremities may be required; patient comfort and compliance may be a factor in length of each spot)

Whole Body

- 512 × 1024 matrix, 10 cm/min or longer (minimum 30 minutes) head to pelvis

Single Photon Emission Computed Tomography (SPECT)

- 360°, 64 stops, 45–60 sec/stop, 64 × 64 word matrix. Butterworth, cutoff 0.4, power 5, slice thickness 1–2 mm

Procedure *(time: blood draw, ~15 minutes; spots, ~30–60 minutes; whole-body, ~30 minutes; SPECT, ~30 minutes)*

Blood Preparation

- Order a blood sample collection kit from the radiopharmacy.
- Arrange for time of pickup (takes ~4 hours for turnaround time).
- Optional collection: Using a large enough syringe (60–100 mL) for collection, add ~4–8 mL of ADC or heparin.
- Withdraw 50–80 mL of blood from patient (100 mL if patient's WBC count is low). Use a large-gauge needle.
- Invert gently for ~1 minute to mix.
- Fill out all necessary paperwork; label syringe and patient.
- Store collected blood sample in supplied or fabricated container with needle or red cap facing up.
- Send to radiopharmacy for processing. Turnaround is ~4 hours.
- Reinject tagged WBCs slowly, using large-bore needle. Flush IV well, if used.
- Wait for appropriate amount of time to image (see below).

Imaging

- Instruct patient to void; remove attenuating articles from patient's clothing.
- Place patient in supine position.
- Acquire whole-body sweep or statics, or SPECT as per protocol and radiologist's request. Laterals and obliques may also be required, particularly with visualized suspicious areas. Check with radiologist before releasing patients (especially outpatients).

^{111}In-Oxine

- Image at 2–6 hours or 24 hours after reinjection (usually only 24 hours).
- Optional: image at 48 hours.

^{99m}Tc-Ceretec™

- Because of higher photon flux, times for images can be reduced.
- Image at 1–4 hours after reinjection (usually ~2 hours, although optimum time is 1 hour).
- 24-hour delays may be required in cases of chronic infections.

Normal Results

^{111}In-Oxine

- Up to 4 hours, pulmonary uptake.

- Liver, spleen, and bone marrow activity.

- No renal or gastrointestinal activity.

^{99m}Tc-Ceretec™

- Initial uptake in lung, liver, and spleen.

- 1–2 hours: liver, spleen, bladder, and kidney, some gallbladder.

- 4 hours: lung activity reduced, gallbladder brighter, and bowel activity presents.

- 24 hours: colonic activity, others reduced.

Abnormal Results

- Areas of focal activity outside normal areas.

- Activity compared with liver: more than or equal to liver indicates infectious process; less than liver indicates noninfectious process.

- Splenic activity changes may indicate inflammatory bowel disease.

- True-positive results: abscesses communicating with bowel, pseudomembranous colitis, inflammatory bowel disease, or necrotic bowel.

Preparation for Injection

Kits (from the radiopharmacy)

- Included (usually): container, 60-mL syringe, ADC (or other) blood thinner, wrist label and extra number stickers, cap, butterfly, plastic bag, and paperwork.

- Start IV or butterfly.

- Draw ~5 mL of ADC into syringe.

- Draw 50 mL of blood into syringe (more, up to 100 mL in two syringes, if WBC count is known to be low).

- Cap syringe and label with number tag; place into plastic bag.

- Place into shipping container so that cap is up when case is upright (to facilitate settling).

- Fill out paperwork and place a number tag on paper.

- Affix the wrist band onto the patient's arm.

- Send blood sample back to radiopharmacy. The turnaround time varies but may be ~3–4 hours.

- Upon return, reinject patient with tagged WBCs after checking number tags and paperwork.

- Wait specified time for particular scan and image.

For the "Do-It-Yourselfers" (home-spun injections)

- Withdraw 50–100 mL of whole blood with 1–8 mL of blood thinner.

- Clamp syringe at 10°–30° angle, needle side (or red cap side) up.

- Add 5 mL of 6% hetastarch to settle RBCs or let sit for 30–60 minutes.

- Reclamp syringe straight up.

- Remove upper layer containing leukocyte-rich plasma and place slowly into sterile plastic tubes or one 50-mL centrifuge tube.

- Centrifuge at 300g for 15 minutes or at 450g for 5 minutes. (Makes leukocyte "button" at bottom.)

- Remove leukocyte-poor plasma layer(s) and place into fresh plastic tube(s).

- Centrifuge tube(s) at 100g for 15 minutes. (Separates out platelets.)

- Remove and save all platelet-poor plasma.

- Combine leukocyte buttons and add 5 mL of normal saline to resuspend.

- At this point, some wash buttons by centrifuging again at 450g for 5 minutes, remove and discard supernatant, then resuspend with 5 mL of normal saline.

- Add 0.5–1 mCi (18.5–37 MBq) ^{111}In-oxine or 30 mCi (1110 MBq) ^{99m}Tc-HMPAO slowly to suspension while swirling tube, then incubate at room temperature for 15–30 minutes.

- Add 5 mL of the previously saved platelet-poor plasma to suspension to bind any free indium or ^{99m}Tc-HMPAO.

- Centrifuge at 300g for 5 minutes, remove, assay, and save supernatant layer for quality control.

- Add 2 mL of the platelet-poor plasma to wash labeled WBCs without resuspending, then remove, assay, and discard.

- Add 5 mL of the platelet-poor plasma and resuspend labeled WBCs; assay.

$$\% \text{ bound} = \frac{\mu\text{Ci or mCi in WBCs}}{\mu\text{Ci or mCi in WBCs} + \mu\text{Ci or mCi in supernatant}} \times 100$$

- Check with microscope for clumps and foreign particles.

- Perform trypan blue exclusion test to determine cell viability.

- Draw 500 μCi (18.5 MBq) ^{111}In-oxine or 24 mCi (888 MBq) ^{99m}Tc-HMPAO of labeled WBCs into syringe; assay.

- It is now ready for injection. Reinject patient and wait specified time for particular scan for imaging.

Artifacts

- Attenuation from clothing or articles.

- False-positive results: inflammation from tracheal tubes, pneumonia, emphysema, sinusitis, pulmonary embolism, congestive heart failure, adult respiratory distress syndrome, ulcers, diverticula, tumors, metastases, IV catheters, colostomies, postsurgical wounds, hematomas, or fractures.

Note

Donor WBCs (ABO matched) can be used in leukopenic patients.

[99m]Tc-sulfur colloid (5 mCi or 185 MBq) can be injected after the ^{111}In-oxine study is com-

plete with a standard liver/spleen study taken to compare and help evaluate upper abdomen for abscesses.

^{99m}Tc-Ceretec™ is particularly useful for osteomyelitis detection in extremities.

SUGGESTED READINGS

Datz FL. Handbook of Nuclear Medicine. 2nd ed. St. Louis: Mosby, 1993.

Early PJ, Sodee DB. Principles and Practice of Nuclear Medicine. 2nd ed. St. Louis: Mosby, 1995.

Murray IPC, Ell PJ, eds. Nuclear Medicine in Clinical Diagnosis and Treatment. Vols. 1 and 2. New York: Churchill Livingstone, 1994.

Wilson, MA. Textbook of Nuclear Medicine. Philadelphia: Lippincott-Raven, 1998.

Ceretec™ is a trademark of Amersham International Plc, Amersham, UK.

Notes

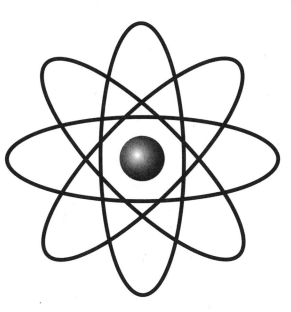

SECTION | TWO

Quick Reference

Conversion Tables

lb/kg

in/cm

Target Heart Rates (Cardiac Studies)

mCi/MBq

Conversion Table for Pounds to Kilograms

Weight (in lb) ÷ 2.2 = kg (rounded off to nearest number)

lb	kg	lb	kg	lb	kg	lb	kg	lb	kg	lb	kg	lb	kg	lb	kg
65	30	90	41	115	52	140	64	165	75	190	86	215	98	240	109
66	30	91	41	116	53	141	64	166	75	191	87	216	98	241	110
67	31	92	42	117	53	142	64	167	76	192	87	217	99	242	110
68	31	93	42	118	54	143	65	168	76	193	88	218	99	243	110
69	31	94	43	119	54	144	65	169	77	194	88	219	100	244	111
70	32	95	43	120	55	145	66	170	77	195	89	220	100	245	111
71	32	96	44	121	55	146	66	171	78	196	89	221	100	246	112
72	33	97	44	122	55	147	67	172	78	197	90	222	101	247	112
73	33	98	45	123	56	148	67	173	79	198	90	223	101	248	113
74	34	99	45	124	56	149	68	174	79	199	90	224	102	249	113
75	34	100	46	125	57	150	68	175	80	200	91	225	102	250	114
76	35	101	46	126	57	151	69	176	80	201	91	226	103	251	114
77	35	102	46	127	58	152	69	177	80	202	92	227	103	252	115
78	36	103	47	128	58	153	70	178	81	203	92	228	104	253	115
79	36	104	47	129	59	154	70	179	81	204	93	229	104	254	115
80	36	105	48	130	59	155	70	180	82	205	93	230	105	255	116
81	37	106	48	131	60	156	71	181	82	206	94	231	105	256	116
82	37	107	49	132	60	157	71	182	83	207	94	232	105	257	117
83	38	108	49	133	60	158	72	183	83	208	95	233	106	258	117
84	38	109	50	134	61	159	72	184	84	209	95	234	106	259	118
85	39	110	50	135	61	160	73	185	84	210	95	235	107	260	118
86	39	111	50	136	62	161	73	186	85	211	96	236	107	261	119
87	40	112	51	137	62	162	74	187	85	212	96	237	108	262	119
88	40	113	51	138	63	163	74	188	85	213	97	238	108	263	120
89	41	114	52	139	63	164	75	189	86	214	97	239	109	264	120

Conversion Table for Inches to Centimeters

Height (inches) $\times$ 2.54 = cm

Feet	Inches	Centimeters (rounded off)
4' 9"	57"	145 cm
4' 10"	58"	147 cm
4' 11"	59"	150 cm
5'	60"	152 cm
5' 1"	61"	155 cm
5' 2"	62"	157 cm
5' 3"	63"	160 cm
5' 4"	64"	163 cm
5' 5"	65"	165 cm
5' 6"	66"	168 cm
5' 7"	67"	170 cm
5' 8"	68"	173 cm
5' 9"	69"	175 cm
5' 10"	70"	178 cm
5' 11"	71"	180 cm
6'	72"	183 cm
6' 1"	73"	185 cm
6' 2"	74"	188 cm
6' 3"	75"	191 cm
6' 4"	76"	193 cm
6' 5"	77"	196 cm
6' 6"	78"	198 cm
6' 7"	79"	200 cm
6' 8"	80"	203 cm
6' 9"	81"	206 cm
6' 10"	82"	208 cm

Conversion Table for Target Heart Rates (Cardiac Studies)

220 − age = 100% target rate

Age	100%	85%	Age	100%	85%	Age	100%	85%
18	202	172	42	178	151	66	154	131
19	201	171	43	177	150	67	153	130
20	200	170	44	176	150	68	152	129
21	199	169	45	175	149	69	151	128
22	198	168	46	174	148	70	150	128
23	197	167	47	173	147	71	149	127
24	196	167	48	172	146	72	148	126
25	195	166	49	171	145	73	147	125
26	194	165	50	170	145	74	146	124
27	193	164	51	169	144	75	145	123
28	192	163	52	168	143	76	144	122
29	191	162	53	167	142	77	143	122
30	190	162	54	166	141	78	142	121
31	189	161	55	165	140	79	141	120
32	188	160	56	164	139	80	140	119
33	187	159	57	163	139	81	139	118
34	186	158	58	162	138	82	138	117
35	185	157	59	161	137	83	137	116
36	184	156	60	160	136	84	136	116
37	183	156	61	159	135	85	135	115
38	182	155	62	158	134	86	134	114
39	181	154	63	157	133	87	133	113
40	180	153	64	156	133	88	132	112
41	179	152	65	155	132	89	131	111

Conversion Table for Millicuries (mCi) to Megabecquerels (MBq)

mCi × 37 = MBq

µCi	MBq	mCi	MBq	mCi	MBq	mCi	MBq
1 (0.001 mCi)	0.037	1	37	26	962	350	12,950
2	0.074	2	74	27	999	400	14,800
5	0.185	3	111	28	1,036	450	16,650
10	0.370	4	148	29	1,073	500	18,500
25	0.925	5	185	30	1,110	550	20,350
50	1.85	6	222	31	1,147	600	22,200
75	2.775	7	259	32	1,184	650	24,050
100	3.70	8	296	33	1,221	700	25,900
150	5.55	9	333	34	1,258	750	27,750
200	7.40	10	370	35	1,295	800	29,600
250	9.25	11	407	36	1,332	850	31,450
300	11.10	12	444	37	1,369	900	33,300
350	12.95	13	481	38	1,406	950	35,150
400	14.80	14	518	39	1,443	1,000	37,000
450	16.65	15	555	40	1,480	1,500	55,500
500	18.50	16	592	50	1,850	2,000	74,000
550	20.35	17	629	60	2,220	2,500	92,500
600	22.20	18	666	70	2,590	3,000	111,000
650	24.05	19	703	80	2,960	3,500	129,500
700	25.90	20	740	90	3,330	4,000	148,000
750	27.75	21	777	100	3,700	4,500	166,500
800	29.60	22	814	150	5,550	5,000	185,000
850	31.45	23	851	200	7,400	7,500	277,500
900	33.30	24	888	250	9,250	10,000	370,000
950	35.15	25	925	300	11,100	50,000	1,850,000

Radiopharmaceuticals

Standard Adult Nuclear Medicine Dose Ranges

Routine Medical Radionuclides

Equations

Kit Preparations (Overview)

Pediatric Dosing in Nuclear Medicine

Radioactive Isotopes

Standard Adult Nuclear Medicine Dose Ranges

Procedure	Radiopharmaceutical	Standard Dose ± 10%	Range ± 10%
Adrenocortical Scan	^{131}I-Iodomethylnorcholesterol	2 mCi	2 mCi
Bone scan	^{99m}Tc-MDP, -HDP	25 mCi	20–30 mCi
Bone marrow scan	^{99m}Tc-SC	15 mCi	10–20 mCi
Brain scan	^{99m}Tc-O$_4$$^-$, -DTPA, -GH	25 mCi	20–30 mCi
Brain scan-SPECT	^{99m}Tc-Ceretec® or Neurolite®	25 mCi	20–30 mCi
Cardiac first pass	^{99m}Tc, Cardiolite® or Myoview®	25 mCi	7–30 mCi
Cardiac rest/stress			
1-day, first study	^{99m}Tc, Cardiolite® or Myoview®	8 mCi	7–10 mCi
second study	^{99m}Tc, Cardiolite® or Myoview®	25 mCi	20–30 mCi
2-day	^{99m}Tc, Cardiolite® or Myoview®	25 mCi	20–30 mCi
Cardiac stress/redistribution: stress	^{201}Tl	0.5 mCi	2.5–3.5 mCi
Redistribution and/or 24-hour delay	Reinjection	1 mCi	1 mCi
Cardiac dual-isotope: Rest	^{201}Tl	3.0 mCi	2.5–3.5 mCi
Stress	^{99m}Tc, Cardiolite® or Myoview®	25 mCi	20–30 mCi
CEA-Scan®	^{99m}Tc-arcitumomab	20 mCi	20–30 mCi
Cisternogram	^{111}In-DTPA	1 mCi	0.5–1.5 mCi
Cystogram (voiding)	^{99m}Tc-SC, ^{99m}Tc-O$_4$$^-$	500 μCi	0.5–1 mCi
Gallium scan (infection)	^{67}Ga	7 mCi	5–10 mCi
Gallium scan (tumor)	^{67}Ga	10 mCi	5–10 mCi
Gastric emptying	^{99m}Tc-SC	500 μCi	0.5–1 mCi
GI bleed	^{99m}Tc-pyp-RBCs	25 mCi	20–30 mCi
HIDA (hepatobiliary scan)	^{99m}Tc-Choletec®	8 mCi	5–10 mCi
Liver/spleen scan	^{99m}Tc-SC	4 mCi	2–7 mCi
Liver SPECT (hemangioma)	^{99m}Tc-pyp-RBCs	25 mCi	20–30 mCi
Lung perfusion scan	^{99m}Tc-MAA	4 mCi	3–5 mCi
Lung ventilation scan	^{133}Xe	10 mCi	10–20 mCi
Lung ventilation scan	^{99m}Tc-DTPA (aerosol)	35 mCi	25–40 mCi
Lymphoscintigraphy	^{99m}Tc-SC	500 μCi	100–800 μCi
Meckel's diverticulum	^{99m}Tc-O$_4$$^-$	10 mCi	10–15 mCi
MUGA scan	^{99m}Tc-pyp-RBCs	25 mCi	20–30 mCi
Myocardial (MI) scan	^{99m}Tc-pyp	25 mCi	20–30 mCi
OctreoScan®	^{111}In-pentetriotide	6 mCi	6 mCi
OncoScint®	^{111}In-satumomab pendetide	5 mCi	4–6 mCi

Procedure	Radiopharmaceutical	Standard Dose ± 10%	Range ± 10%
Parathyroid scan	^{99m}Tc-Cardiolite®	25 mCi	16–30 mCi
Subtraction:	^{201}Tl	2 mCi	2–3 mCi
	^{99m}Tc-O$_4^-$	5 mCi	5–12 mCi
Pheochromocytoma scan	^{123}I and ^{131}I-mIBG ^{123}I	5 mCi	3–10 mCi
	^{131}I	500 μCi	0.5–1 mCi
ProstaScint®	^{111}In-CYT-356	5 mCi	5–17 mCi
Renal scan	^{99m}Tc-DTPA	10 mCi	10–15 mCi
Renal scan	^{99m}Tc-DMSA	5 mCi	3–10 mCi
Renal scan	^{99m}Tc-MAG$_3$®	7 mCi	3–10 mCi
Renogram	^{131}I-OIH	300 μCi	150–300 μCi
Schilling	B$_{12}$-^{57}Co	0.3 μCi	0.3–0.5 μCi
Scintimammography	^{99m}Tc-Cardiolite®	20 mCi	20 mCi
Testicular scan	^{99m}Tc-O$_4^-$	20 mCi	0–25 mCi
Thyroid ablation	^{131}I	150 mCi	30–300 mCi
Thyroid hyperthyroid therapy	^{131}I diffuse	10 mCi	1–10 mCi
	nodular	29 mCi	< 30 mCi
Thyroid scan	^{99m}Tc-O$_4^-$	10 mCi	5–10 mCi
Thyroid uptake and scan	^{123}I	140 μCi	100–350 μCi
	^{131}I	50 μCi	15–100 μCi
Thyroid scan (substernal)	^{131}I	50 μCi	15–100 μCi
WBC scan	^{99m}Tc-WBC	10 mCi	10–15 mCi
	^{99m}Tc-Ceretec®	10 mCi	10–24 mCi
	^{111}In-WBC	500 μCi	500 μCi
Whole-body ^{131}I carcinoma work-up	^{131}I	1 mCi	1–5 mCi

Routine Medical Radionuclides

Name	$t_{1/2}$	Emitter	Energies (keV)	Medical Uses
C-14	5730 y	β^-	156.5	*Helicobacter pylori* breath test
H-3	12.26 y	β^-	18.6	Body composition: total body water, intracellular and extracellular water
P-32	14.3 d	β^-	1710	RBCs for polycythemia vera or sodium phosphate solution for bone metastases
Sr-89	50.5 d	β^-	1463	Bone pain and metastases
Sr-90	28.6 y	β^-	546	Therapy
Cs-137	30 y	β^-, γ	662	Calibration of machines
Fe-59	45 d	β^-, γ	1100, 1290	Ferrokinetics, formation of RBCs
Mo-99	66 h	β^-, γ	740, 780	Generators for Tc only
I-131	8.1 d	β^-, γ	606, 364	Thyroid therapy, uptake 1–10 μCi, hyperthyroid ~30 mCi, follicular cancer 100–300 mCi
Sm-153	46.7 h	β^-, γ	632, 702, 805, 103, γ	Bone pain and metastases
Xe-133	5.3 d	β^-, γ	81, 32, x-ray	Pulmonary ventilation
Au-195^m	30.6 s	IT, γ	200, 262	First-pass angiography
Kr-81^m	13.1 s	IT, γ	191	Pulmonary ventilation
Tc-99^m	6 h	IT, γ	140	General imaging
Co-57	270 d	EC, γ	122	"Mock Tc," markers, vitamin B-12 Schilling test
Cr-51	28 d	EC, γ	320	RBC survival
Ga-67	78 h	EC, γ	93, 184, 300	Tumors, infections, lymphomas, hepatomas, bronchogenic carcinomas
I-123	13.1 h	EC, γ	159	Thyroid uptake, imaging
I-125	60 d	EC, γ	30 × + γ	In vitro therapy, seed implants, radioimmunoassay
In-111	2.8 d	EC, γ	173, 247	Tag WBCs for infections, MoAbs, tumors, cisternography-DTPA
Pd-103	16.9 d	EC, γ	21	Seed implant therapy
Rb-81	4.7 h	EC, γ, β^+	190, 446, 511	Generators for Kr
Se-75	120 d	EC, γ	265	Pancreatic imaging
Tl-201	73 h	EC, γ	135, 167, γ 68–80 Hg k x-rays	Myocardial perfusion
Xe-127	36 d	EC, γ	202	Pulmonary ventilation
Yb-169	32 d	EC, γ	177, 198	Cisternography
C-11	20 m	β^+	511	Brain PET, cardiac PET
F-18	110 m	β^+	511	Brain PET, cardiac PET (fluorodeoxyglucose FDG)
N-13	10 m	β^+	511	Brain PET, myocardial perfusion
O-15	2.1 m	β^+	511	Brain PET, cardiac PET

Equations

1. Pediatric doses: $\dfrac{\text{wt. in kg} \times \text{adult dose}}{70 \text{ kg}} = \text{pediatric dose}$

2. Drawing doses: $\dfrac{\text{what you want}}{\text{what you have}} = \text{what you will get}$

   Or: $\dfrac{\text{dose needed (mCi)}}{C_1 \text{ (concentration on hand in mCi/mL)}} = V_1 \text{ (volume to draw up in mL)}$

3. Weight: weight in lb $\div$ 2.2 = kg; weight in kg $\times$ 2.2 = lb

4. Height: height in inches $\times$ 2.54 = cm; height in cm $\div$ 2.54 = inches

5. Activity: mCi $\times$ 37 = MBq; MBq $\div$ 37 = mCi

6. Cardiac functions:

   Target heart rates: 220 $-$ age = 100% target heart rate (HR)

   % Ejection fraction: $\dfrac{ED - ES}{ED} \times 100,$

   where ED is end-diastolic volume, and ES is end-systolic volume

   SV (stroke volume) = ED $-$ ES

   CO (cardiac output in mL) = SV $\times$ HR

7. Decay: $A_t = A_0 \, e^{-\frac{.693}{t_{1/2}}(t)}$

8. Inverse square law: $I_1 D_1^{\,2} = I_2 D_2^{\,2}$ (I = intensity in mR/time, D = distance)

9. Concentrations: $C_1 V_1 = C_2 V_2$ (C = concentration in mCi/mL, V = volume in mL)

10. Doses from concentrations:

    Decay concentration: $C_2 = C_1 \, e^{-\frac{.693}{t_{1/2}}(t)}$

    Draw from concentration: $C_1 = \dfrac{A_0}{V_1}$

11. Shielding: $I_2 = I_1 \, e^{-\frac{.693}{HVL}(x)}$ (X = thickness of material)

    (HVL = half value layer of radionuclide)

    (I = intensity of radionuclide)

12. Effective/biologic half-lives: $t_e = \dfrac{t_{1/2} \times t_b}{t_{1/2} + t_b}$

    $t_b = \dfrac{t_{1/2} \times t_e}{t_{1/2} - t_e}$

Kit Preparations (Overview)

General Considerations

- Most kit preparations are for use with ^{99m}Tc-pertechnetate, which is usually supplied in bulk form from the radiopharmacy or from department generators.

- Check to make sure you have the proper kit or vial with an unexpired date on the label.

- If more than one is being prepared at the same time, label each lead container properly.

- When adding the ^{99m}Tc-pertechnetate to the kit(s), it is important not to introduce any O_2 from the syringe into the vial as this may oxidize the ^{99m}Tc or seriously affect the stannous ions. If you add, e.g., 2 mL of ^{99m}Tc-pertechnetate or normal saline to a kit vial, withdraw the 2 mL of air before removing syringe. This will help to remove any unwanted O_2 and leave the vial with negative pressure. This is a desired result.

- Use only normal nonbacteriostatic 0.9% NaCl without preservatives to dilute the pertechnetate and kits for dilution to proper concentration.

- Follow instructions on kit package inserts if available, paying close attention to suggested mCi, volumes, and incubation time before injection.

- On the label, note the name of the kit, total activity, total volume, specific activity (mCi/mL), date, time made, expiration date, and time.

- Record this information as well as lot numbers from the kit and pertechnetate, into the computer or log book.

- Perform quality control on the product before injection.

Rules of Thumb

- Never use < 30 mCi in a kit. Some require or suggest more (30–100 or more mCi per kit).

- Most are brought up to a total of about 2–4 mL with normal saline after the pertechnetate is added for a good and workable concentration.

- If you are needing ~25 mCi and a small bolus is preferred, use 50–70 mCi of pertechnetate and bring up to 2–3 mL for concentration. If you are needing 5 mCi, use less pertechnetate and 3–4 mL of saline. Most institutions have established protocols to follow for each type of kit.

- Always remember to label the lead container.

Example: Say you get bulk ^{99m}Tc, 100 mCi/2 mL. Dose calibrate vial, it is now 72 mCi/2 mL (36 mCi/mL). You want 40 mCi for a Choletec® kit. What you want ÷ what you have = what you will get; or 40 mCi ÷ 36 mCi/mL = 1.1 mL. Draw 1.1 mL into a 3-mL (or 5-mL) syringe. Dose calibrate syringe. It comes out to 38 mCi. Say you want to bring it up to 3 mL. Draw 1.9 mL normal saline. It is now 38 mCi/3 mL (12.6 mCi/mL). Inject into kit, withdraw air, swirl, run quality control, and incubate for proper time. Say your protocol calls for 5 mCi of Choletec®. What you want ÷ what you have = what you will get; or 5 mCi ÷ 12.6 mCi/mL = 0.39 or 0.4 mL. In a fresh syringe, draw ~0.4 mL from kit. Dose calibrate your syringe, it should be 5 mCi ± 10%. If you do not like the math, common sense and eye balling will get you pretty much to the same place.

Note

Chromatography

Thin-layer chromatography is usually the recommended quality control. Protocols for each kit, supplies on hand, and specific instructions vary slightly among institutions. Most kits on hand are for routine on-call procedures or radiopharmacy after-hours routine procedures. Most of these involve ^{99m}Tc-pertechnetate and must have 90–95% radiochemical purity for their use. Most need to incubate (reconstitute) for about 5 minutes after radioactivity and normal saline are added to the vial. Follow protocols supplied by the department or hospital (or package insert if none are available).

Here is just one example of a hospital protocol for mixing up kit preparations.

Bone	Osteolite®	up to 200 mCi	2–8 mL	stand for 2 min
Lung	diethylenetriaminepentaacetic acid	up to 100 mCi	2–8 mL	stand for 2 min
	Pulmolite®*	up to 50 mCi	2–8 mL	stand for 2 min
Liver/spleen	Microlite®	up to 75 mCi	2–8 mL	stand for 2 min
Gallbladder	Choletec®	up to 100 mCi	1–5 mL	stand for 15 min
Tagged RBC	Cold Pyp		1.5–2.5 mL	stand for 3–5 min

Protocols

There are many protocols and supply companies with different products and kits that may be used at various institutions. Most have a list with specific instructions in the hot lab.

*One that must be handled with care is the macroaggregated albumin kit. If a kit is made up early in the evening and more out of the same vial is needed much later, care must be taken not to inject the patient with too many particles.

Particles in Kits

- Particles in kits range from 2–8 million/vial. Average, 5 million.

- Accepted range of particles injected per dose, 200,000 to 700,000. Average, 450,000.

- Accepted range of activity is 3–5 mCi (111–185 MBq). Average, 4 mCi (148 MBq).

- A workable concentration for this scenario (assuming an uncompromised adult patient):

    - Pull 50 mCi from bulk ^{99m}Tc; it is (for instance) in 1 mL.

    - Add 4 mL (or whatever to bring to 5 mL) normal saline. Inject into macroaggregated albumin vial.

    - Results: 50 mCi/5 mL or 10 mCi/mL.

- Particle number is now (on average) 5,000,000/5 mL or 1,000,000/mL.

- A 4-mCi dose drawn immediately is 0.4 mL, having 400,000 particles (on average). Well within accepted limits.

- In 6 hours, the kit has decayed to 25 mCi/5 mL or 5 mCi/mL. These concentration ratios remain pretty much the same whether the kit has been used earlier or not. A 4-mCi dose then is 0.8 mL and 800,000 particles (on average) and at the upper recommended limit of particles per dose.

- 75–100 mCi at the start is not unlikely for busy departments.

- A rule of thumb in the case of using aging kits is to never draw up more than 1 mL into the injection syringe. It's better to give a low dose than to jeopardize the patient's mortality. Better yet, if more bulk ^{99m}Tc is available, make a new kit.

Choletec® is a registered trademark of Bracco Diagnostics, Inc., Princeton, NJ.
Microlite® is a registered trademark of DuPont Merck, Wilmington, DE.
Osteolite® is a registered trademark of DuPont Merck, Wilmington, DE.
Pulmolite® is a registered trademark of DuPont Merck, Wilmington, DE.

Notes

Pediatric Dosing in Nuclear Medicine

Standard Pediatric Dose *(Clark's Rule)*

(Patient weight in kg × standard adult dose) ÷ 70 kg = pediatric dose.

(Patient weight in lb × standard adult dose) ÷ 154 lb = pediatric dose.

The standard adult dose assumes a 70 kg or 154 lb person ÷ 20% (56−84 kg, 123−185 lb).

Dose by body surface area (modified Talbot's nomogram)

kg	lb	Surface Area (m^2)	% of Adult Dose
1	2.2	0.09	5
2	4.4	0.15	8
3	6.6	0.20	11
4	8.8	0.24	13
5	11.0	0.28	16
6	13.2	0.32	18
7	15.4	0.35	20
8	17.6	0.39	22
9	19.8	0.42	24
10	22.0	0.46	26
11	24.2	0.49	27
12	26.4	0.52	29
13	28.6	0.55	31
14	30.8	0.58	32
15	33.0	0.61	34
20	44.0	0.74	42
25	55.0	0.87	49
30	66.0	0.98	55
35	77.0	1.10	62
40	88.0	1.20	68
45	99.0	1.31	73
50	110.0	1.41	79
55	121.0	1.50	84
60	132.0	1.60	90
65	143.0	1.69	95
70	154.0	1.78	100

body surface area (BSA) = $(body\ weight)^{0.7}/11$

For 70 kg adult, BSA = 1.779 m^2

% of adult dose = $BSA/1.779 × 100$

(from the Mayo Clinic Manual of Nuclear Medicine)

Note

A child's physiology and metabolism is not a miniature adult's; uptake of radiopharmaceuticals vary greatly. For instance, a child's thyroid is perhaps 50% smaller than an adult's but has the same uptake. Bone uptake in children is ~80% compared with that of adults at ~40%. The weight of a 1-year-old child's brain may be 80% of the adult weight, whole body ~15%, and liver ~25%. Many methods to calculate proper doses have been considered.

As well as the standard weight method and body surface area methods above, others have considered the mass of target organs.

Weight/Metabolic Rule

$$\text{Pediatric dose} = \frac{(Mp)^{2/3}}{(Ma)^{2/3}} \times \text{adult dose}$$

where Mp = mass of pediatric organ, and Ma = mass of adult organ

Webster's rule (age/mass approximation)

$$\text{Pediatric dose} = \frac{x + 1}{x + 7} \times \text{adult dose}$$

where x is the age of the child

Adjusted Webster's or Wellman

< 5 years old:	25% of adult dose
5–10 years old:	50% of adult dose
10–15 years old:	75% of adult dose
> 15 years old:	adult dose

Young's Rule

$$\text{Pediatric dose} = \frac{\text{age (in yrs)}}{\text{age} + 12} \times \text{adult dose}$$

Modified Wright's formula *(old formula and radiotracers but it is based in kilograms)*

Child Dose

Study	Radiotracer	Amount	Minimum/Patient
Bone	^{99m}Tc-PP	0.240 mCi/kg	
Bone marrow	^{99m}Tc-SC	0.100 mCi/kg	
Cardiac	^{99m}Tc-O$_4^-$	0.240 mCi/kg	
Cerebral	^{99m}Tc-O$_4^-$	0.240 mCi/kg	2 mCi
Cerebral	^{99m}Tc-DTPA	0.280 mCi/kg	2 mCi
Cisternogram	^{131}I-IHSA-H	1.5 µCi/kg	25 µCi/max = 100 µCi
Cisternogram	^{111}In-DTPA	0.030 mCi/kg	
GI bleed	^{99m}Tc-O$_4^-$	0.240 mCi/kg	2 mCi
Hepatic	^{99m}Tc-SC	0.050 mCi/kg	200 µCi

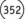

Study	Radiotracer	Amount	Minimum/Patient
Pulmonary	^{99m}Tc-MS	0.030 mCi/kg	
Pulmonary	^{133}Xe	0.147 mCi/kg	
Renal	^{131}I-OIH	1.5 µCi/kg per kidney:	25 µCi/max = 200 µCi
Renal	^{99m}Tc-DTPA	0.070 mCi/kg per kidney	
Thyroid	^{123}I-sodium iodide	1.5 µCi/kg	
Thyroid	^{99m}Tc-O$_4^-$	0.030 mCi/kg	0.5 mCi/max = 2.0 mCi
Spleen	^{99m}Tc-SC	0.050 mCi/kg	

$$\text{child dose} + \frac{(\text{child weight in kg} \times \text{standard adult dose})}{\text{adult weight in kg*}}$$

*63.63 kg for hepatic study; 58.18 kg for cerebral study; 72.72 kg for all other studies

As indicated in the above table, there are minimum doses to consider (to ensure enough counts [photon flux] for a diagnostic examination). Here is a more current list based in pounds from the Children's Memorial Hospital in Chicago:

Procedure	Radiotracer	Dose	Minimum	Maximum
Angiogram	^{99m}Tc-O$_4^-$	200 µCi/lb	2.5 mCi	15 mCi
Bone scan	^{99m}Tc-MDP/HDP	300 µCi/lb	5 mCi	20 mCi
LTD bone scan	^{99m}Tc-MDP/HDP	200 µCi/lb	5 mCi	20 mCi
Brain scan	^{99m}Tc-DTPA	400 µCi/lb	10 mCi	20 mCi
Cystogram	^{99m}Tc-O$_4^-$	1 mCi	1 mCi	1 mCi
Dacryoscintigraphy	^{99m}Tc-O$_4^-$	200 µCi/drop	400 µCi	800 µCi
Gallium scan	^{67}Ga-citrate	3–10 mCi	3 mCi	10 mCi
GE reflux	^{99m}Tc-SC	150 µCi	150 µCi	150 µCi
GI bleed	^{99m}Tc-SC	5 mCi	1 mCi	5 mCi
HIDA	^{99m}Tc-disofenin	1.0–8.0 mCi	1 mCi	8 mCi
Liver scan	^{99m}Tc-SC	25 µCi/lb	500 µCi	2 mCi
Lung scan	^{99m}Tc-MAA	25 µCi/lb	500 µCi	2 mCi
Meckel's	^{99m}Tc-O$_4^-$	100 µCi/lb	2.5 mCi	15 mCi
mIBG scan	^{131}I-mIBG		500 µCi	2 mCi
MUGA	^{99m}Tc-RBCs	350 µCi/lb	10 mCi	20 mCi
Plasma volume	^{123}I-HSA	3 µCi	1 µCi	3 µCi
Renal scan	^{99m}Tc-DTPA	50 µCi/lb	2.5 mCi	15 mCi
	^{99m}Tc-MAG$_3$	22 µCi/lb	1 mCi	5 mCi
Renogram	^{131}I-IOH	100 µCi	50 µCi	100 µCi
Subarachnoid scan	^{111}In-DTPA	300 µCi	100 µCi	300 µCi
Testicular scan	^{99m}Tc-O$_4^-$	200 µCi/lb	5.0 mCi	15 mCi
Thyroid uptake	^{123}I-sodium iodide	100 µCi	2 µCi	100 µCi
Thyroid scan	^{99m}Tc-O$_4^-$	1–2 mCi	1 mCi	2 mCi

And as more proof that printed data vary from source to source, the following scans and minimum doses are taken from the Mayo Clinic Manual of Nuclear Medicine:

Procedure	Radiopharmaceutical	Minimum Dose
Central nervous system		
Brain SPECT	^{99m}Tc-HMPAO or ECD	2 mCi (74 MBq)
CSF imaging (cisternography/ventriculography)	^{111}In-DTPA	100 µCi (3.7 MBq)
Recurrent brain tumor	^{201}Tl-thallous chloride	50 µCi (1.85 MBq)
Brain death	^{99m}Tc-HMPAO	2 mCi (74 MBq)
Cardiovascular system		
Cardiac left to right shunt	^{99m}Tc-DTPA	2 mCi (74 MBq)
Angiography	^{99m}Tc-RBCs	5 mCi (185 MBq)
Perfusion study	^{99m}Tc-sestamibi/tetrafosmin	3 mCi (111 MBq)
	^{201}Tl-thallous chloride	300 µCi (11.1 MBq)
MI study	^{99m}Tc-pyp	4 mCi (148 MBq)
Endocrine system		
Substernal thyroid	^{131}I-sodium iodide	20 µCi (0.740 MBq)
	^{123}I-sodium iodide	30 µCi (1.11 MBq)
Thyroid scan	^{99m}Tc-O$_4^-$	1 mCi (37 MBq)
^{131}I Uptake	^{131}I-sodium iodide	2 µCi (0.074MBq)
^{131}I Neck scan	^{131}I-sodium iodide	150 µCi (5.55 MBq)
^{131}I Total body scan	^{131}I-sodium iodide	150 µCi (5.55 MBq)
Parathyroid scan	^{99m}Tc-O$_4^-$	250 µCi (9.25 MBq)
	^{99m}Tc-sestamibi/tetrafosmin	3 mCi (111 MBq)
Adrenal medulla scan	^{131}I-mIBG	500 µCi (18.5 MBq)
	^{123}I-mIBG	2 mCi (74 MBq)
Adrenal cortex scan	^{131}I-NP-59	500 µCi (18.5 MBq)
Gastrointestinal system		
Salivary gland scan	^{99m}Tc-O$_4^-$	1 mCi (37 MBq)
Esophageal study	^{99m}Tc-sulfur colloid	150 µCi (5.55 MBq)
GE reflux	^{99m}Tc-sulfur colloid	500 µCi (18.5 MBq)
Gastric empty	^{99m}Tc-sulfur colloid	500 µCi (18.5 MBq)
	^{111}In-DTPA	250 µCi (9.25 MBq)
GI bleed	^{99m}Tc-RBCs	2 mCi (74 MBq)
Meckel's	^{99m}Tc-O$_4^-$	2 mCi (74 MBq)
Protein-losing enteropathy	^{99m}Tc-human serum albumin	2 mCi (74 MBq)
Liver/spleen scan	^{99m}Tc-sulfur colloid	500 µCi (18.5 MBq)
Liver SPECT	^{99m}Tc-RBCs	2 mCi (74 MBq)
HIDA	^{99m}Tc-disofenin	1 mCi (37 MBq)

Procedure	Radiopharmaceutical	Minimum Dose
Genitourinary system		
Renal scan	^{99m}Tc-MAG$_3$	1 mCi (37 MBq)
	^{99m}Tc-DTPA	2.5 mCi (9.25 MBq)
Renal cortical scan	^{99m}Tc-DMSA	500 μCi (18.5 MBq)
Cystography	^{99m}Tc-DTPA Age 0–1	1 mCi (37 MBq)
	Age > 1	2 mCi (74 MBq)
Residual urine study	^{99m}Tc-DTPA	500 μCi (18.5 MBq)
Testicular scan	^{99m}Tc-O$_4^-$	2 mCi (74 MBq)
Infection/bone		
WBC scan	^{111}In-WBCs	50 μCi (1.85 MBq)
	^{99m}Tc-HMPAO	1 mCi (37 MBq)
Gallium scan	^{67}Ga-gallium citrate	1 mCi (37 MBq)
Bone marrow scan	^{99m}Tc-sulfur colloid	500 μCi (18.5 MBq)
Bone scan	^{99m}Tc-MDP	4 mCi (148 MBq)
Joint scan	^{99m}Tc-O$_4^-$	1 mCi (37 MBq)
Respiratory system		
Lung ventilation	^{133}Xe gas	1 mCi (37 MBq)
aerosol	^{99m}Tc-DTPA	100 μCi (3.7 MBq)
pertechnegas	^{99m}Tc-pertechnegas	none established
Lung perfusion	^{99m}Tc-MAA	500 μCi (18.5 MBq)
Tumor imaging		
Gallium scan	^{67}Ga-gallium citrate	1 mCi (37 MBq)
Oncoscint®	^{111}In-Oncoscint®	none established
Special imaging		
Dacryoscintigraphy	^{99m}Tc-O$_4^-$	200 μCi (7.4 MBq)/eye
LeVeen shunt	^{99m}Tc-MAA (into shunt tubing)	100 μCi (3.7 MBq)
	(intraperitoneal)	1 mCi (37 MBq)

SUGGESTED READINGS

Bernier, DR, Christian PE, Langan JK, eds. Nuclear Medicine: Technology and Techniques. 3rd ed. St. Louis: Mosby, 1994.

O'Connor, MK. The Mayo Clinic Manual of Nuclear Medicine. New York: Churchill Livingstone, 1996.

Murray IPC, Ell PJ, eds. Nuclear Medicine in Clinical Diagnosis and Treatment. Vols. 1 and 2. New York: Churchill Livingstone, 1994.

Wilson, MA. Textbook of Nuclear Medicine. Philadelphia: Lippincott-Raven, 1998.

OncoScint® is a registered trademark of Cytogen Corporation, Princeton, NJ.

Radioactive Isotopes

(highest % of significant energies)   ✓ = emissions but no significant % or energies

Isotope	Name	$T_{1/2}$	α MeV	%	β⁻ Max MeV	β⁻ Ave MeV	%	β⁺ Max MeV	β⁺ Ave MeV	%	γ MeV	%
Ac-225	Actinium	10.00 d	5.731	10							0.12	22
			5.792	18								
			5.829	52								
Ac-227	Actinium	21.77 y	✓		0.0344	0.0087	35				✓	
					0.0437	0.0111	54					
Ac-228	Actinium	6.130 h			1.168	0.3860	32				0.338	11
					1.741	0.6110	12				0.911	28
											0.969	17
Ag-106m	Silver	8.460 d									0.451	28
											0.512	88
											0.616	22
											0.717	29
											1.05	30
Ag-108	Silver	2.370 min			1.650	0.6290	96	✓			✓	
Ag-108m	Silver	127.0 y									0.434	90
											0.614	90
											0.723	91
Ag-109m	Silver	39.60 s									0.022	19
Ag-110	Silver	24.57 s			2.893	1.199	95				✓	
Ag-110m	Silver	249.9 d			0.0839	0.0218	67				0.658	94
					0.5307	0.1656	31				0.764	22
											0.885	73
											0.937	34
											1.38	24
Ag-111	Silver	7.460 d			1.028	0.3604	92				✓	
Al-26	Aluminum	7.20×10^5 y						1.174	0.5439	82	0.511	166
											1.81	99
Al-28	Aluminum	2.240 min			2.864	1.242	100				1.78	100
Am-241	Americium	432.2 y	5.486	85							0.014	43
											0.060	36
Am-242	Americium	16.02 h			0.6190	0.1848	42				0.015	20
					0.6612	0.1990	41					

Isotope	Name	$T_{1/2}$	α MeV	%	β^- Max MeV	β^- Ave MeV	%	β^+ Max MeV	β^+ Ave MeV	%	γ MeV	%
Am-242m	Americium	152.0	✓								0.015	30
Am-243	Americium	7.380×10^3 y	5.275	88							0.014	39
											0.075	66
Am-244	Americium	10.10 h			0.3870	0.1096	100				0.015	117
											0.746	67
											0.900	28
Am-245	Americium	122.4 min			0.8961	0.2810	77				✓	
Am-246	Americium	25.00 min			1.221	0.4000	38				0.015	39
											0.799	25
											1.08	28
Ar-37	Argon	35.02 d									0.003	9
Ar-39	Argon	269.0 y			0.5650	0.2188	100					
Ar-41	Argon	1.827 h			1.198	0.4593	99				1.29	99
As-72	Arsenic	26.00 h						2.495	1.115	65	0.511	176
											0.834	80
As-73	Arsenic	80.30 d									0.010	90
As-74	Arsenic	17.77 d			1.353	0.5309	19	0.9445	0.4080	27	0.511	59
											0.596	60
As-76	Arsenic	26.32 h			2.410	0.9963	35				0.559	45
					2.969	1.267	51					
As-77	Arsenic	38.80 h			0.6904	0.2318	97				✓	
At-211	Astatine	7.214 h	5.867	42							0.079	21
At-217	Astatine	0.032 s	7.066	100							✓	
Au-194	Gold	39.50 h						✓			0.328	64
Au-195	Gold	183.0 d									0.065	29
											0.067	50
											0.076	22
Au-195m	Gold	30.60 s									0.262	68
Au-196	Gold	6.183 d			✓						0.065	22
											0.067	38
											0.333	23
											0.355	88
Au-198	Gold	2.696 d			0.9607	0.3146	99				0.412	96
Au-199	Gold	3.139 d			0.2448	0.0673	21				0.158	37
					0.2946	0.0824	66					

Isotope	Name	$T_{1/2}$	α MeV	%	β⁻ Max MeV	β⁻ Ave MeV	%	β⁺ Max MeV	β⁺ Ave MeV	%	γ MeV	%
Ba-131	Barium	11.80 d									0.123	29
											0.216	20
											0.496	47
Ba-133	Barium	10.50 y									0.031	97
											0.035	23
											0.081	33
											0.356	61
Ba-133m	Barium	38.90 h									0.032	28
Ba-135m	Barium	28.70 h									0.032	28
Ba-137m	Barium	2.552 min									0.662	90
Ba-139	Barium	83.10 min			2.140	0.8370	22				0.166	17
					2.306	0.9120	78					
Ba-140	Barium	12.79 d			0.4539	0.1360	26				0.537	26
					0.9912	0.3400	37					
					1.005	0.3570	22					
Ba-141	Barium	18.27 min			2.382	0.9470	25				0.190	49
					2.563	1.029	19				0.277	25
											0.304	27
Ba-142	Barium	10.70 min			0.9960	0.3400	40				0.255	18
Be-7	Beryllium	53.44 d									0.478	10
Be-10	Beryllium	1.6×10^6 y			0.5558	0.2025	100					
Bi-206	Bismuth	6.24 d									0.011	49
											0.073	32
											0.075	54
											0.085	24
											0.344	23
											0.516	41
											0.538	31
											0.803	99
											0.881	66
											1.72	32
Bi-207	Bismuth	33.40 y									0.011	36
											0.073	22
											0.075	37
											0.570	98
											1.06	75

Isotope	Name	$T_{1/2}$	α MeV	%	β⁻ Max MeV	β⁻ Ave MeV	%	β⁺ Max MeV	β⁺ Ave MeV	%	γ MeV	%
Bi-208	Bismuth	368.0×10^3 y									0.011	31
											0.075	21
											2.62	100
Bi-210	Bismuth	5.013 d			1.161	0.3890	100					
Bi-211	Bismuth	2.130 min	6.279	16	✓						0.351	13
			6.623	84								
Bi-212	Bismuth	60.55 min	6.051	25	2.246	0.8316	48				0.727	12
Bi-213	Bismuth	45.65 min	✓		0.9796	0.3190	32				0.440	28
					1.420	0.4910	64					
Bi-214	Bismuth	19.90 min			1.506	0.5250	18					
					1.540	0.5390	18					
					3.270	1.269	17				0.609	46
Bk-249	Berkelium	320.0 d			0.1264	0.0330	100					
Bk-250	Berkelium	3.222 h			0.7483	0.2280	83				0.989	45
											1.03	35
Bk-251	Berkelium	57.0 min			1.120	0.3611	100					
Br-77	Bromine	57.04 h						✓			0.239	23
											0.521	22
Br-80	Bromine	17.40 min			2.006	0.8050	85	✓			✓	
Br-80m	Bromine	4.420 h									0.037	39
Br-82	Bromine	35.30 h			0.4443	0.1378	98				0.554	71
											0.619	43
											0.698	28
											0.776	83
											0.828	24
											1.04	27
											1.32	27
Br-83	Bromine	2.390 h			0.9184	0.3230	99				✓	
Br-84	Bromine	31.80 min			4.673	2.072	32				0.882	42
Br-85	Bromine	172.0 s			2.495	1.030	96				✓	
C-11	Carbon	20.48 min						0.9601	0.3856	100	0.511	200
C-14	Carbon	5.730×10^3 y			0.1565	0.0495	100					
C-15	Carbon	2.449 s			4.510	2.000	68				✓	
					9.820	4.354	32					
Ca-41	Calcium	103.0×10^3 y									0.003	12

Isotope	Name	$T_{1/2}$	α MeV	%	β⁻ Max MeV	β⁻ Ave MeV	%	β⁺ Max MeV	β⁺ Ave MeV	%	γ MeV	%
Ca-45	Calcium	162.7 d			0.2569	0.0772	100				✓	
Ca-47	Calcium	4.536 d			0.6905	0.2409	82				1.30	75
Ca-49	Calcium	8.719 min			2.184	0.9086	92				3.08	92
Cd-109	Cadmium	464.0 d									0.022	35
Cd-111m	Cadmium	48.70 min									0.151	31
											0.245	94
Cd-113	Cadmium	9.3 × 10¹⁵ y			0.3220	0.0933	100					
Cd-113 m	Cadmium	13.70 y			0.5857	0.1854	100					
Cd-115	Cadmium	53.46 h			0.5834	0.1846	35				0.528	29
					1.111	0.3944	60					
Cd-115m	Cadmium	44.60 d			1.621	0.6150	98				✓	
Cd-117	Cadmium	2.490 h			0.6361	0.2040	32				0.273	28
					2.213	0.8820	21					
Cd-117 m	Cadmium	3.360 h			0.5694	0.1790	26				1.07	23
					0.6671	0.2160	47				2.00	26
Ce-139	Cerium	137.7 d									0.166	80
Ce-141	Cerium	32.50 d			0.4346	0.1296	71				0.145	48
					0.5800	0.1807	30					
Ce-143	Cerium	33.0 h			1.104	0.3846	48				0.036	32
					1.398	0.5075	38				0.293	42
Ce-144	Cerium	284.3 d			0.3182	0.0911	77				✓	
Cf-248	Californium	333.5 d	6.260	83							✓	
Cf-249	Californium	350.6 y	5.814	84							0.388	66
Cf-250	Californium	13.08 y	6.031	83							✓	
Cf-251	Californium	900.0 y	5.677	35							0.015	60
			5.852	27							0.109	25
Cf-252	Californium	2.639 y	6.118	82							✓	
Cf-253	Californium	17.81 d	✓		0.2870	0.0790	100				✓	
Cf-254	Californium	60.50 d	✓								✓	
Cl-36	Chlorine	301.0 × 10³ y			0.7096	0.2513	99				✓	
Cl-38	Chlorine	37.21 min			1.107	0.4203	33				1.64	33
					4.917	2.244	56				2.17	44
Cm-242	Curium	163.2 d	6.070	26							✓	
			6.113	74								
Cm-243	Curium	28.50 y	5.785	73							0.104	23

Isotope	Name	$T_{1/2}$	α MeV	%	β⁻ Max MeV	β⁻ Ave MeV	%	β⁺ Max MeV	β⁺ Ave MeV	%	γ MeV	%
Cm-244	Curium	18.11 y	5.763	24							✓	
			5.805	76								
Cm-245	Curium	8.50×10^3 y	5.362	93							0.104	22
Cm-246	Curium	4.750×10^3 y	5.343	21								
			5.386	79							✓	
Cm-247	Curium	15.60×10^6 y	4.868	71							0.402	72
Cm-248	Curium	339.0×10^3 y	5.079	75							✓	
Cm-249	Curium	64.15 min			0.8912	0.2790	96				✓	
Cm-250	Curium	6.90×10^3 y	5.190	25	0.0370	0.0090	14					
Co-56	Cobalt	78.76 d						1.461	0.6319	19	0.511	40
											0.847	100
											1.24	67
Co-57	Cobalt	270.9 d									0.122	86
Co-58	Cobalt	70.80 d						0.4750	0.2012	15	0.511	30
											0.811	99
Co-58m	Cobalt	9.150 h									✓	
Co-60	Cobalt	5.271 y			0.3179	0.0958	100				1.17	100
											1.33	100
Co-60m	Cobalt	10.47 min			✓						✓	
Co-61	Cobalt	1.650 h			1.255	0.4744	96				0.067	85
Cr-49	Chromium	42.09 min						1.453	0.6255	46	0.091	53
								1.515	0.6537	35	0.153	30
											0.511	184
Cr-51	Chromium	27.70 d									✓	
Cs-126	Cesium	1.640 min			3.419	1.560	24				0.389	38
					3.808	1.740	51				0.511	164
Cs-129	Cesium	32.06 h									0.372	31
											0.412	23
Cs-131	Cesium	9.688 d									0.030	60
Cs-132	Cesium	6.475 d			✓			✓			0.668	97
Cs-134	Cesium	2.062 y			0.0885	0.0231	27				0.605	98
					0.6578	0.2101	70				0.796	85
Cs-134 m	Cesium	2.90 h									✓	

Isotope	Name	$T_{1/2}$	α MeV	%	β⁻ Max MeV	β⁻ Ave MeV	%	β⁺ Max MeV	β⁺ Ave MeV	%	γ MeV	%
Cs-135	Cesium	2.30×10^6 y			0.2050	0.0563	100					
Cs-136	Cesium	13.16 d			0.3410	0.0988	95				0.341	49
											0.819	100
											1.05	80
Cs-137	Cesium	30.17 y			0.5115	0.1568	95					
Cs-138	Cesium	32.20 min			2.884	1.179	44				0.463	31
											1.01	30
											1.44	76
Cs-139	Cesium	9.40 min			4.204	1.794	84				✓	
Cu-61	Copper	3.408 h						1.216	0.5242	51	0.511	123
Cu-62	Copper	9.740 min						2.927	1.316	98	0.511	196
Cu-64	Copper	12.70 h			0.5782	0.1902	37	0.6529	0.2781	18	0.511	36
Cu-67	Copper	61.88 d			0.3904	0.1210	57				0.185	49
					0.4817	0.1540	22					
					0.5750	0.1890	20					
Dy-157	Dysprosium	8.060 h									0.326	94
Dy-165	Dysprosium	2.334 h			1.285	0.4531	83				✓	
Dy-166	Dysprosium	81.60 h			0.4015	0.1175	92				0.047	37
Er-169	Erbium	9.40 d			0.3418	0.0979	45				✓	
					0.3502	0.1006	55					
Er-171	Erbium	7.520 h			1.066	0.3622	94				0.112	21
											0.296	29
											0.308	64
Es-253	Einsteinium	20.47 d	6.633	90							✓	
Es-254	Einsteinium	275.7 d	6.429	93							✓	
Es-254m	Einsteinium	39.30 h	✓		0.4373	0.1247	19				0.649	34
					0.4772	0.1373	67				0.694	29
Es-255	Einsteinium	39.80 d	✓		0.2800	0.0767	92				✓	
Eu-152	Europium	13.60 y			✓						0.122	28
											0.344	27
											1.41	21
Eu-152m	Europium	9.320 h			1.865	0.7041	67				✓	
Eu-154	Europium	8.80 y			0.2474	0.0688	27				0.123	41
					0.5694	0.1757	37				1.28	36

Isotope	Name	$T_{1/2}$	α MeV	%	β⁻ Max MeV	β⁻ Ave MeV	%	β⁺ Max MeV	β⁺ Ave MeV	%	γ MeV	%
Eu-155	Europium	4.960 y			0.1407	0.0374	46				0.087	31
					0.1595	0.0428	26				0.105	21
Eu-156	Europium	15.19 d			0.4871	0.1470	32				✓	
					2.453	0.9660	27					
F-18	Fluorine	109.7 min						0.6335	0.2498	97	0.511	194
Fe-52	Iron	8.275 h						0.8036	0.3400	56	0.169	97
											0.511	112
Fe-55	Iron	2.70 y									✓	
Fe-59		44.63 d			0.2734	0.0810	45				1.10	57
					0.4658	0.1492	53				1.29	43
Fm-254	Fermium	3.240 h	7.189	85							✓	
Fm-255	Fermium	20.07 h	7.022	93							✓	
Fm-256	Fermium	157.6 min	✓									
Fr-221	Francium	2.80 min	6.340	83							✓	
Fr-223	Francium	21.80 min			1.098	0.3611	57				0.050	32
Ga-66	Gallium	9.40 h						4.153	1.904	49	0.511	115
											1.04	39
											2.75	24
Ga-67	Gallium	3.261 d									0.093	36
											0.185	20
											0.300	16
Ga-68	Gallium	68.0 min						1.899	0.8630	88	0.511	178
Ga-72	Gallium	14.10 h			0.6666	0.2235	22				0.630	24
					0.9561	0.3418	28				0.834	96
											2.20	26
Gd-152	Gadolinium	1.1 × 10¹⁴ y	2.150	100								
Gd-153	Gadolinium	241.6 d									0.097	31
											0.103	22
Gd-159	Gadolinium	18.56 h			0.9167	0.3057	21				✓	
					0.9747	0.3286	70					
Gd-162	Gadolinium	9.70 m			0.9584	0.3200	100				0.403	46
											0.411	53
Ge-68	Germanium	288.0 d									✓	
Ge-71	Germanium	11.80 d									✓	

Isotope	Name	$T_{1/2}$	α MeV	%	β⁻ Max MeV	β⁻ Ave MeV	%	β⁺ Max MeV	β⁺ Ave MeV	%	γ MeV	%
Ge-77	Germanium	11.30 h			1.512	0.5835	19				0.211	31
					2.070	0.8389	21				0.216	28
					2.226	0.9117	17				0.264	53
											0.416	22
H-3	Hydrogen	12.28 y			0.0186	0.0057	100					
Hf-181	Hafnium	42.39 d			0.4072	0.1187	93				0.133	42
											0.482	83
Hg-197	Mercury	64.14 h									✓	
Hg-197m	Mercury	23.80 h									0.134	34
Hg-203	Mercury	46.60 d			0.2122	0.0577	100				0.279	77
Ho-166	Holmium	26.80 h			1.774	0.6511	48				✓	
					1.854	0.6938	51					
Ho-166m	Holmium	1.20×10^3 y			0.0724	0.0187	73				0.184	73
											0.281	30
											0.712	54
											0.810	57
I-122	Iodine	3.620 min						3.118	1.414	63	0.511	152
											0.564	21
I-123	Iodine	13.13 h									0.159	83
I-124	Iodine	4.180 d						✓			0.511	47
											0.603	59
I-125	Iodine	60.14 d									0.027	112
											0.031	25
I-126	Iodine	12.93 d			0.8624	0.2897	27	✓			0.389	29
											0.666	40
I-128	Iodine	24.99 min			2.127	0.8357	80				✓	
I-129	Iodine	15.70×10^6 y			0.1524	0.0409	100				✓	
I-130	Iodine	12.36 h			0.6219	0.1970	47				0.418	34
					1.034	0.3610	48				0.536	99
											0.669	96
											0.740	82
I-131	Iodine	8.040 d			0.6063	0.1916	89				0.365	81
I-132	Iodine	2.30 h			1.185	0.4220	19				0.668	99
					2.140	0.8410	17				0.773	76

Isotope	Name	$T_{1/2}$	α MeV	%	β⁻ Max MeV	β⁻ Ave MeV	%	β⁺ Max MeV	β⁺ Ave MeV	%	γ MeV	%
I-133	Iodine	20.80 h			1.230	0.4410	84				0.530	86
I-134	Iodine	52.60 min			1.283	0.4600	33				0.847	95
											0.884	65
I-135	Iodine	6.610 h			1.033	0.3590	22				1.13	23
					1.451	0.5350	24				1.26	29
I-136	Iodine	83.0 s			4.366	1.880	36				1.31	69
					5.687	2.500	30				1.32	26
In-111	Indium	2.830 d									0.171	90
											0.245	94
In-113m	Indium	1.658 h									0.392	65
In-114	Indium	71.90 s			1.984	0.7769	99				✓	
In-114m	Indium	49.51 d									✓	
In-115	Indium	4.6×10^{15} y			0.4950	0.1520	100					
In-115m	Indium	4.360 h			✓						0.336	47
In-116m	Indium	54.15 min			0.8711	0.2950	33				0.417	28
					1.009	0.3510	51				1.10	55
											1.29	89
In-117	Indium	43.80 min			0.7435	0.2450	100				0.159	86
											0.553	99
In-117m	Indium	116.5 min			1.770	0.6800	35				0.315	19
Ir-190	Iridium	11.78 d									0.187	50
											0.371	22
											0.407	23
											0.519	32
											0.558	29
											0.569	27
											0.605	38
Ir-190m1	Iridium	1.20 h									✓	
Ir-190m2	Iridium	3.20 h									0.063	35
Ir-192	Iridium	74.02 d			0.5361	0.1612	41				0.296	29
					0.6724	0.2089	48				0.309	30
											0.317	83
											0.468	48
Ir-193m	Iridium	11.90 d									✓	
Ir-194	Iridium	19.15 h			2.251	0.8475	85				✓	

Isotope	Name	$T_{1/2}$	α MeV	%	β⁻ Max MeV	β⁻ Ave MeV	%	β⁺ Max MeV	β⁺ Ave MeV	%	γ MeV	%
Ir-194m	Iridium	171.0 d			0.2525	0.0697	100				0.329	93
											0.339	55
											0.391	35
											0.483	97
											0.562	70
											0.601	62
											0.689	59
K-40	Potassium	1.277×10^9 y			1.312	0.5085	89				✓	
K-42	Potassium	12.36 h			3.521	1.564	82				1.53	18
K-43	Potassium	22.60 h			0.8267	0.2980	92				0.373	87
											0.618	81
Kr-79	Krypton	35.04 h						✓			0.511	14
Kr-81	Krypton	210.0×10^3 y									✓	
Kr-83m	Krypton	1.830 h									✓	
Kr-85	Krypton	10.72 y			0.6870	0.2514	100				✓	
Kr-85m	Krypton	4.480 h			0.8407	0.2904	79				0.151	75
Kr-87	Krypton	76.30 min			3.486	1.502	47				0.403	50
					3.889	1.695	30					
Kr-88	Krypton	2.480 h			0.5209	0.1560	67				0.196	26
											2.39	35
Lr-89	Krypton	3.160 min			4.970	2.210	23				0.221	20
Kr-90	Krypton	32.32 s			2.610	1.086	62				0.122	32
					4.390	1.935	29				0.540	30
											1.12	37
La-140	Lanthanum	40.22 h			1.348	0.4874	45				0.329	21
					1.677	0.6295	21				0.487	46
											0.816	24
											1.60	96
La-141	Lanthanum	3.940 h			2.430	0.9670	97				✓	
La-142	Lanthanum	95.40 min			1.974	0.7610	20					
					2.119	0.8260	22					
Lu-177	Lutetium	6.710 d			0.4971	0.1489	79				✓	
Lu-177m	Lutetium	160.1 d			0.1518	0.405	79				0.113	22
											0.208	61
											0.228	37

Isotope	Name	$T_{1/2}$	α MeV	%	β^- Max MeV	β^- Ave MeV	%	β^+ Max MeV	β^+ Ave MeV	%	γ MeV	%
											0.379	28
											0.419	20
Mg-27	Magnesium	9.458 min			1.595	0.6457	29				0.844	72
					1.765	0.7244	71				1.01	28
Mg-28	Magnesium	20.91 h			0.4589	0.1559	95				0.401	37
											0.942	38
											1.34	53
Mn-52	Manganese	5.591 d						0.5753	0.2416	29	0.511	59
											0.744	90
											0.936	95
											1.43	100
Mn-52m	Manganese	21.40 min						2.633	1.174	96	0.511	193
											1.43	98
Mn-53	Manganese	3.70×10^6 y									✓	
Mn-54	Manganese	312.7 d									0.835	100
Mn-56	Manganese	2.578 h			1.038	0.3819	28				0.847	99
					2.849	1.217	56				1.81	27
Mn-57	Manganese	1.470 min			2.678	1.135	81				✓	
Mo-91	Molybdenum	15.49 min						3.416	1.553	93	0.511	188
Mo-93	Molybdenum	3.50×10^3 y									✓	
Mo-99	Molybdenum	66.02 h			0.4360	0.1330	17					
					1.214	0.4427	83				0.740	13
Mo-101	Molybdenum	14.61 min			0.7633	0.2560	21				0.192	19
N-13	Nitrogen	9.970 min			1.199	0.4918	100				0.511	200
N-16	Nitrogen	7.13 s			4.288	1.941	68				6.13	69
Na-22	Sodium	2.602 y						0.5455	0.2155	90	0.511	180
											1.28	100
Na-24	Sodium	15.0 h			1.390	0.5539	100				1.37	100
											2.75	100
Nb-90	Niobium	14.60 h						1.500	0.6622	53	0.141	69
											0.511	106
											1.13	92
											2.32	82
Nb-91	Niobium	10.0×10^3 y						✓			✓	

Isotope	Name	$T_{1/2}$	α MeV	%	β^- Max MeV	β^- Ave MeV	%	β^+ Max MeV	β^+ Ave MeV	%	γ MeV	%
Nb-91m	Niobium	61.0 d									✓	
Nb-92	Niobium	36.0×10^6 y									0.561	100
											0.935	100
Nb-92m	Niobium	10.15 d									0.935	99
Nb-93m	Niobium	14.60 y									✓	
Nb-94	Niobium	20.30×10^3 y			0.4715	0.1458	100				0.703	100
											0.871	100
Nb-94m	Niobium	6.260 min			✓						✓	
Nb-95	Niobium	35.06 d			0.1598	0.0434	100				0.766	100
Nb-95m	Niobium	86.60 h			✓						0.236	25
Nb-96	Niobium	23.35 h			0.7486	0.2406	96				0.460	28
											0.569	56
											0.778	97
											0.850	21
											1.09	49
											1.20	20
Nb-97	Niobium	72.10 min			1.275	0.4698	98				0.658	98
Nb-97m	Niobium	60.0 s									0.743	98
Nd-147	Neodymium	10.98 d			0.8047	0.2640	81				0.091	28
Nd-149	Neodymium	1.730 h			1.151	0.4024	24				0.211	27
					1.478	0.5398	26					
Ni-56	Nickel	6.10 d									0.158	99
											0.270	37
											0.480	37
											0.750	50
											0.812	86
Ni-57	Nickel	36.08 h						0.8434	0.3590	33	0.511	80
											1.38	78
Ni-59	Nickel	75.0×10^3 y									✓	
Ni-63	Nickel	100.1 y			0.0659	0.0171	100					
Ni-65	Nickel	2.520 h			0.6552	0.2209	28				1.48	24
					2.137	0.8757	61					
Np-235	Neptunium	396.1 d									✓	

Isotope	Name	$T_{1/2}$	α MeV	%	β⁻ Max MeV	β⁻ Ave MeV	%	β⁺ Max MeV	β⁺ Ave MeV	%	γ MeV	%
Np-236	Neptunium	115.0 + 10³ y			✓						0.094	21
											0.098	34
											0.160	28
Np-236m	Neptunium	22.50 h			0.5360	0.1580	40				✓	
Np-237	Neptunium	2.140 × 10⁶ y	4.771	25							✓	
			4.788	47								
Np-238	Neptunium	2.117 d			0.2634	0.0722	42				0.985	24
					1.248	0.4124	45					
Np-239	Neptunium	2.355 d			0.3298	0.0921	35				0.104	24
					0.4360	0.1253	52				0.106	23
Np-240	Neptunium	65.0 min			0.7814	0.2410	100				0.566	27
											0.601	20
											0.974	21
Np-240m	Neptunium	7.40 min			1.513	0.5140	32					
					2.067	0.7330	52				0.554	22
O-15	Oxygen	122.24 s						1.732	0.7352	100	0.511	200
Os-185	Osmium	93.60 d									0.646	80
Os-186	Osmium	2.0 × 10¹⁵ y	2.756	100								
Os-190m	Osmium	9.90 min									0.187	70
											0.361	95
											0.503	98
											0.616	99
Os-191	Osmium	15.40 d			0.1388	0.0367	100				0.129	26
Os-191m	Osmium	13.03 h									✓	
Os-193	Osmium	30.00 h			1.132	0.3831	53				✓	
P-32	Phosphorus	14.29 d			1.710	0.6949	100					
P-33	Phosphorus	25.40 d			0.2490	0.0766	100					
Pa-230	Protactinium	17.40 d			✓						0.093	31
											0.952	29
Pa-231	Protactinium	32.76 × 10³ y	4.950	23							✓	
			5.011	25								
			5.028	20								

Isotope	Name	$T_{1/2}$	α MeV	%	β⁻ Max MeV	β⁻ Ave MeV	%	β⁺ Max MeV	β⁺ Ave MeV	%	γ MeV	%
Pa-233	Protactinium	27.00 d			0.1565	0.0415	24				0.312	39
					0.2318	0.0630	28					
					0.2604	0.0714	33					
Pa-234	Protactinium	6.70 h			0.6887	0.1410	24				0.098	25
											0.131	20
Pa-234m	Protactinium	1.170 min			2.281	0.8254	99				✓	
Pb-203	Lead	52.02 h									0.279	77
Pb-204m	Lead	66.90 min									0.375	94
											0.899	99
											0.912	91
Pb-205	Lead	15.10 × 10⁶ y									0.010	23
Pb-209	Lead	3.253 h			0.6646	0.1976	100					
Pb-210	Lead	22.26 y			0.0165	0.0041	80				0.011	24
					0.0630	0.0161	20					
Pb-211	Lead	36.10 min			1.373	0.4733	93				✓	
Pb-212	Lead	10.64 h			0.3342	0.0944	85				0.239	45
Pb-214	Lead	26.80 min			0.6721	0.2070	48				0.352	37
					0.7288	0.2270	43					
Pd-103	Palladium	16.96 d									✓	
Pd-107	Palladium	6.5 × 10⁶ y			0.0331	0.0093	100					
Pd-109	Palladium	13.45 h			1.028	0.3610	100				✓	
Pm-143	Promethium	265.0 d									0.742	38
Pm-144	Promethium	363.0 d									0.477	42
											0.618	99
											0.697	100
Pm-145	Promethium	17.70 y									✓	
Pm-146	Promethium	5.534 y			0.7949	0.2599	34				0.454	63
											0.736	22
											0.747	36
Pm-147	Promethium	2.623 y			0.2247	0.0620	100				✓	
Pm-148	Promethium	5.370 d			0.9989	0.3400	33				0.550	22
					2.464	0.9750	56				1.47	22
Pm-148m	Promethium	41.30 d			0.4072	0.1200	54				0.550	95
					0.6953	0.2220	22				0.630	89

Isotope	Name	$T_{1/2}$	α MeV	%	β⁻ Max MeV	β⁻ Ave MeV	%	β⁺ Max MeV	β⁺ Ave MeV	%	γ MeV	%
											0.726	33
											1.01	20
Pm-149	Promethium	53.08 h			1.071	0.3690	96				✓	
Pm-151		28.40 h			0.8431	0.2780	43				0.340	23
Po-209	Polonium	102.0 y	4.882	99							✓	
Po-210	Polonium	138.4 d	5.305	100							✓	
Po-211	Polonium	0.5160 s	7.450	99							✓	
Po-212	Polonium	0.000 s	8.785	100								
Po-213	Polonium	0.000 s	8.377	100							✓	
Po-214	Polonium	0.000 s	7.687	100							✓	
Po-215	Polonium	0.001 s	7.386	100							✓	
Po-216	Polonium	0.146 s	6.779	100							✓	
Po-218	Polonium	3.050 min	6.003	100								
Pr-142	Praseody-mium	19.13 h			2.159	0.8328	96				✓	
Pr-143	Praseody-mium	13.56 d			0.9353	0.3156	100				✓	
Pr-144	Praseody-mium	17.28 min			2.996	1.221	98				✓	
Pr-144m	Praseody-mium	7.20 min									✓	
Pt-191	Platinum	2.710 d									0.065	65
Pt-193	Platinum	50.00 y									✓	
Pt-193m	Platinum	4.330 d									✓	
Pt-195m	Platinum	4.020 d									0.067	38
Pt-197	Platinum	18.30 h			0.6417	0.1977	82				✓	
Pt-197m	Platinum	94.40 min			✓						0.067	23
Pu-236	Plutonium	2.851 y	5.722	32							✓	
			5.770	68								
Pu-237	Plutonium	45.30 d									0.101	21
Pu-238	Plutonium	87.75 y	5.457	28							✓	
			5.499	72								
Pu-239	Plutonium	24.131 × 10³ y	5.155	73							✓	
Pu-240	Plutonium	6.537 × 10³ y	5.123	26							✓	
			5.168	74								

Isotope	Name	T$_{1/2}$	α MeV	%	β⁻ Max MeV	β⁻ Ave MeV	%	β⁺ Max MeV	β⁺ Ave MeV	%	γ MeV	%
Pu-241	Plutonium	14.40 y			0.208	0.0052	100					
Pu-242	Plutonium	375.80 × 10³ y	4.856	22							✓	
			4.901	78								
Pu-243	Plutonium	4.956 h			0.4980	0.1451	29				0.084	23
					0.5820	0.1727	59					
Pu-244	Plutonium	82.60 × 10⁶ y	4.546	20							✓	
			4.589	81								
Pu-245	Plutonium	10.57 h			0.9326	0.2950	57				0.327	27
PU-246	Plutonium	10.85 d			0.1503	0.0400	73				0.224	28
					0.3302	0.0920	27					
Ra-222	Radium	38.00 s	6.556	97							✓	
Ra-223	Radium	11.43 d	5.606	24							0.084	25
			5.715	53								
Ra-224	Radium	3.620 d	5.686	95							✓	
Ra-225	Radium	14.80 d			0.3220	0.0900	72					
					0.3620	0.1030	28				✓	
Ra-226	Radium	1.60 × 10³ y	4.785	95							✓	
Ra-228	Radium	5.750 y			0.0389	0.0099	100				✓	
Rb-81	Rubidium	4.580 h						1.050	0.4580	31	0.190	66
											0.511	66
Rb-82	Rubidium	1.250 min						3.356	1.524	83	0.511	191
Rb-83	Rubidium	86.20 d									0.520	46
											0.530	30
Rb-84	Rubidium	32.90 d			✓			✓			0.511	54
											0.882	68
Rb-86	Rubidium	18.66 d			1.774	0.7093	91				✓	
Rb-87	Rubidium	4.7 × 10¹⁰ y			0.2733	0.0788	100					
Rb-88	Rubidium	17.80 min			5.315	2.372	78				1.84	21
Rb-89	Rubidium	15.44 min			1.275	0.4736	33				1.03	58
					2.223	0.9031	34				1.25	42
					4.503	1.987	25					
Rb-90	Rubidium	157.0 s			6.553	2.976	37				0.832	33

Isotope	Name	$T_{1/2}$	α MeV	%	β⁻ Max MeV	β⁻ Ave MeV	%	β⁺ Max MeV	β⁺ Ave MeV	%	γ MeV	%
Rb-90m	Rubidium	258.0 s			✓						0.832	93
Re-182	Rhenium	64.0 h									0.059	87
											1.12	21
Re-182m	Rhenium	12.70 h						✓			0.059	52
											1.21	32
											1.22	25
Re-183	Rhenium	70.00 d									0.059	60
											0.162	23
Re-184	Rhenium	38.00 d									0.059	44
											0.792	37
											0.903	38
Re-184m	Rhenium	169.0 d									0.061	24
Re-186	Rhenium	90.64 h			0.9394	0.3088	22				✓	
					1.077	0.3620	71					
Re-187	Rhenium	4.7 × 10¹⁰ y			0.0026	0.0006	100					
Re-188	Rhenium	16.98 h			1.965	0.7286	25				✓	
					2.120	0.7951	71					
Rh-103m	Rhodium	56.12 min									✓	
Rh-105	Rhodium	35.36 h			0.2480	0.0699	20					
					0.5669	0.1794	75				0.319	19
Rh-105m	Rhodium	45.00 s									0.130	20
Rh-106	Rhodium	29.92 s			3.541	1.509	79				0.512	21
Rn-218	Radon	0.035 s	7.133	100							✓	
Rn-219	Radon	3.960 s	6.819	80							✓	
Rn-220	Radon	55.61 s	6.288	100							✓	
Rn-222	Radon	3.823 d	5.490	100							✓	
Ru-97	Ruthenium	2.90 d									0.216	86
Ru-103	Ruthenium	39.35 d			0.2261	0.0632	90				0.497	89
Ru-105	Ruthenium	4.440 h			1.112	0.3975	20				0.725	49
					1.193	0.4322	50					
Ru-106	Ruthenium	368.2 d			0.0394	0.0100	100					
S-35	Sulfur	87.44 d			0.1675	0.0488	100					
Sb-117	Antimony	2.800 h						✓			0.159	86
Sb-122	Antimony	2.700 d			1.417	0.5224	67				0.564	71
					1.981	0.7721	26					

Isotope	Name	$T_{1/2}$	α MeV	%	β⁻ Max MeV	β⁻ Ave MeV	%	β⁺ Max MeV	β⁺ Ave MeV	%	γ MeV	%
Sb-124	Antimony	60.20 d			0.6113	0.1940	53				0.603	98
					2.302	0.9186	22				1.69	49
Sb-125	Antimony	2.770 y			0.3034	0.0870	40				0.428	29
Sb-126	Antimony	12.40 d			0.3714	0.1090	29				0.415	83
					1.068	0.3740	16				0.666	97
					1.789	0.6890	19				0.695	100
											0.697	29
											0.721	54
Sb-126	Antimony	19.00 min			1.807	0.6940	81				0.415	86
											0.666	86
											0.695	86
Sb-127	Antimony	3.850 d			0.8959	0.3041	35				0.473	25
					1.108	0.3909	22				0.685	36
Sb-128	Antimony	4.400 h			0.5344	0.1660	23				0.813	46
					0.6497	0.2080	27				0.915	21
Sc-44	Scandium	3.927 h						1.476	0.6329	94	0.511	189
Sc-46	Scandium	83.80 d			0.3573	0.1120	100				0.889	100
											1.12	100
Sc-46m	Scandium	18.72 s									0.142	63
Sc-47	Scandium	3.422 d			0.4411	0.1427	68				0.159	68
					0.6005	0.2040	32					
Sc-48	Scandium	43.67 h			0.6569	0.2265	90				0.984	100
											1.04	98
											1.31	100
Sc-49	Scandium	54.40 min			2.004	0.8231	100				✓	
Sc-73	Selenium	7.150 h						1.290	0.5620	65	0.067	77
											0.361	97
											0.511	132
Se-75	Selenium	119.8 d									0.136	59
											0.264	60
											0.280	25
Se-79	Selenium	65.00 × 10³ y			0.1490	0.0522	100					
Si-31	Silicon	157.3 min			1.491	0.5956	100				✓	
Si-32	Silicon	330.0 y			0.2130	0.0647	100					

Isotope	Name	$T_{1/2}$	α MeV	%	β^- Max MeV	β^- Ave MeV	%	β^+ Max MeV	β^+ Ave MeV	%	γ MeV	%
Sm-147	Samarium	6.900×10^9 y	2.248	100								
Sm-151	Samarium	90.00 y			0.0761	0.0197	99				✓	
Sm-153	Samarium	46.70 h			0.634	0.1986	34				0.103	28
					0.7020	0.2244	44					
					0.8052	0.2634	21					
Sn-113	Tin	115.1 d									✓	
Sn-117m	Tin	13.60 d									0.159	86
Sn-119m	Tin	293.0 d									✓	
Sn-123	Tin	129.2 d			1.397	0.5231	99				✓	
Sn-125	Tin	1.640 d			2.350	0.9380	83				✓	
Sn-126	Tin	100.0×10^3 y			0.2501	0.0700	100				0.088	37
Sr-82	Strontium	25.00 d									✓	
Sr-85	Strontium	64.84 d									0.514	99
Sr-85m	Strontium	67.66 min									0.232	85
Sr-87m	Strontium	2.805 h									0.388	82
Sr-89	Strontium	50.55 d			1.491	0.5830	100				✓	
Sr-90	Strontium	28.60 y			0.5460	0.1958	100					
Sr-91	Strontium	9.500 h			1.104	0.3989	34				0.750	23
					1.379	0.5180	24				1.02	33
					2.684	1.121	31					
Sr-92	Strontium	2.710 h			0.5461	0.1740	96				1.38	90
Sr-93	Strontium	7.30 min			1.692	0.6600	18				0.710	22
					2.733	1.140	16				0.876	24
											0.888	22
Ta-182	Tantalum	114.7 d			0.2581	0.716	29				0.068	42
					0.4375	0.1286	21				1.12	35
					0.5222	0.1572	41				1.22	27
Tb-157	Terbium	150.0 y									✓	
Tb-160	Terbium	72.30 d			0.5687	0.1750	46				0.299	27
					0.8673	0.2860	25				0.879	29
											0.966	24
Tb-162	Terbium	7.760 min			1.382	0.4900	96				0.808	42
											0.888	38
Tc-95	Technetium	20.00 h									0.766	94

Isotope	Name	T$_{1/2}$	α MeV	%	β$^-$ Max MeV	β$^-$ Ave MeV	%	β$^+$ Max MeV	β$^+$ Ave MeV	%	γ MeV	%
Tc-95m	Technetium	61.00 d						✓			0.204	62
											0.582	29
											0.835	26
Tc-96	Technetium	4.280 d									0.778	100
											0.813	82
											0.850	98
Tc-96m	Technetium	51.50 min									✓	
Tc-97	Technetium	2.600 × 10^6 y									0.018	36
Tc-97m	Technetium	89.00 d									0.018	27
Tc-98	Technetium	4.200 × 10^6 y			0.3942	0.1180	100				0.652	100
											0.745	100
Tc-99	Technetium	213.0 × 10^3 y			0.2936	0.0846	100				✓	
Tc-99m	Technetium	6.020 h									0.140	89
Tc-101	Technetium	14.20 min			1.318	0.4870	89				0.307	88
Te-121	Tellurium	16.80 d									0.573	80
Te-121m	Tellurium	154.0 d									0.212	81
Te-123	Tellurium	1.0 × 10^{13} y									0.026	38
Te-123m	Tellurium	119.7 d									0.159	84
Te-125m	Tellurium	58.00 d									0.027	92
Te-127	Tellurium	9.350 h			0.6940	0.2247	99				✓	
Te-127m	Tellurium	109.0 d	✓								0.027	29
Te-129	Tellurium	69.60 min			1.470	0.5445	90				✓	
Te-129m	Tellurium	33.60 d			1.604	0.6073	33				✓	
Te-131	Tellurium	25.00 min			1.687	0.6220	22				0.150	69
					2.099	0.8250	59					
Te-131m	Tellurium	30.00 h			0.4510	0.1362	37				0.774	38
Te-132	Tellurium	78.20 h			0.2151	0.0594	100				0.228	88
Te-133	Tellurium	12.45 min			2.250	0.8900	33				0.312	71
					2.658	1.080	29				0.408	30
Te-133m	Tellurium	55.40 min			1.528	0.5700	20				0.864	20
					1.744	0.6700	29				0.913	87
					2.392	0.9600	38					

Isotope	Name	$T_{1/2}$	α MeV	%	β⁻ Max MeV	β⁻ Ave MeV	%	β⁺ Max MeV	β⁺ Ave MeV	%	γ MeV	%
Te-134	Tellurium	41.80 min			0.3766	0.1108	43				0.079	21
					0.4533	0.1370	41				0.210	22
											0.278	21
											0.767	30
Th-226	Thorium	30.90 min	6.234	23							✓	
			6.338	76								
Th-227	Thorium	18.72 d	5.757	20							✓	
			5.978	23								
			6.038	25								
Th-228	Thorium	1.913 y	5.341	27							✓	
			5.423	73								
Th-229	Thorium	7.340×10^3 y	4.845	56							0.089	27
Th-230	Thorium	77.00×10^3 y	4.621	23							✓	
			4.688	76								
Th-231	Thorium	25.52 h			0.2876	0.0796	41				✓	
					0.3047	0.0848	35					
Th-232	Thorium	1.4×10^{10} y	3.953	23							✓	
			4.010	77								
Th-233	Thorium	22.30 min			1.239	0.4121	51				✓	
					1.245	0.4146	30					
Th-234	Thorium	24.10 d			0.1886	0.0506	73				✓	
Ti-44	Titanium	47.30 y									0.068	92
											0.078	98
Ti-45	Titanium	3.080 h						1.041	0.4391	85	0.511	170
Ti-51	Titanium	5.752 min			2.146	0.8882	92				0.320	93
Tl-200	Thallium	26.10 h						✓			0.069	24
											0.071	40
											0.368	87
											1.21	30
Tl-201	Thallium	73.06 h									0.069	27
											0.71	47
											0.080	21
											0.167	10

Isotope	Name	$T_{1/2}$	α MeV	%	β⁻ Max MeV	β⁻ Ave MeV	%	β⁺ Max MeV	β⁺ Ave MeV	%	γ MeV	%
Tl-202	Thallium	12.23 d									0.069	23
											0.071	39
											0.440	92
Tl-204	Thallium	3.779 y			0.7634	0.2439	97				✓	
Tl-207	Thallium	4.770 min			1.422	0.4941	100				✓	
Tl-208	Thallium	3.053 min			1.284	0.4387	23				0.511	22
					1.517	0.5325	23				0.583	84
					1.794	0.6465	49				2.62	100
Tl-209	Thallium	2.200 min			1.825	0.6590	100				0.117	77
											0.465	97
											1.57	100
Tl-210	Thallium	1.300 min			1.317	0.4500	25				0.298	79
					1.867	0.6800	56				0.800	99
					2.337	0.8700	19				1.31	21
Tm-170	Thulium	128.6 d			0.8837	0.2904	24				✓	
					0.9679	0.3231	76					
Tm-171	Thulium	1.920 y			0.0967	0.0252	98				✓	
U-230	Uranium	20.80 d	5.818	32							✓	
			5.889	67								
U-231	Uranium	4.200 d									0.096	28
U-232	Uranium	72.00 y	5.264	31							✓	
			5.320	69								
U-233	Uranium	159.20 10^3 y	4.824	84							✓	
U-234	Uranium	244.50 × 10^3 y	4.724	27							✓	
			4.776	72								
U-235	Uranium	703.80 × 10^6 y	4.396	55							0.184	54
U-236	Uranium	3.415 × 10^6 y	4.445	26								
			4.494	74							✓	
U-237	Uranium	6.750 d			0.2381	0.0648	53				0.060	34
					0.2519	0.0688	44				0.101	26
											0.208	22

Isotope	Name	$T_{1/2}$	α MeV	%	β^- Max MeV	β^- Ave MeV	%	β^+ Max MeV	β^+ Ave MeV	%	γ MeV	%
U-238	Uranium	4.468×10^9 y	4.147	23							✓	
			4.196	77								
U-239	Uranium	23.40 min			1.191	0.3920	68				0.075	48
					1.266	0.4206	28					
U-240	Uranium	14.10 h			0.4360	0.1250	100				✓	
V-48	Vanadium	15.97 d						0.6974	0.2914	50	0.511	100
											0.984	100
											1.31	98
V-49	Vanadium	330.0 d									✓	
V-52	Vanadium	3.750 min			2.542	1.074	99				1.43	100
W-181	Tungsten	121 d									0.057	33
W-185	Tungsten	75.10 d			0.4324	0.1268	100				✓	
W-187	Tungsten	23.83 h			0.6267	0.1935	59				0.480	23
					1.313	0.4571	25				0.686	29
W-188	Tungsten	69.40 d			0.3490	0.0997	99				✓	
Xe-122	Xenon	20.10 h									0.028	63
Xe-123	Xenon	2.140 h						1.505	0.6740	17	0.028	60
											0.149	48
											0.511	45
Xe-125	Xenon	16.80 h						✓			0.028	81
											0.188	55
											0.243	29
Xe-127	Xenon	36.41 d									0.028	71
											0.172	25
											0.203	68
Xe-129m	Xenon	8.890 d									0.029	103
											0.034	24
Xe-131m	Xenon	11.84 d									0.029	43
Xe-133	Xenon	5.245 d			0.3463	0.1006	99				0.030	38
											0.081	36
Xe-133m	Xenon	2.190 d									0.029	45
Xe-135	Xenon	9.110 h			0.9092	0.3080	96				0.250	90
Xe-135m	Xenon	15.36 min									0.527	81

Isotope	Name	$T_{1/2}$	α MeV	%	β⁻ Max MeV	β⁻ Ave MeV	%	β⁺ Max MeV	β⁺ Ave MeV	%	γ MeV	%
Xe-137	Xenon	3.830 min			3.889	1.649	30				0.456	31
					4.344	1.862	67					
Xe-138	Xenon	14.13 min			0.7133	0.2310	33				0.258	32
					2.290	0.9080	20				0.435	20
Y-86	Yttrium	14.74 h						1.254	0.5500	12	0.511	66
											0.628	33
											0.777	22
											1.08	83
											1.15	31
											1.92	21
Y-87	Yttrium	80.30 h						✓			0.485	94
Y-88	Yttrium	106.6 d						✓			0.898	93
											1.84	99
Y-90	Yttrium	64.10 h			2.284	0.9348	100					
Y-90m	Yttrium	3.190 h									0.203	97
											0.480	91
Y-91	Yttrium	58.51 d			1.543	0.6038	100				✓	
Y-91m	Yttrium	49.71 min									0.558	95
Y-92	Yttrium	3.540 h			3.634	1.563	86				0.935	14
Y-93	Yttrium	10.10 h			2.890	1.214	90				✓	
Yb-169	Ytterbium	31.97 d									0.050	53
											0.051	93
											0.058	38
											0.063	44
											0.177	21
											0.198	35
Yb-175	Ytterbium	4.190 d			0.4679	0.1392	87				✓	
Zn-62	Zinc	9.260 h						✓			0.041	27
											0.597	28
Zn-65	Zinc	244.4 d						✓			1.12	51
Zn-69	Zinc	55.60 min			0.9045	0.3209	100				✓	
Zn-69m	Zinc	13.76 h									0.439	95
Zr-86	Zirconium	16.50 h									0.243	96

Isotope	Name	$T_{1/2}$	α MeV	%	β⁻ Max MeV	β⁻ Ave MeV	%	β⁺ Max MeV	β⁺ Ave MeV	%	γ MeV	%
Zr-88	Zirconium	83.40 d									0.393	97
Zr-89	Zirconium	78.43 h						0.9047	0.3969	23	0.511	46
											0.909	99
Zr-93	Zirconium	1.530×10^6 y			0.0615	0.0195	100					
Zr-95	Zirconium	64.02 d			0.3664	0.1093	55				0.724	44
					0.3989	0.1204	44				0.757	55
Zr-97	Zirconium	16.90 h			1.914	0.7566	86				✓	

Excerpted from Hacker C. *Radiation Decay: Emissions Tables and Spectra.* 3.5-inch floppy disk program, Rockville, MD: Grove Engineering, 1995. Most isotopes have many more emissions than are listed. For a complete list, please refer to the program mentioned or one that is similar. If discrepancies are noted, be aware that published energy and half-life values vary slightly from source to source.

Decay Tables of Common Radionuclides

^{137}Cs

^{57}Co

^{67}Ga

^{111}In

^{123}I

^{131}I

^{99}Mo

^{99m}Tc

^{201}Tl

^{133}Xe

Cesium-137 Decay Table

Radionuclide: ^{137}Cs

$t_{1/2}$: 30.17 years

Energies: Beta (maximums): 511.6 keV (94.6%), 1173.2 keV (5.4%)

             Gamma: 661.7 keV (89.98% from ^{137m}Ba, $t_{1/2}$ 2.55 minutes)

Type: β^-, γ emitter, fission product

Decays to: ^{137m}Ba $\rightarrow$ ^{137}Ba (100%)

Original amount $\times$ decay factor (DF) for years and/or days = factored amount

Ex: 10 mCi after 6 years 35 days: 10 $\times$ 0.8713 (6 years) $\times$ 0.9978 (35 days) = 8.69 mCi

Days	DF	Days	DF	Days	DF	Years	DF	Years	DF	Years	DF	Years	DF
1	0.9999	13	0.9992	50	0.9968	2	0.9551	14	0.7250	26	0.5503	50	0.3171
2	0.9999	14	0.9991	60	0.9962	3	0.9334	15	0.7085	27	0.5378	55	0.2827
3	0.9998	15	0.9991	70	0.9956	4	0.9122	16	0.6925	28	0.5256	60	0.2520
4	0.9997	16	0.9990	80	0.9950	5	0.8915	17	0.6767	29	0.5137	65	0.2247
5	0.9997	17	0.9989	90	0.9943	6	0.8713	18	0.6614	30	0.5020	70	0.2003
6	0.9996	18	0.9989	100	0.9937	7	0.8515	19	0.6463	32	0.4795	75	0.1786
7	0.9996	19	0.9988	150	0.9906	8	0.8321	20	0.6317	34	0.4580	80	0.1592
8	0.9995	20	0.9987	200	0.9875	9	0.8132	21	0.6173	36	0.4374	85	0.1419
9	0.9994	25	0.9984	250	0.9844	10	0.7948	22	0.6033	38	0.4178	90	0.1265
10	0.9994	30	0.9981	300	0.9813	11	0.7767	23	0.5896	40	0.3990	95	0.1128
11	0.9993	35	0.9978	350	0.9782	12	0.7591	24	0.5762	42	0.3811	100	0.1006
12	0.9992	40	0.9975	365	0.9773	13	0.7419	25	0.5631	45	0.3557	150	0.0319

Values for $t_{1/2}$, energies, and percentages vary from data source to data source.

These numbers were derived from the following formulas (1 year = 365.24 days):

$$e^{-\frac{.693}{11019.2908} \times \text{time in days}} \quad \text{for days}$$

$$e^{-\frac{.693}{30.17} \times \text{time in years}} \quad \text{for years}$$

Cobalt-57 Decay Table

Radionuclide: ^{57}Co

$t_{1/2}$: 271.8 days

Energies: 14.4 keV (9.5%), 122.1 keV (85.5%), 136.5 keV (10.6%)

Type: electron capture, γ emitter, accelerator

Decays to: ^{57}Fe (100%)

Original amount $\times$ decay factor (DF) for days and/or hours = factored amount

Ex: 10 mCi after 60 days 15 hours: 10×0.8581 (60 days) $\times 0.9984$ (15 hours) = 8.57 mCi

Hours	DF	Hours	DF	Days	DF	Days	DF	Days	DF	Days	DF	Days	DF
1	0.9999	13	0.9986	2	0.9949	14	0.9649	26	0.9359	70	0.8365	160	0.6650
2	0.9998	14	0.9985	3	0.9924	15	0.9625	27	0.9335	75	0.8259	170	0.6483
3	0.9997	15	0.9984	4	0.9899	16	0.9600	28	0.9311	80	0.8155	180	0.6320
4	0.9996	16	0.9983	5	0.9873	17	0.9576	29	0.9287	85	0.8052	190	0.6160
5	0.9995	17	0.9982	6	0.9848	18	0.9551	30	0.9264	90	0.7950	200	0.6005
6	0.9994	18	0.9981	7	0.9823	19	0.9527	35	0.9146	95	0.7849	250	0.5286
7	0.9993	19	0.9980	8	0.9798	20	0.9503	40	0.9030	100	0.7749	275	0.4960
8	0.9992	20	0.9979	9	0.9773	21	0.9479	45	0.8916	110	0.7554	300	0.4654
9	0.9990	21	0.9978	10	0.9748	22	0.9455	50	0.8803	120	0.7364	365	0.3943
10	0.9989	22	0.9977	11	0.9723	23	0.9430	55	0.8692	130	0.7179	400	0.3606
11	0.9988	23	0.9976	12	0.9699	24	0.9406	60	0.8581	140	0.6998	450	0.3175
12	0.9987	24	0.9975	13	0.9674	25	0.9382	65	0.8473	150	0.6822	500	0.2795

Values for $t_{1/2}$, energies, and percentages vary from data source to data source.

These numbers were derived from the following formulas:

$$e^{-\frac{.693}{6523.2} \times \text{time in hours}} \text{ for hours}$$

$$e^{-\frac{.693}{271.8} \times \text{time in days}} \text{ for days}$$

Gallium-67 Decay Table

Radionuclide: ^{67}Ga

$t_{1/2}$: 78.24 hours or 3.26 days

Energies: 93.3 keV (35.7%), 184.6 keV (19.7%), 300.2 keV (16%), 393.5 keV (4.5%)

Type: electron capture, γ emitter, accelerator

Decays to: ^{67}Zn (100%)

Original amount $\times$ decay factor (DF) for days, hours, and/or minues = factored amount

Ex: 8.5mCi after 6 h 35 min: 8.5 $\times$ 0.9482 (6 h) $\times$ 0.9948 (35 min) = 8.02 mCi

Min	DF	Hours	DF	Hours	DF	Hours	DF	Hours	DF	Hours	DF	Hours	DF
5	0.9993	2	0.9824	14	0.8834	26	0.7943	38	0.7142	52	0.6309	78	0.5011
10	0.9985	3	0.9738	15	0.8756	27	0.7873	39	0.7079	54	0.6198	80	0.4923
15	0.9978	4	0.9652	16	0.8679	28	0.7804	40	0.7017	56	0.6090	85	0.4710
20	0.9971	5	0.9567	17	0.8602	29	0.7735	41	0.6955	58	0.5983	90	0.4506
25	0.9963	6	0.9482	18	0.8526	30	0.7667	43	0.6833	60	0.5878	95	0.4311
30	0.9956	7	0.9399	19	0.8451	31	0.7599	44	0.6772	62	0.5774	100	0.4124
35	0.9948	8	0.9316	20	0.8377	32	0.7532	45	0.6713	64	0.5673	105	0.3945
40	0.9941	9	0.9234	21	0.8303	33	0.7465	46	0.6654	68	0.5476	110	0.3775
45	0.9934	10	0.9152	22	0.8229	34	0.7400	47	0.6595	70	0.5379	115	0.3611
50	0.9926	11	0.9072	23	0.8157	35	0.7334	48	0.6537	72	0.5285	120	0.3455
55	0.9919	12	0.8982	24	0.8085	36	0.7270	49	0.6479	74	0.5192	125	0.3305
60	0.9912	13	0.8912	25	0.8014	37	0.7206	50	0.6422	76	0.5101	130	0.3162

Values for $t_{1/2}$, energies, and percentages vary from data source to data source.

These numbers were derived from the following formulas:

$$e^{-\frac{.693}{4694.4} \times \text{time in minutes}} \text{ for minutes}$$

$$e^{-\frac{.693}{78.24} \times \text{time in hours}} \text{ for hours}$$

Indium-111 Decay Table

Radionuclide: ^{111}In

$t_{1/2}$: 67.92 hours or 2.83 days

Energies: 23 keV (68.2%), 171.3 keV (90.2%), 245.4 keV (94%)

Type: electron capture, γ emitter, accelerator

Decays to: ^{111}Cd (100%)

Original amount $\times$ decay factor (DF) for days, hours, and/or minutes = factored amount

Ex: 0.450 mCi after 6 h 35 min: 0.450 $\times$ 0.9406 (6 h) $\times$ 0.9941 (35 min) = 0.421 mCi

Min	DF	Hours	DF	Hours	DF	Hours	DF	Hours	DF	Hours	DF	Hours	DF
5	0.9992	2	0.9798	14	0.8669	26	0.7670	38	0.6786	52	0.5883	78	0.4512
10	0.9983	3	0.9699	15	0.8581	27	0.7592	39	0.6717	54	0.5764	80	0.4421
15	0.9975	4	0.9600	16	0.8494	28	0.7515	40	0.6649	56	0.5675	85	0.4201
20	0.9966	5	0.9503	17	0.8408	29	0.7439	41	0.6581	58	0.5533	90	0.3992
25	0.9958	6	0.9406	18	0.8322	30	0.7363	43	0.6449	60	0.5416	95	0.3793
30	0.9949	7	0.9311	19	0.8238	31	0.7288	44	0.6383	62	0.5312	100	0.3605
35	0.9941	8	0.9216	20	0.8154	32	0.7214	45	0.6318	64	0.5205	105	0.3426
40	0.9932	9	0.9123	21	0.8071	33	0.7141	46	0.6254	68	0.4997	110	0.3255
45	0.9924	10	0.9030	22	0.7989	34	0.7069	47	0.6191	70	0.4896	115	0.3092
50	0.9915	11	0.8938	23	0.7908	35	0.6997	48	0.6128	72	0.4797	120	0.2939
55	0.9907	12	0.8848	24	0.7828	36	0.6926	49	0.6066	74	0.4700	125	0.2793
60	0.9898	13	0.8758	25	0.7749	37	0.6856	50	0.6004	76	0.4605	130	0.2654

Values for $t_{1/2}$, energies, and percentages vary from data source to data source.

These numbers were derived from the following formulas:

$$e^{-\frac{.693}{4075.2} \times \text{time in minutes}} \text{ for minutes}$$

$$e^{-\frac{.693}{67.92} \times \text{time in hours}} \text{ for hours}$$

Iodine-123 Decay Table

Radionuclide: ^{123}I

$t_{1/2}$: 13.13 hours

Energies: 159 keV (83.3%), 27.5 keV (45.9%), 27.2 keV (24.7%)

Type: electron capture, γ emitter, accelerator

Decays to: ^{123}Te (100%)

Original amount $\times$ decay factor (DF) for days, hours, and/or minutes = factored amount

Ex: 0.250 mCi after 6 h 35 min; 0.250 $\times$ 0.7286 (6 h) $\times$ 0.9697 (35 min) = 0.177 mCi or: 0.250 mCi after 6 h 35 min: 0.250 $\times$ 0.7065 (6 h + 35 min) = 0.177 mCi.

Min	DF	2 h + DF	4 h + DF	6 h + DF	8 h + DF	10 h + DF	Hours	DF
0	1.0000	0.89982	0.80968	0.72856	0.65557	0.58990	-	-
5	0.9956	0.8959	0.8061	0.7254	0.6527	0.5873	12	0.5308
10	0.9912	0.8919	0.8026	0.7222	0.6498	0.5847	14	0.4776
15	0.9869	0.8880	0.7991	0.7190	0.6470	0.5822	16	0.4298
20	0.9826	0.8841	0.7956	0.7159	0.6441	0.5796	18	0.3867
25	0.9782	0.8802	0.7921	0.7127	0.6413	0.5771	20	0.3480
30	0.9739	0.8764	0.7886	0.7096	0.6385	0.5745	22	0.3131
35	0.9697	0.8725	0.7851	0.7065	0.6357	0.5720	24	0.2818
40	0.9654	0.8687	0.7817	0.7034	0.6329	0.5695	26	0.2535
45	0.9612	0.8649	0.7783	0.7003	0.6301	0.5670	28	0.2281
50	0.9670	0.8611	0.7748	0.6972	0.6274	0.5645	30	0.2053
55	0.9528	0.8573	0.7714	0.6942	0.6246	0.5620	48	0.0794
60	0.9486	0.8536	0.7681	0.6911	0.6219	0.5596	60	0.0421

Values for $t_{1/2}$, energies, and percentages vary from data source to data source.

These numbers were derived from the following formulas:

$$e^{-\frac{.693}{787.8} \times \text{time in minutes}} \text{ for minutes}$$

$$e^{-\frac{.693}{13.13} \times \text{time in hours}} \text{ for hours}$$

Iodine-131 Decay Table

Radionuclide: ^{131}I

$t_{1/2}$: 192.96 hours or 8.04 days

Energies: Beta (maximums): 606.3 keV (89.3%)

               Gamma: 364.5 keV (81.2%), 636.9 keV (7.3%)

Type: β^-, γ emitter, fission product

Decays to: ^{131}Xe (100%)

Original amount $\times$ decay factor (DF) for days, hours, and/or minutes = factored amount

Ex: 29 mCi after 6 h 35 min: 29 $\times$ 0.9787 (6 h) $\times$ 0.9979 (35 min) = 28.3 mCi

Min	DF	Hours	DF	Hours	DF	Hours	DF	Hours	DF	Hours	DF	Days	DF
5	0.9997	2	0.9928	14	0.9510	26	0.9108	38	0.8724	52	0.8296	4	0.7084
10	0.9994	3	0.9893	15	0.9476	27	0.9076	39	0.8630	54	0.8237	5	0.6499
15	0.9991	4	0.9857	16	0.9442	28	0.9043	40	0.8662	56	0.8178	6	0.5962
20	0.9988	5	0.9822	17	0.9408	29	0.9011	41	0.8631	58	0.8120	7	0.5470
25	0.9985	6	0.9787	18	0.9374	30	0.8979	43	0.8569	60	0.8062	8	0.5018
30	0.9982	7	0.9752	19	0.9340	31	0.8946	44	0.8538	62	0.8004	9	0.4604
35	0.9979	8	0.9717	20	0.9307	32	0.8914	45	0.8508	64	0.7947	10	0.4223
40	0.9976	9	0.9682	21	0.9274	33	0.8882	46	0.8477	68	0.7833	15	0.2745
45	0.9973	10	0.9641	22	0.9240	34	0.8851	47	0.8447	70	0.7777	20	0.1784
50	0.9970	11	0.9613	23	0.9207	35	0.8819	48	0.8416	72	0.7721	25	0.1159
55	0.9967	12	0.9578	24	0.9174	36	0.8787	49	0.8386	74	0.7666	30	0.0753
60	0.9964	13	0.9544	25	0.9141	37	0.8756	50	0.8352	76	0.7611	40	0.0318

Values for $t_{1/2}$, energies, and percentages vary from data source to data source.

These numbers were derived from the following formulas:

$$e^{-\frac{.693}{11577.6} \times \text{time in minutes}} \quad \text{for minutes}$$

$$e^{-\frac{.693}{192.96} \times \text{time in hours}} \quad \text{for hours}$$

Molybdenum-99 Decay Table

Radionuclide: ^{99}Mo

$t_{1/2}$: 66.02 hours or 2.75 days

Energies: Beta (maximums): 436 keV (17.3%), 1214 keV (82.7%)

Gamma: 140.5 keV (3.8%), 181 keV (6.2%), 739.6 keV (12.8%), 778 keV (4.5%)

Type: β^-, γ emitter, fission product

Decays to: ^{99}Tc (11%), ^{99m}Tc → ^{99}Tc (89%)

Original amount × decay factor (DF) for days, hours, and/or minutes = factored amount

Ex: 120 mCi after 6 h 35 min: 120 × 0.9390 (6 h) × 0.9939 (35 min) = 111.99 mCi

Min	DF	Hours	DF	Hours	DF	Hours	DF	Hours	DF	Hours	DF	Hours	DF	Hours	DF
5	0.9991	2	0.9792	14	0.8633	26	0.7612	38	0.6711	52	0.5794	78	0.4410
10	0.9983	3	0.9690	15	0.8543	27	0.7532	39	0.6641	54	0.5673	80	0.4318
15	0.9973	4	0.9589	16	0.8454	28	0.7453	40	0.6571	56	0.5555	85	0.4097
20	0.9965	5	0.9489	17	0.8366	29	0.7376	41	0.6503	58	0.5440	90	0.3888
25	0.9956	6	0.9390	18	0.8378	30	0.7299	43	0.6368	60	0.5327	95	0.3689
30	0.9948	7	0.9292	19	0.8192	31	0.7288	44	0.6301	62	0.5216	100	0.3500
35	0.9939	8	0.9195	20	0.8106	32	0.7147	45	0.6235	64	0.5108	105	0.3322
40	0.9930	9	0.9099	21	0.8022	33	0.7072	46	0.6170	68	0.4898	110	0.3152
45	0.9922	10	0.9004	22	0.7938	34	0.6998	47	0.6106	70	0.4796	115	0.2991
50	0.9913	11	0.8910	23	0.7855	35	0.6925	48	0.6042	72	0.4696	120	0.2838
55	0.9904	12	0.8816	24	0.7773	36	0.6853	49	0.5979	74	0.4599	125	0.2693
60	0.9896	13	0.8724	25	0.7692	37	0.6782	50	0.5916	76	0.4503	130	0.2555

Values for $t_{1/2}$, energies, and percentages vary from data source to data source.

These numbers were derived from the following formulas:

$$e^{-\frac{.693}{3961.2} \times \text{time in minutes}} \text{ for minutes}$$

$$e^{-\frac{.693}{66.02} \times \text{time in hours}} \text{ for hours}$$

Technetium-99m Decay Table

Radionuclide: ^{99m}Tc

$t_{1/2}$: 6.01 hours

Energies: 140.5 keV (89.1%), 18 keV (6%), 20.6 keV (1%)

Type: isomeric transition, γ emitter, generator

Decays to: ^{99}Tc (100%)

Original amount $\times$ decay factor (DF) for days, hours, and/or minutes = factored amount

Ex: 25 mCi after 2 h 35 min: 25 $\times$ 0.7940 (2 h) $\times$ 0.9349 (35 min) = 18.56 mCi or: 25 mCi after 2 h 35 min: 25 $\times$ 0.7424 (2 h + 35 min) = 18.56 mCi.

. . . .

Min	DF	1h + DF	2 h + DF	3 h + DF	4 h + DF	5 h + DF	Hours	DF
5	0.9904	0.8826	0.7865	0.7008	0.6245	0.5565	7	0.4461
10	0.9809	0.8741	0.7789	0.6941	0.6185	0.5511	8	0.3975
15	0.9716	0.8658	0.7715	0.6875	0.6126	0.5459	9	0.3542
20	0.9623	0.8575	0.7641	0.6809	0.6067	0.5407	10	0.3157
25	0.9531	0.8493	0.7568	0.6744	0.6009	0.5355	11	0.2813
30	0.9439	0.8412	0.7496	0.6679	0.5952	0.5304	12	0.2507
35	0.9349	0.8331	0.7424	0.6615	0.5895	0.5253	13	0.2234
40	0.9260	0.8252	0.7353	0.6552	0.5839	0.5203	14	0.1990
45	0.9172	0.8173	0.7283	0.6489	0.5783	0.5153	15	0.1774
50	0.9084	0.8096	0.7213	0.6427	0.5727	0.5104	16	0.1580
55	0.8997	0.8017	0.7144	0.6366	0.5673	0.5055	17	0.1408
60	0.8911	0.7940	0.7076	0.6305	0.5618	0.5006	18	0.1255

Values for $t_{1/2}$, energies, and percentages vary from data source to data source.

These numbers were derived from the following formulas:

$$e^{-\frac{.693}{360.6} \times \text{time in minutes}} \quad \text{for minutes}$$

$$e^{-\frac{.693}{6.01} \times \text{time in hours}} \quad \text{for hours}$$

Thallium-201 Decay Table

Radionuclide: ^{201}Tl

$t_{1/2}$: 73.06 hours or 3.04 days

Energies: 68.9 to 80.3 keV (94.3%), 135.3 keV (2.6%), 167.4 keV (10%)

Type: electron capture, γ emitter, accelerator

Decays to: ^{201}Hg (100%)

Original amount $\times$ decay factor (DF) for days, hours, and/or minutes = factored amount

Ex: 3.5 mCi after 6 h 35 min: 3.5×0.9447 (6 h) $\times 0.9945$ (35 min) = 3.29 mCi

Min	DF	Hours	DF	Hours	DF	Hours	DF	Hours	DF	Hours	DF	Hours	DF	Hours	DF
5	0.9992	2	0.9812	14	0.8756	26	0.7814	38	0.6974	52	0.6106	78	0.4772		
10	0.9984	3	0.9719	15	0.8674	27	0.7741	39	0.6908	54	0.5992	80	0.4682		
15	0.9976	4	0.9628	16	0.8592	28	0.7668	40	0.6843	56	0.5879	85	0.4465		
20	0.9968	5	0.9537	17	0.8511	29	0.7591	41	0.6778	58	0.5769	90	0.4258		
25	0.9961	6	0.9447	18	0.8404	30	0.7523	43	0.6651	60	0.5660	95	0.4178		
30	0.9953	7	0.9358	19	0.8351	31	0.7452	44	0.6588	62	0.5554	100	0.3873		
35	0.9945	8	0.9269	20	0.8272	32	0.7382	45	0.6526	64	0.5449	105	0.3694		
40	0.9937	9	0.9182	21	0.8194	33	0.7312	46	0.6464	68	0.5247	110	0.3523		
45	0.9929	10	0.9095	22	0.8117	34	0.7243	47	0.6403	70	0.5148	115	0.3359		
50	0.9921	11	0.9009	23	0.8040	35	0.7175	48	0.6343	72	0.5051	120	0.3204		
55	0.9913	12	0.8924	24	0.7964	36	0.7107	49	0.6283	74	0.4956	125	0.3055		
60	0.9906	13	0.8840	25	0.7889	37	0.7040	50	0.6223	76	0.4863	130	0.2914		

Values for $t_{1/2}$, energies, and percentages vary from data source to data source.

These numbers were derived from the following formulas:

$$e^{-\frac{.693}{4380.6} \times \text{time in minutes}} \text{ for minutes}$$

$$e^{-\frac{.693}{73.06} \times \text{time in hours}} \text{ for hours}$$

Xenon-133 Decay Table

Radionuclide: ^{133}Xe

$t_{1/2}$: 126 hours or 5.25 days

Energies: Beta (maximums): 346.3 keV (99.3%)

    Gamma: 81 keV (36.5%)

Type: β^-, γ emitter, fission product

Decays to: ^{133}Cs (100%)

Original amount $\times$ decay factor (DF) for days, hours, and/or minutes = factored amount

Ex: 10 mCi after 6 h 35 min: 10 $\times$ 0.9675 (6 h) $\times$ 0.9968 (35 min) = 9.6 mCi

Min	DF	Hours	DF	Hours	DF	Hours	DF	Hours	DF	Hours	DF	Hours	DF	Hours	DF
5	0.9995	2	0.9891	14	0.9259	26	0.8715	38	0.8114	52	0.7513	78	0.6512
10	0.9990	3	0.9836	15	0.9208	27	0.8620	39	0.8069	54	0.7430	80	0.6440
15	0.9986	4	0.9782	16	0.9158	28	0.8715	40	0.8025	56	0.7349	85	0.6266
20	0.9982	5	0.9729	17	0.9107	29	0.8526	41	0.7981	58	0.7269	90	0.6096
25	0.9977	6	0.9675	18	0.9057	30	0.8479	43	0.7894	60	0.7189	95	0.5930
30	0.9973	7	0.9622	19	0.9008	31	0.8432	44	0.7851	62	0.7111	100	0.5769
35	0.9968	8	0.9570	20	0.8958	32	0.8386	45	0.7808	64	0.7033	105	0.5613
40	0.9963	9	0.9517	21	0.8909	33	0.8340	46	0.7765	68	0.6880	110	0.5461
45	0.9959	10	0.9465	22	0.8803	34	0.8294	47	0.7722	70	0.6805	115	0.5313
50	0.9954	11	0.9413	23	0.8812	35	0.8249	48	0.7680	72	0.6730	120	0.5169
55	0.9950	12	0.9361	24	0.8763	36	0.8204	49	0.7638	74	0.6656	125	0.5028
60	0.9945	13	0.9310	25	0.8715	37	0.8159	50	0.7596	76	0.6584	130	0.4892

Values for $t_{1/2}$, energies, and percentages vary from data source to data source.

These numbers were derived from the following formulas:

$$e^{-\frac{.693}{7560} \times \text{time in minutes}} \text{ for minutes}$$

$$e^{-\frac{.693}{126} \times \text{time in hours}} \text{ for hours}$$

Standard Drug Interventions

Calculations, Preparations, and Administration

Infusion Rate Tables

Side Effects of Common Drugs

Drugs and Studies Affecting [123]I Uptake

Calculations, Preparations, and Administration

Pediatric Dose

(Patient weight in kg $\times$ adult dose) $\div$ 70 kg = pediatric dose.

(Patient weight in lb $\times$ adult dose) $\div$ 154 lb = pediatric dose.

See Pediatric Doses in Reference Section.

Drip Conversions

15 drops = 1 mL. Some tubing has drip factor (on package) of 10, microtubing at 60.

Amount of mL in bag $\div$ time to drip into patient in minutes = mL/min.

mL/min $\times$ 15 = drops per minute. (Or divide by 2 for drops per 30 seconds, etc.)

Kinevac® *(Sincalide, Cholecystokinin, CCK; HIDA/gallbladder studies)*

Weight in lb _____ ÷ 2.2 = _____ kg × 0.02 µg/kg = _____ µg ÷ 1 µg/mL = _____ mL.

Administer IV, slowly for 3 minutes.

Vials supplied with 5 µg. Add 5 mL of sterile water. Some administer 1.5 µg for gallbladder studies or 1.5 mL in a 3-mL syringe.

Morphine Sulfate *(HIDA/gallbladder studies)*

Weight in lb _____ ÷ 2.2 = _____ kg × 0.04 mg/kg = _____ mg ÷ 10 mg/mL = _____ mL.

Weight in lb _____ ÷ 2.2 = _____ kg × 0.04 mg/kg = dose

Dilute with saline to 10 mL. Administer IV, slowly for 3 minutes. Some administer between 2 and 4 mg per patient as a standard dose.

Dipyridamole *(Persantine®; cardiac stress test)*

Weight in lb _____ ÷ 2.2 = _____ kg × 0.57 mg/kg = _____ mg ÷ 5 mg/mL = _____ mL.

Maximum dose per patient: 60 mg.   Maximum patient size per vial: 105.5 kg or 232 lb.

0.57 mg × weight in kg = patient dose.

0.259 mg × weight in lb = patient dose.

10-mL vials at 5 mg/mL.

8-minute protocol: Dilute with saline to total of 50 mL. Administer IV slowly for 8 minutes.

4-minute protocol: Dilute with saline to total of 30 mL. Administer IV slowly for 4 minutes.

Antidote is aminophylline.

Adenosine *(cardiac stress test)*

Weight in lb _____ ÷ 2.2 = _____ kg × 140 µg/min = _____ kg/µg/min × 6 min = _____ µg × 1000 (to convert to mg) = _____ mg ÷ 3 mg/mL = _____ mL.

or: weight in kg × 0.83 (already converted to mg) ÷ 3 = _____ mL to draw up.

or: weight in kg × 0.28 = _____ mL to draw up × 3 = total mg given to patient.

Usually diluted to 30 mL with saline or 60 mL if weight is more than 235.7 lb.

Administer slowly for 6 minutes. Although the half-life is less than 10 seconds, the antidote, if needed, is aminophylline.

Dobutamine *(cardiac stress test)*

Administer in increments of 3 minutes, IV, based on patient weight and age (maximal and submaximal heart rates). Cardiologist directs the changes.

Start with 250 mg of dobutamine mixed in 250 mL of normal saline in a final solution of 1000 µg/mL.

5 µg/kg/min for 3 minutes.

10 µg/kg/min for 3 minutes.

Continue increasing by 5 µg/kg/min to 40 µg.

Antidote is Inderol® (atropine, Lopressor®, and Proventil® are also used).

Propranolol or Lopressor® may be administered (0.1 mg/kg) IV to interrupt ischemia.

Atropine may be administered (0.6 mg) IV to increase heart rate if dobutamine is failing.

Furosemide *(Lasix®; renal studies)*

Weight in lb _____ ÷ 2.2 = _____ kg × 0.3 mg/kg = _____ mg ÷ 10 mg/mL = _____ mL.

20–40 mg given in some renal studies as standard dose.

Vials supplied with 40 mg in 4 mL.

Administer IV slowly.

Captopril *(Capoten®; renal studies)*

50-mg capsule or tablet, usually given PO for some renal studies as standard dose.

Enalaprilat *(Vasotec®) ACE inhibitor (renal studies)*

Weight in lb _____ ÷ 2.2 = _____ kg × 0.04 mg/kg = _____ mg ÷ 1.25 mg/mL = _____ mL.

(Maximum 2.5 mg/2 mL) Administer IV slowly.

Pyrolite® *(pyp or pyrophosphate; RBC tagged studies)*

Warm to room temperature.

Inject 2–3 mL of normal saline into bottle.

Mix, let sit for 5 minutes.

Draw back into syringe (some draw only the equivalent of 1.2 mg pyp), administer IV.

UltraTag®

Draw 0.3–1 mL heparin into 3- to 6-mL syringe (10–15 U/mL).

Draw 2–3 mL patient blood into syringe (more if RBC count is low); mix well.

Inject contents into package vial, let sit for 5 minutes, swirl once or twice.

Inject package syringe I, swirl; inject package syringe II, swirl.

Inject $^{99m}TcO_4^-$ (amount as per protocol, 20–50 mCi) into vial, let sit for 20 minutes.

Reinject into patient.

Metaclopramide *(Reglan®; gastric emptying)*

Supply: 10 mg/2 mL ampule.

Adult dose: 10 mg IV.

Administer slowly for 2 minutes by nurse or doctor.

Response occurs 1–3 minutes after injection.

Pentagastrin *(Peptavlon®; Meckel's diverticulum study)*

Supply: 0.25 mg/mL (2.0 mL volume) = 250 μg/mL. Total in one vial = 500 μg.

Dosage: Patient weight in lb ÷ 2.2 = _____ kg × 6 μg pentagastrin = dose.

Administer IV.

Diamox® *(acetazolamide; brain SPECT)*

Potent cerebral vasodilator. Shows affected area as regional decreased perfusion in patients suffering from transient ischemic attacks (frequently a precursor to cerebral infarction).

A normal brain will show shunting and is referred to as the "reversed Robin Hood" effect.

Dosage: 1.0 g, administer IV or orally before radiotracer injection.

SUGGESTED READINGS

Chohan N, ed. Nursing 99 Drug Handbook. Springhouse, PA: Springhouse, 1999.

Datz FL. Handbook of Nuclear Medicine. 2nd ed. St. Louis: Mosby, 1993.

Duffy MA, ed. Physicians' Desk Reference. 46th ed. Montvale, NJ: Medical Economics Company, 1992.

Early PJ, Sodee DB. Principles and Practice of Nuclear Medicine. 2nd ed. St. Louis: Mosby, 1995.

Murray IPC, Ell PJ, eds. Nuclear Medicine in Clinical Diagnosis and Treatment. Vols. 1 and 2. New York: Churchill Livingstone, 1994.

Wilson, MA. Textbook of Nuclear Medicine. Philadelphia: Lippincott-Raven, 1998.

Notes

Adenosine Infusion Table

lb	kg	mg/6	mL/6	lb	kg	mg/6	mL/6	lb	kg	mg/6	mL/6	lb	kg	mg/6	mL/6	lb	kg	mg/6	mL/6
95	43	36.1	12.0	128	58	48.9	16.3	161	73	61.5	20.5	194	88	74.1	24.7	227	103	86.7	28.9
96	44	36.7	12.2	129	59	49.3	16.4	162	74	61.9	20.6	195	89	74.5	24.8	228	104	87.1	29.0
97	44	37.0	12.3	130	59	49.6	16.5	163	74	62.2	20.7	196	89	74.8	24.9	229	104	87.4	29.1
98	45	37.4	12.5	131	60	50.0	16.7	164	75	62.6	20.9	197	90	75.2	25.1	230	105	87.8	29.3
99	45	37.8	12.6	132	60	50.4	16.8	165	75	63.0	21.0	198	90	75.6	25.2	231	105	88.2	29.4
100	45	38.2	12.7	133	60	50.8	16.9	166	75	63.4	21.1	199	90	76.0	25.3	232	105	88.6	29.5
101	46	38.6	12.9	134	61	51.2	17.1	167	76	63.8	21.3	200	91	76.4	25.5	233	106	89.0	29.7
102	46	38.9	13.0	135	61	51.5	17.2	168	76	64.1	21.4	201	91	76.7	25.6	234	106	89.3	29.8
103	47	39.3	13.1	136	62	51.9	17.3	169	77	64.5	21.5	202	92	77.1	25.7	235	107	89.7	29.9
104	47	39.7	13.2	137	62	52.3	17.4	170	77	64.9	21.6	203	92	77.5	25.8	236	107	90.1	30.0
105	48	40.1	13.4	138	63	52.7	17.6	171	78	65.3	21.8	204	93	77.9	26.0	237	108	90.5	30.2
106	48	40.5	13.5	139	63	53.1	17.7	172	78	65.7	21.9	205	93	78.3	26.1	238	108	90.9	30.3
107	49	40.9	13.6	140	64	53.5	17.8	173	79	66.1	22.0	206	94	78.7	26.2	239	109	91.3	30.4
108	49	41.2	13.7	141	64	53.8	17.9	174	79	66.4	22.1	207	94	79.0	26.3	240	109	91.6	30.5
109	50	41.6	13.9	142	65	54.2	18.1	175	80	66.8	22.3	208	95	79.4	26.5	241	110	92.0	30.7
110	50	42.0	14.0	143	65	54.6	18.2	176	80	67.2	22.4	209	95	79.8	26.6	242	110	92.4	30.8
111	50	42.4	14.1	144	65	55.0	18.3	177	80	67.6	22.5	210	95	80.2	26.7	243	110	92.8	30.9
112	51	42.8	14.3	145	66	55.4	18.5	178	81	68.0	22.7	211	96	80.6	26.9	244	111	93.2	31.1
113	51	43.1	14.4	146	66	55.7	18.6	179	81	68.3	22.8	212	96	80.9	27.0	245	111	93.5	31.2
114	52	43.5	14.5	147	67	56.1	18.7	180	82	68.7	22.9	213	97	81.3	27.1	246	112	93.9	31.3
115	52	43.9	14.6	148	67	56.5	18.8	181	82	69.1	23.0	214	97	81.7	27.2	247	112	94.3	31.4
116	53	44.3	14.8	149	68	56.9	19.0	182	83	69.5	23.2	215	98	82.1	27.4	248	113	94.7	31.6
117	53	44.7	14.9	150	68	57.3	19.1	183	83	69.9	23.3	216	98	82.5	27.5	249	113	95.1	31.7
118	54	45.1	15.0	151	69	57.7	19.2	184	84	70.3	23.4	217	99	82.9	27.6	250	114	95.5	31.8
119	54	45.4	15.1	152	69	58.0	19.3	185	84	70.6	23.5	218	99	83.2	27.7	251	114	95.8	31.9
120	55	45.8	15.3	153	70	58.4	19.5	186	85	71.0	23.7	219	100	83.6	27.9	252	115	96.2	32.1
121	55	46.2	15.4	154	70	58.8	19.6	187	85	71.4	23.8	220	100	84.0	28.0	253	115	96.6	32.2
122	55	46.6	15.5	155	70	59.2	19.7	188	85	71.8	23.9	221	100	84.4	28.1	254	115	97.0	32.3
123	56	47.0	15.7	156	71	59.6	19.9	189	86	72.2	24.1	222	101	84.8	28.3	255	116	97.4	32.5
124	56	47.3	15.8	157	71	59.9	20.0	190	86	72.5	24.2	223	101	85.1	28.4	256	116	97.7	32.6
125	57	47.7	15.9	158	72	60.3	20.1	191	87	72.9	24.3	224	102	85.5	28.5	257	117	98.1	32.7
126	57	48.1	16.0	159	72	60.7	20.2	192	87	73.3	24.4	225	102	85.9	28.6	258	117	98.5	32.8
127	58	48.5	16.2	160	73	61.1	20.4	193	88	73.7	24.6	226	103	86.3	28.8	259	118	98.9	33.0

Total mg given: mg/6 min = weight in kg $\times$ 0.14 $\times$ 6 min
Total adenosine to withdraw: mL/6 min = (kg $\times$ 0.14 $\times$ 6) $\div$ 3

Dobutamine Drip Infusion Table

lb	kg	mg/3	mL/h	lb	kg	mg/3	mL/h	lb	kg	mg/3	mL/h	lb	kg	mg/3	mL/h	lb	kg	mg/3	mL/h
95	43	64.8	77.8	128	58	87.3	105	161	73	109.8	132	194	88	132.3	159	227	103	154.8	186
96	44	65.5	78.5	129	59	88.0	106	162	74	110.5	133	195	89	133.0	160	228	104	155.5	187
97	44	66.1	79.4	130	59	88.6	106	163	74	111.1	133	196	89	133.6	160	229	104	156.1	187
98	45	66.8	80.2	131	60	89.3	107	164	75	111.8	134	197	90	134.3	161	230	105	156.8	188
99	45	67.5	81.0	132	60	90.0	108	165	75	112.5	135	198	90	135.0	162	231	105	157.5	189
100	45	68.2	81.8	133	60	90.7	109	166	75	113.2	136	199	90	135.7	163	232	105	158.2	190
101	46	68.9	82.6	134	61	91.4	110	167	76	113.9	137	200	91	136.4	164	233	106	158.9	191
102	46	69.5	83.5	135	61	92.0	110	168	76	114.5	137	201	91	137.0	164	234	106	159.5	191
103	47	70.2	84.3	136	62	92.7	111	169	77	115.2	138	202	92	137.7	165	235	107	160.2	192
104	47	70.9	85.1	137	62	93.4	112	170	77	115.9	139	203	92	138.4	166	236	107	160.9	193
105	48	71.6	85.9	138	63	94.1	113	171	78	116.6	140	204	93	139.1	167	237	108	161.6	194
106	48	72.3	86.7	139	63	94.8	114	172	78	117.3	141	205	93	139.8	168	238	108	162.3	195
107	49	73.0	87.5	140	64	95.5	115	173	79	118.0	142	206	94	140.5	169	239	109	163.0	196
108	49	73.6	88.4	141	64	96.1	115	174	79	118.6	142	207	94	141.1	169	240	109	163.6	196
109	50	74.3	89.2	142	65	96.8	116	175	80	119.3	143	208	95	141.8	170	241	110	164.3	197
110	50	75.0	90.0	143	65	97.5	117	176	80	120.0	144	209	95	142.5	171	242	110	165.0	198
111	50	75.7	90.8	144	65	98.2	118	177	80	120.7	145	210	95	143.2	172	243	110	165.7	199
112	51	76.4	91.6	145	66	98.9	119	178	81	121.4	146	211	96	143.9	173	244	111	166.4	200
113	51	77.0	92.5	146	66	99.5	119	179	81	122.0	146	212	96	144.5	173	245	111	167.0	200
114	52	77.7	93.3	147	67	100.2	120	180	82	122.7	147	213	97	145.2	174	246	112	167.7	201
115	52	78.4	94.1	148	67	100.9	121	181	82	123.4	148	214	97	145.9	175	247	112	168.4	202
116	53	79.1	94.9	149	68	101.6	122	182	83	124.1	149	215	98	146.6	176	248	113	169.1	203
117	53	79.8	95.7	150	68	102.3	123	183	83	124.8	150	216	98	147.3	177	249	113	169.8	204
118	54	80.5	96.5	151	69	103.0	124	184	84	125.5	151	217	99	148.0	178	250	114	170.5	205
119	54	81.1	97.4	152	69	103.6	124	185	84	126.1	151	218	99	148.6	178	251	114	171.1	205
120	55	81.8	98.2	153	70	104.3	125	186	85	126.8	152	219	100	149.3	179	252	115	171.8	206
121	55	82.5	99.0	154	70	105.0	126	187	85	127.5	153	220	100	150.0	180	253	115	172.5	207
122	55	83.2	99.8	155	70	105.7	127	188	85	128.2	154	221	100	150.7	181	254	115	173.2	208
123	56	83.9	101	156	71	106.4	128	189	86	128.9	155	222	101	151.4	182	255	116	173.9	209
124	56	84.5	101	157	71	107.0	128	190	86	129.5	155	223	101	152.0	182	256	116	174.5	209
125	57	85.2	102	158	72	107.7	129	191	87	130.2	156	224	102	152.7	183	257	117	175.2	210
126	57	85.9	103	159	72	108.4	130	192	87	130.9	157	225	102	153.4	184	258	117	175.9	211
127	58	86.6	104	160	73	109.1	131	193	88	131.6	158	226	103	154.1	185	259	118	176.6	212

mg/3 min = kg × 0.5 mg × 3 min
mL/h = (kg × 0.5 × 3) ÷ 0.83

Persantine® Infusion Table

lb	kg	mg/4	lb	kg	mg/4	lb	kg	mg/4	lb	kg	mg/4
96	44	24.8	131	60	33.8	166	75	42.9	201	91	51.9
97	44	25.0	132	60	34.1	167	76	43.1	202	92	52.2
98	45	25.3	133	60	34.3	168	76	43.4	203	92	52.4
99	45	25.6	134	61	34.6	169	77	43.6	204	93	52.7
100	45	25.8	135	61	34.9	170	77	43.9	205	93	52.9
101	46	26.1	136	62	35.1	171	78	44.1	206	94	53.2
102	46	26.3	137	62	35.4	172	78	44.4	207	94	53.4
103	47	26.6	138	63	35.6	173	79	44.7	208	95	53.7
104	47	26.9	139	63	35.9	174	79	44.9	209	95	54.0
105	48	27.1	140	64	36.1	175	80	45.2	210	95	54.2
106	48	27.4	141	64	36.4	176	80	45.4	211	96	64.5
107	49	27.6	142	65	36.7	177	80	45.7	212	96	54.7
108	49	27.9	143	65	36.9	178	81	46.0	213	97	55.0
109	50	28.1	144	65	37.2	179	81	46.2	214	97	56.3
110	50	28.4	145	66	37.4	180	82	46.6	215	98	55.5
111	50	28.7	146	66	37.7	181	82	46.7	216	98	55.8
112	51	28.9	147	67	38.0	182	83	47.0	217	99	56.0
113	51	29.2	148	67	38.2	183	83	47.2	218	99	56.3
114	52	29.4	149	68	38.5	184	84	47.5	219	100	56.5
115	52	29.7	150	68	38.7	185	84	47.8	220	100	56.8
116	53	29.9	151	69	39.0	186	85	48.0	221	100	57.1
117	53	30.2	152	69	39.2	187	85	48.3	222	101	57.3
118	54	30.5	153	70	39.5	188	85	48.5	223	101	57.6
119	54	30.7	154	70	39.8	189	86	48.8	224	102	57.8
120	55	31.0	155	70	40.0	190	86	49.1	225	102	58.1
121	55	31.2	156	71	40.3	191	87	49.3	226	103	58.3
122	55	31.5	157	71	40.5	192	87	49.6	227	103	58.6
123	56	31.8	158	72	40.8	193	88	49.8	228	104	58.9
124	56	32.0	159	72	41.1	194	88	50.1	229	104	59.1
125	57	32.3	160	73	41.3	195	89	50.3	230	105	59.4
126	57	32.6	161	73	41.6	196	89	60.6	231	105	59.6
127	58	32.8	162	74	41.8	197	90	50.9	232	105	59.9
128	58	33.0	163	74	42.1	198	90	51.1	233	106	60
129	59	33.3	164	75	42.3	199	90	51.4	234	106	60
130	59	33.6	165	75	42.6	200	91	51.6	235	107	60

Reverse with aminophylline: 100–125 mg at 50 mg/min
Maximum dose = 60 mg
mg/4 = kg $\times$ 0.142 $\times$ 4 min

Urokinase Infusion Table

Rate (mL/h)	Dosage (U/min)	Dosage (U/h)	Rate (mL/h)	Dosage (U/min)	Dosage (U/h)
1	83.3333	5,000	31	2583.33	155,000
2	166.667	10,000	32	2666.67	160,000
3	250	15,000	33	2750	165,000
4	333.333	20,000	34	2833.33	170,000
5	416.667	25,000	35	2916.67	175,000
6	500	30,000	36	3000	180,000
7	583.333	35,000	37	3083.33	185,000
8	666.667	40,000	38	3166.67	190,000
9	750	45,000	39	3250	195,000
10	833.333	50,000	40	3333.33	200,000
11	916.667	55,000	41	3416.67	205,000
12	1000	60,000	42	3500	210,000
13	1083.33	65,000	43	3583.33	215,000
14	1166.67	70,000	44	3666.67	220,000
15	1250	75,000	45	3750	225,000
16	1333.33	80,000	46	3833.33	230,000
17	1416.67	85,000	47	3916.67	235,000
18	1500	90,000	48	4000	240,000
19	1583.33	95,000	49	4083.33	245,000
20	1666.67	100,000	50	4166.67	250,000
21	1750	105,000	51	4250	255,000
22	1833.33	110,000	52	4333.33	260,000
23	1916.67	115,000	53	4416.67	265,000
24	2000	120,000	54	4500	270,000
25	2083.33	125,000	55	4583.33	275,000
26	2166.67	130,000	56	4666.67	280,000
27	2250	135,000	57	4750	285,000
28	2333.33	140,000	58	4833.33	290,000
29	2416.67	145,000	59	4916.67	295,000
30	2500	150,000	60	5000	300,000

For lysis of pulmonary emboli, usually 4400 IU/kg for 10 minutes, then 4400 IU/kg per hour for 12–24 hours.

Side Effects of Common Drugs

Adrenergics: nausea and vomiting, anorexia, headache, anaphylaxis, hypotension, hypertension, insomnia, angina, anxiety, dizziness, pallor, flushing, dysuria, bradycardia, tachycardia, asthmatic episodes.

Adrenocortical steroids: nausea and vomiting, headache, pancreatitis, seizures, hypertension, congestive heart failure, rash, poor wound healing, glaucoma, shock, weakness.

Antacids: nausea, vomiting, and diarrhea, constipation, fecal impactions, Ca^{2+} imbalance, anorexia, encephalopathy, mental depression, osteomalacia, muscle weakness.

Antianginals: nausea, vomiting, and diarrhea, headache, rash, arrhythmia, abdominal pain, tachycardia, hypotension, dizziness, weakness, dyspnea.

Antiarrhythmics: nausea and vomiting, headache, abdominal pain, liver disorders, bitter taste, rash, CHF, hypotension, flushing, blurred vision, chest pressure, dyspnea.

Antibiotics or antibacterials: nausea, vomiting, and diarrhea, headache, anorexia, skin disorders, respiratory disorders, dizziness, weakness.

Antidiabetics: nausea, vomiting, and diarrhea, headache, abdominal pain, dizziness, jaundice, rash, weakness, anemia, hematologic changes, anaphylaxis.

Antiemetics: nausea, vomiting, and diarrhea, headache, dry mouth, dizziness, confusion, blurred vision, drowsiness, hypotension, palpitations, tachycardia, wheezing, anaphylaxis.

Antihistamines: nausea, vomiting, and diarrhea, headache, drowsiness, dizziness, dry mouth, epigastric pain, anorexia, constipation, urinary frequency or retention, nervousness, palpitations, hypotension, tachycardia, anaphylaxis.

Antihypertensives: nausea, vomiting, and diarrhea, headache, congestive heart failure, constipation, abdominal pain, tachycardia, bradycardia, orthostatic hypotension, angina, rash.

Antilipemics: nausea, vomiting, and diarrhea, headache, constipation, flatulence, dizziness, fatigue, syncope, tinnitus, GI bleed, abdominal pain, hematuria, dysuria, rash.

Antineoplastics: nausea, vomiting, and diarrhea, headache, dizziness, abdominal pain, renal & hepatic disorders, hematologic changes, rash, alopecia.

Electrolytes, vitamins, or minerals: nausea, vomiting, and diarrhea, headache, confusion, arrhythmia, abdominal pain, hypotension, palpitations, hematologic and hepatic changes, weakness, anaphylaxis, wheezing, rash, diaphoresis.

Inotropics or cardiac glycosides: nausea, vomiting, and diarrhea, headache, fatigue, anorexia, cramps, confusion, visual disturbance, dizziness, arrhythmia, muscular weakness.

Laxatives or stool softeners: nausea, vomiting, and diarrhea, dizziness, cramps, weakness, dehydration.

Muscle relaxants: nausea, vomiting, and diarrhea, headache, dizziness, fatigue, hypo/hypertension, constipation, tachycardia, bradycardia, arrhythmia, blurred vision, diaphoresis, urinary frequency or retention.

Narcotic analgesics: nausea and vomiting, headache, dry mouth, constipation, urinary retention, dyspnea, bradycardia, tachycardia, hypertension, dizziness, sedation.

Nonnarcotic analgesics: nausea, vomiting, and diarrhea, headache, anorexia, GI bleed, rash, leukopenia, increased prothrombin time, tinnitus, dizziness, confusion, thirst, thrombocytopenia, hepatitis, shortness of breath.

Side Effects of Common Drugs *(continued)*

Anticholinergics: nausea and vomiting, headache, heartburn, constipation, blurred vision, urinary hesitancy and retention, tachycardia, rash, nervousness.	**Antiparkinsons:** nausea, vomiting, and diarrhea, headache, constipation, hallucinations, confusion, blurred vision, GI cramps, insomnia, weakness, nervousness, anxiety, tachycardia, orthostatic hypotension.	**Sedatives or hypnotics:** nausea, vomiting, and diarrhea, headache, abdominal pain, rash, dizziness, delirium, excitement, confusion, hypotension, apnea.
Anticoagulants: nausea, vomiting, and diarrhea, headache, fever, hemorrhage, liver disorders, GI bleed, rash, thrombocytopenia, decreased renal flow.	**Bronchodilators:** nausea, vomiting, and diarrhea, headache, hypertension, seizures, anorexia, restlessness, tachycardia, arrhythmia, anxiety, tremor, bronchospasms.	**Thyroid hormones:** nausea, vomiting, and diarrhea, headache, palpitations, arrhythmia, angina, tachycardia, tremors, insomnia, depression, nervousness, anorexia, weight loss, edema.
Anticonvulsants: nausea, vomiting, and diarrhea, nystagmus, constipation, confusion, dizziness, rash, fatigue, nervousness, palpitations, hypotension, hypertension.	**Cholinergics:** nausea, vomiting, and diarrhea, headache, blurred vision, dizziness, weakness, abdominal cramps, rash, urinary urgency, hypotension, bradycardia, diaphoresis.	**Tranquilizers or antipsychotics:** nausea, vomiting, and diarrhea, anorexia, psychosis, dry mouth, constipation, liver disorders, postural hypotension, hypertension, tachycardia, cardiac arrest, urine retention, diaphoresis, rash.
Antidepressants: nausea, vomiting, and diarrhea, headache, seizures, delusions, constipation, orthostatic hypotension, hypertension, arrhythmia, tachycardia, confusion, anxiety, dry mouth, rash.	**Diuretics:** nausea, vomiting, and diarrhea, headache, confusion, syncope, weakness, dizziness, orthostatic hypotension, dysuria, hematuria, constipation, abdominal pain, pancreatitis, dehydration, rash.	**Vasodilators:** nausea and vomiting, dizziness, weakness, abdominal pain, hypotension, tachycardia, rash.

These are excerpts. See complete listings in Nursing 98 Drug Handbook, Springhouse, PA, 1998.

Drugs and Studies Affecting ^{123}I Uptake: Suggested Withholding Times

Treatment	Off	Treatment	Off
Butizalidine (Butisol)	3 weeks	Theragram M	10 days
Levoxine	3 weeks	Combid	1 week
Progesterone	1 month	Multivitamins	10 days
Renografin: kidney	2 months	Antiarrhythmics: Amiodarone HCl, Aratac, Cordarone, Pacerone	3 to 6 months
Resorcinol		Thyroid Hormones	
Salpingography	2 months	Proloid (thyroid)	2 weeks
Salpix	1 month	Synthroid (thyroid)	3 weeks
Seafood	3 days	Thyrolar (main hormone)	2 weeks
Kelp	3 days	Cytomel	2 weeks
Ekiodan, acocia	30 days	Propylthiouracil (PTU)	2 weeks
Sulfonamides	1 week	Thyroglobulin	3 weeks
Tapazole (methimazole)	1 month	Thyronine	3 weeks
Telepaque: gallbladder	2 months	TSH	increases uptake
Thiocyanates	10 days	Dessicated thyroid grains	6 weeks
Thioxolon	3 weeks	Birth control pills (↓ uptake)	2 weeks
Urokon	30 days	CT scan with contrast	6 weeks
Visciodol	1 year or more	IVP	6 weeks
Vitamin preps M	1 week	Upper and lower GI	No iodine
Vaginal suppositories with iodine		Gallbladder with contrast	3 months
Ornade	1 week	Therapeutic dose ^{131}I	3 months
Cough medicines	1 week	CT brain with contrast	3 months
Myelogram	up to 6 months	Heart catheterization	3 months
Arteriography	up to 3 months	Thypinone: normal pretreatment (TRH) before thyroid scan and uptake	
Perchlorate	up to 6 weeks		
Large doses of aspirin	1 week		
Antihistamines	1 week		
Large doses of penicillin (antibiotics)			

Times vary. These are only suggested suspensions. Check with endocrinologist or radiologist.

Laboratory Tests

Normal Ranges

Enzymes and Hormones

Laboratory Tests: Normal Ranges Commonly Associated With Nuclear Medicine

Test	Normal Range	Clinical Significance
ACID PHOSPHATASE	0–11 U/L	High: carcinoma of the prostate, advanced Paget's disease, hyperparathyroidism, Gaucher's disease (lipid accumulation in the reticuloendothelial system)
ALKALINE PHOSPHATASE	30–126 U/L	High: increased osteoblastic activity of bone, rickets, hyperparathyroidism, liver disease
AMYLASE	30–296 U/L	High: acute pancreatitis, mumps, duodenal ulcer, carcinoma of pancreas, drugs like morphine, codeine, cholinergics Low: chronic pancreatitis, pancreatic fibrosis and atrophy, cirrhosis of liver, pregnancy
BUN (BLOOD UREA NITROGEN)	7–21 mg/dL	High: decreased kidney function, acute glomerulonephritis, obstructive uropathy, nephrotic syndrome, dehydration, high protein diet or strenuous exercise, mercury poisoning Low: liver damage, pregnancy, low-protein–high-carbohydrate diet
CA-15-3 TUMOR MARKER	< 22 IU/mL	increased in breast cancer
CA-19-9 TUMOR MARKER	< 37 IU/mL	increased in pancreatic, hepatobiliary, gastric, and colorectal cancer, gallstones, and cirrhosis
CA-125	0–35 IU/mL	increased in colon, upper gastrointestinal, and ovarian and other gynecologic cancers, pregnancy, peritonitis
CALCIUM	8.5–10.6 mg/dL	High: tumor or hyperplasia of parathyroid, hypervitaminosis D, multiple myeloma, nephritis with uremia, malignant tumors, sarcoidosis, hyperthyroidism, skeletal immobilization, excess calcium intake Low: hypoparathyroidism, diarrhea, celiac disease, vitamin D deficiency, acute pancreatitis, nephrosis
CEA (CARCINO-EMBRYONIC ANTIGEN)	0.0–2.5 ng/mL (nonsmoker) 0.0–5 ng/mL (smoker)	High: repeated elevated levels indicate possible carcinoma of colon, rectum, pancreas, stomach
CHOLESTEROL	150–210 mg/dL	High: increased risk of coronary heart disease, lipemia, obstructive jaundice, diabetes, hypothyroidism Low: pernicious anemia, hemolytic anemia, hyperthyroidism, severe infection, terminal stage illnesses
CREATINE	0.2–0.8 mg/mL	High: skeletal muscle necrosis or atrophy, pregnancy, starvation, hyperthyroidism
CREATININE	0.7–1.5 mg/dL	High: renal dysfunction, nephritis, destruction of muscle tissue, hyperthyroidism, active rheumatoid arthritis Low: kidney diseases
GASTRIN (FASTING) (POSTPRANDIAL)	50–155 ng/L 80–170 ng/L	High: Zollinger-Ellison syndrome, peptic ulcer of the duodenum, pernicious anemia

Test	Normal Range	Clinical Significance
GGTP (γ-GLUTAMYL TRANSPEPTIDASE)	8–78 U/L Males: < 45 U/L Females: < 30 U/L	High: hepatobiliary disease, anicteric alcoholics, drug-therapy damage, myocardial infarction, renal infarction
GLUCOSE (FASTING)	65–110 mg/dL	High: diabetes, nephritis, hyperthyroidism, early hyperpituitarism, cerebral lesions, infections, pregnancy, uremia Low: hypoglycemia, hyperinsulinism, hypothyroidism, late hyperpituitarism, pernicious vomiting, Addison's disease, severe hepatic damage
GUAIAC TEST	positive/negative	Positive: occult blood present in stool
O_2 SAT	94–100%	Low: cardiac obstruction, chronic obstructive pulmonary disease
PHOSPHOROUS	2.4–4.5 mg/dL	High: chronic nephritis, hypoparathyroidism Low: hyperparathyroidism, vitamin D deficiency
TOTAL PROTEIN	6.3–8.2 g/dL	High: hemoconcentration Low: malnutrition
PROTEIN/ALBUMIN	3.5–5.0 g/dL	High: shock Low: malnutrition, hemorrhage, proteinuria
PROTEIN/GLOBULIN	1.5–3.0 g/dL	High: multiple myeloma, chronic infections, liver disease Low: malnutrition, hemorrhage, proteinuria
$P_A O_2$	95–100 mm Hg	High: polycythemia, anhydremia Low: anemia, cardiac obstruction
$P_A CO_2$	35–45 mm Hg	High: respiratory acidosis, metabolic alkalosis Low: respiratory alkalosis, metabolic acidosis
pH	7.35–7.45	High: vomiting, hyperpnea, fever, intestinal obstruction Low: uremia, diabetic acidosis, hemorrhage, nephritis
PSA (PROSTATE SERUM ANTIGEN)	0.0–6.0 ng/mL	High: indication of prostate cancer, benign prostatic hyperplasia, prostatitis
PO_4 (INORGANIC PHOSPHORUS)	2.5–4.5 mg/dL	High: chronic nephritis, hypoparathyroidism Low: hyperparathyroidism, vitamin D deficiency
RENIN (PLASMA)	Normal diet: 0.3–3.6 ng/mL/h Low-salt diet: 0.9–9.1 ng/mL/h	High: renovascular hypertension, malignant hypertension, untreated Addison's disease, primary salt-losing nephropathy, low-salt diet, diuretic therapy, hemorrhage Low: primary aldosteronism, high salt intake, salt-retaining steroid therapy, antidiuretic hormone therapy, blood transfusion
SGOT (AST; SERUM GLUTAMIC-OXALOACETATE TRANSAMINASE)	5–40 U/mL	High: liver disease, myocardial infarction, skeletal muscle disease
SGPT (ALT; SERUM GLUTAMATE PYRUVATE TRANSAMINASE)	7–56 U/mL	High: liver disease (better marker), myocardial infarction, skeletal muscle disease
TOTAL BILIRUBIN	0.1–1.3 mg/dL	High: biliary obstruction and disease, hepatocellular damage (hepatitis), pernicious anemia

Test	Normal Range	Clinical Significance
THYROID		
CALCITONIN	400 ng/L	High: medullary carcinoma of the thyroid, some nonthyroid tumors, Zollinger-Ellison syndrome
T_4 (THYROXINE)	4.5–11.5 μg/dL	High: hyperthyroidism, thyroiditis, pregnancy, oral contraceptives Low: hypothyroidism, hypoproteinemia, nephrotic syndrome, androgenic and anabolic steroids
T_3 (TRIIODO-THYRONINE)	uptake: 25–35%	High: hyperthyroidism, thyroxine-binding globulin deficiency, androgens and anabolic steroids Low: hypothyroidism, pregnancy, thyroxine-binding globulin excess, estrogens and antiovulatory drugs
T_3 (TOTAL CIRCULATING)	75–200 ng/dL	High: pregnancy, hyperthyroidism Low: hypothyroidism
T_7 (FREE T_4 INDEX)	1–2.2 ng/dL	High: Euthyroid patients with normal free thyroxine levels may have abnormal T_3 and T_4 levels caused by drug preparations
TSH (THYROID STIM-ULATING HORMONE)	0.3–5 m/IU/L	High: primary hypothyroidism Low: hyperthyroidism
THYROGLOBULIN (SERUM) **NORMAL THYROID** **ATHYROID**	≤ 59.4 ng/mL < 5 ng/mL	High: active thyroid tissue
PTH (PARATHYROID HORMONE)	160–350 ng/L	High: hyperparathyroidism
BLOOD		
WBC (WHITE BLOOD CELLS)	$4.0–10.0 \times 10^9$/L	High: acute infections, acute leukemia, after surgery, trauma, menstruation Low: aplastic anemia, chemotherapy
RBC (RED BLOOD CELLS)	$4.50–6.2 \times 10^{12}$/L	High: severe diarrhea, dehydration, polycythemia, acute poisoning, pulmonary fibrosis Low: anemia, leukemia, after hemorrhage
HGB (HEMO-GLOBIN)	Males: 13.0–18.0 g/dL Females: 12.0–16.0 g/dL	High: chronic obstructive pulmonary diseases, polycythemia, failure of oxygenation because of congestive heart failure, high altitude Low: anemia, pregnancy, hemorrhage, excessive fluid intake
HCT (HEMATOCRIT)	Males: 36.0–54.0% Females: 40.0–48.0%	High: erythrocytosis, dehydration, shock Low: anemia, blood loss, pregnancy
PLATELETS	$0.1–0.4 \times 10^{12}$/L	High: malignancy, myeloproliferative disease, rheumatoid arthritis, postoperative Low: thrombocytopenic purpura, acute leukemic aplastic anemia, infections, drug reactions, during chemotherapy

Test	Normal Range	Clinical Significance
CARDIAC ENZYMES		
CPK (CREATINE PHOSPHOKINASE)	Males: 37–324 mU/mL Females: 37–250 mU/mL	High: (MB band-positive), myocardial infarction, ischemia (MM band), skeletal muscle diseases, intramuscular injections, crush syndrome, hypothyroidism, delirium tremens, alcoholic myopathy, cerebrovascular disease
LDH (LACTATE DEHYDROGENASE)	100–618 U/L	High: myocardial infarction, pulmonary infarction, liver disease, untreated pernicious anemia
TROPONIN	0–0.63 ng/mL	High: myocardial infarction
MYOGLOBIN	0–110 ng/mL	High: myocardial infarction, muscle necrosis

SUGGESTED READINGS

Smeltzer SC, Bare BG. Brunner and Suddarth's Textbook of Medical-Surgical Nursing. 8th ed. Philadelphia: Lippincott-Raven, 1996.

Notes

Enzymes and Hormones

Name	Production Site	Substrate	Action
ENZYMES			
SALIVARY AMYLASE	Salivary glands of the mouth	Starches	Catabolizes starch to polysaccharides
PANCREATIC AMYLASE	Pancreas	Carbohydrates	Released into the small intestine, catabolizes polysaccharides mostly to maltose
MALTASE	Small intestine	Maltose	Hydrolyzes maltose to its constituent two glucoses
LACTASE	Small intestine	Lactose	Hydrolyzes lactose to galactose and glucose
SUCRASE	Small intestine	Sucrose	Hydrolyzes sucrose to fructose and glucose
PEPSIN	Stomach	Proteins	Activated in the stomach by pepsinogen, catabolizes proteins to amino acids
TRYPSIN	Pancreas	Proteins	Cleaves proteins into smaller peptides
CHYMOTRYPSIN	Pancreas	Proteins	Cleaves proteins into smaller peptides
CARBOXYPEPTIDASE	Pancreas and small intestine	Peptides	Splits off one amino acid at a time from end of polypeptide
PANCREATIC LIPASE	Pancreas	Unemulsified fats	In the small intestine, catabolizes fats to monoglycerides, glycerol, and fatty acids
PANCREATIC DEOXYRIBONUCLEASE	Pancreas	Deoxyribonucleic acid	Hydrolyzes DNA to nucleotide monomers
PANCREATIC RIBONUCLEASE	Pancreas	Ribonucleic acid	Hydrolyzes RNA to nucleotide monomers
RENIN	Kidneys (juxtaglomerular cells)	Angiotensinogen	Forms angiotensin I; regulates aldosterone release, extracellular fluid volume, and systemic blood pressure

Name	Production Site	Target	Action
HORMONES			
CHOLECYSTOKININ (CCK)	Duodenal mucosa and small intestine	Liver/pancreas	In the presence of fatty chyme, potentiates secretin's actions on these organs
		Pancreas	Increases output of pancreatic juice
		Gall bladder	Stimulates contraction and expulsion of bile
		Hepatopancreatic sphincter	Relaxes sphincter to allow pancreatic juice into duodenum
		Autonomic nervous system	Invokes feeling of satiety
SECRETIN	Duodenal mucosa and small intestine	Stomach	In the presence of acidic chyme inhibits gastric gland secretion (HCl)
		Pancreas	Increases bicarbonate ions in pancreas, potentiates CCK action
		Liver	Increases bile output
GASTRIN	Stomach mucosa	Stomach	Increases output of gastric glands (HCl)
		Small intestine	Stimulates contraction of intestinal muscle
		Ileocecal valve	Relaxes valve
		Large intestine	Stimulates mass movements
BILE	Hepatocytes in liver	Small intestine	Transports bile salts; emulsifies fats, and facilitates absorption of fats and cholesterol by micelles
hGH (HUMAN GROWTH HORMONE)	Somatotropic cells of adenohypophysis	Bones and skeletal muscles, most body cells	Stimulates growth and cellular uptake of amino acids and sulfur to cartilage, mobilizes stored fat, and inhibits oxidation of glucose

DISORDERS: *Hypersecretion:* In children, results in gigantism or abnormally tall individuals

In adults, when bone growth has stopped, it results in acromegaly, enlargement, and thickening of bony area

Hyposecretion: In children, results in pituitary dwarfism or abnormally small individuals

Name	Production Site	Target	Action
TSH (THYROID-STIMULATING HORMONE)	Thyrotropic cells of adenohypophysis	Thyroid	Stimulates release of thyroid hormones
ACTH (ADRENO-CORTICOTROPIC HORMONE)	Corticotropic cells of adenohypophysis	Adrenal cortex	Stimulates adrenal cortex to release corticosteroid hormones (anti-stressors)

Name	Production Site	Target	Action
ADH (ANTIDIURETIC HORMONE, VASOPRESSIN)	Hypothalamus	Kidney tubules	Controls urine production and reabsorption of water

DISORDERS: *Hypersecretion:* Water retention, weight gain

Hyposecretion: Diabetes insipidus—intense thirst, large urine output

Name	Production Site	Target	Action
MSH (MELANOCYTE-STIMULATING HORMONE)	Pineal gland	Children: hypothalamus, dermis	Inhibits gonadotropin-releasing hormone release, controls pigmentation
THYROXINE	Thyroid	Most cells in follicles	Increases metabolic body rate and body heat, tissue growth, adrenergic receptors

DISORDERS: *Hypothyroidism:* In adults, myxedema—low metabolic rate, chills, constipation, lethargy, water retention

In infants, cretinism—short disproportionate body, thick tongue and neck, mentally retarded

Lack of iodine causes endemic goiter, enlargement of thyroid

Hyperthyroidism: Grave's disease—autoimmune system, hypertension

Name	Production Site	Target	Action
CALCITONIN	Parafollicular cells	Bone	Inhibits Ca^{2+} release
PTH (PARATHYROID HORMONE)	Parathyroid	Bone, kidneys, and intestine	Stimulates release of Ca^{2+} into bloodstream by releasing from bone, and removing from urine and food
ALDOSTERONE (MINERALOCORTICOID)	Zona glomerulosa of adrenal cortex	Kidney tubules	Regulates Na^+ and K^+ in extracellular fluids

DISORDERS: *Hypersecretion:* Aldosteronism—hypertension, edema

Hyposecretion: Addison's syndrome—weight loss, drop in glucose and Na^+ levels, rise in K^+ levels, dehydration, and hypotension

Name	Production Site	Target	Action
CORTISOL (GLUCOCORTICOID)	Zona fasciculata of adrenal cortex	Body cells	Promotes gluconeogenesis, hyperglycemia, mobilizes fat, stimulates protein catabolism, resists stressors, depresses immune system

DISORDERS: *Hypersecretion:* Cushing's syndrome—hyperglycemia, loss of muscle and bone protein, edema, hypertension, and "moon face"

Hyposecretion: Addison's syndrome

Name	Production Site	Target	Action
ANDROGENS (GONADOCORTICOID)	Zona reticulata of adrenal cortex		Women's libido
CATACHOLAMINES:			
EPINEPHRINE	Chromaffin cells of medullary cortex	Organs stimulated by sympathetic nervous system	Intensifies action of sympathetic nervous system, stimulates heart and metabolic activity

Name	Production Site	Target	Action
NOREPINEPHRINE	Chromaffin cells of medullary cortex	Organs stimulated by sympathetic nervous system	Vasoconstricts

DISORDERS: *Hypersecretion:* Hyperglycemia, palpitation, hypertension, sweating

Name	Production Site	Target	Action
GLUCAGON	Alpha cells of pancreas (islets of Langerhans)	Liver	Hyperglycemic agent; raises blood glucose levels by glycogenolysis (glycogen to glucose) and glyco-neogenesis (glucose from fatty acids and amino acids)
INSULIN	Beta cells of pancreas (islets of Langerhans)	Body cells	Hypoglycemic agent; inhibits action of glucagon and uptake of glucose

DISORDERS: *Hyposecretion:* Diabetes mellitus (hyperglycemia)—hypoglycemic state, making even more glucose available by glycogenolysis, lipolysis, and gluco-neogenesis; results in high blood levels (> 200 mg/dL), excess sugar in urine, dehydration, hunger, thirst, frequent urination, dry skin, blurred vision, drowsiness, and nausea

Hypersecretion: Hypoglycemia—low blood sugar (< 70 mg/dL), anxiety, nervousness, hunger, shaking, weakness, tachycardia, sweating, headache, irritability, dizziness, and disorientation

Name	Production Site	Target	Action
THYMOSIN	Thymus	Immune system, targets itself	Responsible for normal development of immune system, T lymphocytes only
FSH (FOLLICLE-STIMULATING HORMONE)	Anterior pituitary (adenohypophysis)	Gonads (testes, ovaries)	Stimulates gamete seminiferous production, ovarian tubules, and follicle development and spermatogenesis
LH OR ICSH (LUTEINIZING HORMONE; INTERSTITIAL CELL–STIMULATING HORMONE)	Anterior pituitary	Gonads (interstitial cells and ovaries)	Promotes production of gonadal hormones, maturation of egg and ovulation, and formation of corpus luteum, stimulates interstitial cells
PROLACTIN	Anterior pituitary lactotrophic cells	Mammary glands (lobules)	Stimulates production of milk, lactation
OXYTOCIN	Hypothalamus neurohypophysis	Uterus (myometrium) and breasts	Stimulates uterine contractions and milk secretion from breasts (milk letdown)
PROGESTERONE	Ovaries, also placenta and corpus luteum	Reproductive organs, endometrial lining	Stimulates breast development and sets menstrual cycle, during pregnancy readies for implantation

Name	Production Site	Target	Action
ESTROGEN	Ovaries	Reproductive organs, endo-metrial lining	Causes maturation of reproductive organs during puberty, breasts, secondary characteristics and shedding and rebuilding endometrial lining
TESTOSTERONE	Testes (interstitial cells)	Male reproductive organs, semin-iferous tubules	Causes maturation of reproductive organs at puberty, promotes sperm production
hCG (HUMAN CHORIONIC GONADOTROPIN)	Blastocyte of early pregnancy	Pituitary gland and corpus luteum	Promotes viability of corpus luteum for 4 months, stops menses
RELAXIN	Placenta	Pelvic ligaments and pubic symphysis	Causes ligaments and symphysis to relax, widen, and become more flexible
INHIBIN	Seminiferous tubules	Anterior pituitary and hypothalamus	Shuts down FSH and LH production

SUGGESTED READINGS

Marieb, Elaine N. Human Anatomy and Physiology. 2nd ed. Redwood City, CA: Benjamin/Cummings, 1992.

Van De Graaf, Kent M. and Stuart Ira Fox. Concepts of Human Anatomy and Physiology. Dubuque, IO: Brown, 1986.

Language Barrier Buster™/Interpretech™

This section is a derivative work in progress, taken from many books and people who speak these languages. It is to be considered only as a stop-gap source for communication where no other alternative is available. Because of variations in accents and dialects, it may or may not serve your specific needs.

Chinese-Mandarin

Introductions	American Phonetics Only
Hello / Good-bye.	Nee how / Jigh-jee-in.
Excuse me.	Mah-fahn nee. Dway-buu-shee.
My name is. . . .	Waw-duh meeng-dzu shir. . . .
I am a technologist.	Waw shir jee-shuu-ywen.
What is your name? / Is your name . . .?	Nee jee-ow shuun-muh meeng-dzu?
How are you?	Neen how mah?
Do you speak English?	Nee jee-ahng Eeng-wun mah?
I cannot speak Chinese.	Waw buu hway jee-ahng Joong-wun (Gwah-ee).
Answer yes or no.	Shir / Buu shir.
Speak slowly.	Cheeng jee-ahng mahn ee-dan.
I do not understand.	Waa buu doong.
Do you understand?	Ne doong mah?
Please.	Cheeng.
Thank you / You're welcome.	Shay shay / Hwahn ee nee (or Boo-ka-see).

Assessment	**Phonetics Only**
What's up? What's going on?	Hey?
Are you okay?	Ne-je et-ta jam yung?
Calm down, it's okay.	Boo yow pop, ma-soo.
Good / Bad.	How / Bu how.
Do you have any pain?	Ne yoe tung mah? Hin-tung?
Where?	Chigh na-ah-lee?
1–10 minutes / hours / days / weeks / months / years.	Ee, err, sahn, suh, wuu, leo, chee, bah, jeo, shuh. Fin / shee-ow-shr / tee-in / sheeng-chee / yeh / nay-in.
Show me.	Cheeng gay waw kahn.
Chest pain?	Shee-ong-koe tuung?
Are you hot / cold?	Ruh? / Lung?
Water, a blanket, a pillow.	Soiy, chwahng tahn-dzu, jing-toe
Would you like to use the bathroom?	Tsuh-swaw?

Directions	**Phonetics Only**
Sign here.	Chen main.
Left / Right.	Jore / Yoe.
Up / Down.	Shahng / She-eh.
Stand up.	Ze-shang.
Come toward me / Back up.	Gan-wa-lie / Twoi-hoe.
Turn around.	Gwie-wahn.
Sit down / here / up.	Jaw se-eh / Jaw-lee / Jaw-shahng.
Let me help.	Cheeng, wo lie bang lee.
Put your head on the pillow.	Ni toe fahn sang, jin-toe.
Lift your feet / head.	Na nee jeo sahn / toe sahn.
Arms up / down.	Na sho shang / fan so she-eh.
Look straight up.	Can ju.
Turn your head to the left / right.	Cheeng ju-ahng jaw / yoe zwahn.
Left / right arm over head.	Jaw show / Yoe show fahn quat toe.
Deep breath. Hold it. Let it out.	Foo-shee. Boo foo-shee. Foo-shee.
Breathe normal.	Foo-shee ping-sher.
Do not move. Hold still.	Poo ya dong!
We are taking a picture.	Wah-mun kuh-ee gay nee jah-oh-shee-ahng.
You are doing great.	Ne chaw ha-now.
Walk faster.	Shee qui-tan.
We are almost done.	Wa man sah-poo-toe how.
You are all done.	Nee ee-ching how.
Wait here.	Cheeng dung ee shee-ah.
You can go home now.	Ne kah-ye whay jee-ah.
You are going back up to your room, now.	Ne kah-ye fahn-jee ne ta fan.

French

Introductions	Translation
Hello / Good-bye.	Bonjour / Au revoir.
Excuse me.	Pardon or Excuse-moi.
My name is. . . .	Je m'appelle. . . .
I am a technologist.	Je suis technologue.
What is your name? / Is your name . . . ?	Comment vous appelez-vous?
How are you?	Comment allez-vous? Comment ça va?
Do you speak English?	Parlez-vous anglais?
I speak very little French.	Je parle très peu le français.
Answer yes or no.	Repondez seulement oui ou non.
Speak slowly.	Parlez plus lentement, s'il vous plaît.
I do not understand.	Je ne comprends pas.
Do you understand?	Comprenez-vous?
Please.	S'il vous plaît.
Thank you / You're welcome.	Merci / De rien.
How do you say [—] in French?	Comment dit-on [—] en français?

Assessment	Translation
What's up? What's going on?	Ça va? Qu'est-ce qu'il y a donc?
Are you okay?	Allez-vous bien?
Calm down, it's okay.	Calmez-vous, c'est bien.
Good / Bad.	Bon / Mal.
Do you have any pain?	Avez-vous mal?
Where?	Où?
How long? 1–10 minutes / hours / days / weeks / months / years.	Depuis combien de temps? un, deux, trois, quatre, cinq, six, sept, huit, neuf, dix.Une minute / une heure / un jour / une semaine / un mois / une année.
Show me.	Montrez-moi.
Chest pain?	Avez-vous mal à la poitrine?
Shortness of breath?	Avez-vous mal à respirer?
Are you hot / cold?	Avez-vous chaud / froid?
Would you like water, a blanket, a pillow, a urinal, a bed pan?	Voulez-vous de l'eau, une couverture, un oreiller, l'urinoir, un bassin (de lit).
Would you like to use the bathroom?	Voulez-vous aller à la toilette?

Directions	Translation
Sign here.	Signez ici.
Left / Right.	À gouche / À droite (ah gōshe / ah dwat).
Up / Down.	Haut / Bas.

Stand up.	Levez-vous.
Come toward me / Back up.	Tout droit / Marchez en renverse.
Turn around	Tournez-vous.
Sit down / here / up.	Asseyez-vous / ici / vertical.
May I help you?	Est-ce que je peux vous aider?
Lay down on your back / on your stomach.	Allongez-vous sur le dos / l'estomac.
Put your head on the pillow.	Ensuite votre tête sur l'oreiller.
Lift your knees / feet / head.	Dácrochez les genous / les pieds / la tête.
Arms up / arms down.	Levez les bras / Baissez les bras.
Look straight up.	Regardez en haut.
Turn your head to the left / right.	Tournez la tête à gouche / à droit.
Left / right arm over head.	Levez le bras gouche / droit sur la tête.
Deep breath. Hold it. Let it out.	Respirez à fond. Retenez. Soufflez (expirez).
Breathe normal.	Respirez normalement.
Do not move. Hold still.	Ne bougez pas. Immobile.
We are taking a picture.	Nous allons prendre un photo.
You are doing great.	Vous faites très bien.
It will go faster soon.	Ça va marcher plus vite.
Walk faster.	Marchez plus vite.
We are almost done.	Nous sommes presque finis.
You are almost / all done.	Vous êtes presque / tout fini.
Wait here.	Attendez ici.
You can go home now.	Vous pouvez rentrer chez vous maintenant.
You are going back up to your room, now.	Vous allez rentrer à votre chambre, maintenant.

German

. . . .

Introductions	**Translation**
Hello / Good-bye.	Guten Morgen / Tag / Gute Nacht / Auf Wiedersehen.
My name is. . . .	Ich heiss(e). . . .
I am a technologist.	Ich bin ein(e) Technologe ♂(. . . login♀)
What is your name? / Is your name . . .?	Wie heissen Sie? / Heissen Sie. . . .?
How are you?	Wie geht es Ihnen? or Wie geht's?
Do you speak English?	Sprechen Sie Englisch?
I speak very little German.	Ich sprech(e) nur ein bisschen Deutsch.
Answer yes or no.	Antworten Sie nur ja (yah) oder nein (nine).
Speak slowly.	Sprechen Sie langsamer, bitte.
I do not understand.	Ich verstehe Sie nicht.
Do you understand?	Verstehen Sie das? or Verstehen Sie mich?
Please.	Bitte.

Thank you / You're welcome.	Danke / Bitte or Dankeschön / Bitteschön.
How do you say [—] in German?	Wie sagt man [—] auf Deutsch?

Assessment	**Translation**
What's up? What's going on?	Was ist los?
Are you okay?	Geht ed Ihnen? Geht's?
Calm down, it's okay.	Beruhigen Sie sich, alles wird klappen.
Good / Bad.	Gut / Schlecht.
Do you have any pain?	Haben Sie schmerzen?
Where?	Wo? (Vo)
How long? 1-10 minutes / hours / days / weeks / months / years	Wie lange? Ein, zwei, drei, vier, fünf, sechs, sieben, achts, neun, zehn. Minuten / Stunden / Tage / Woken / Monate / Jahre.
Show me.	Zeigen Sie es mir.
Chest pain?	Haben Sie schmerzen in der Brust?
Shortness of breath?	Sind Sie atemlos?
Are you hot / cold?	Ist Ihnen heiss / kalt?
Would you like water, a blanket, a pillow, a urinal, a bed pan?	Möchen Sie Wasser, eine Decke, ein Kopfkissen, ein Urinal, eine Bettpfanne.
Would you like to use the bathroom?	Möchten Sie auf die Toilette gehen?

Directions	**Translation**
Sign here.	Unterschreiben Sie bitte hier.
Left / Right.	Links / Rechts.
Up / Down.	Herauf / Herab.
Stand up.	Stehen Sie auf.
Come toward me / Back up.	Kommen Sie hier / Gehen Sie rückwärts.
Turn around.	Drehen Sie Sich bette herum.
Sit down / here / up.	Setzen Sie sich / hier / herauf.
Let me help.	Lassen Sie mich Ihnen helfen.
Lay down on your back / on your stomach.	Legen Sie sich auf den Rücken / auf den Magen.
Put your head on the pillow.	Legen Sie bitte Ihren Kopf auf das Kopfkissen.
Lift your knees / feet / head.	Heben Sie Bitte Ihr(e) Knien / Füße / Kopf.
Arms up / down.	Arme rauf / runter.
Look straight up.	Aufsehen.
Turn your head to the left / right.	Wenden Sie den Kopf nach Links / Rechts.
Left / right arm over head.	Linken / Rechten Arm über den Kopf.
Deep breath. Hold it. Let it out.	Tief Einatmen. Anhalten. Ausatmen.
Breathe normal.	Normal atmen.
Do not move. Hold still.	Bewegen Sie sich nicht. Momentchen.
We are taking a picture.	Wir machen ein Foto.

You are doing great.	Sie machen das ganz gut.
It will go faster soon.	Bald geht es schneller.
Walk faster.	Gehen Sie bitte schneller.
You are almost / all done.	Sie sind fast / ganz fertig.
You can go home now.	Sie können jetze nach Hause gehen.
You are going back up to your room, now.	Jetze gehen Sie wieder in Ihr Zimmer.

Italian

Introductions	Translation
Hello / Good-bye.	Ciao or pronto / Addio (arrivederci).
Excuse me.	Mi scusi.
My name is. . . .	Mi chiamo. . . .
I am a technologist.	Sono un technologo.
What is your name? / Is your name . . . ?	Come ti chiami? / Suo nomeè . . . ?
How are you?	Come va?
Do you speak English?	Parla Ingese?
I speak very little Italian.	Parlo poco Italiano.
Answer yes or no.	Responde si o no.
Speak slowly.	Parla lento.
I do not understand.	No capisco.
Do you understand?	Hai capito?
Please.	Per favore.
Thank you / You're welcome.	Grazie / Prego.
How do you say [—] in Italian?	Como se dice [—] in Italiano?

Assessment	Translation
What's up? What's going on?	Cosa che?
Are you okay?	Stai bene?
Good / Bad.	Buono / Cattivo.
Do you have any pain?	Hai dolore?
Where?	Dove?
How long? 1–10 minutes / hours / days / weeks / months / years	Quanto tempo? Uno, due, tre, quattro, cinque, sei, sette, otto, nove, dieci. Minuto / ora / giorno / settimana / mese / anno.
Show me.	Fa me vedere.
Chest pain?	Dolore del petto?
Shortness of breath?	Respirazione difficile? Difficolta con respiro?
Are you hot / cold?	Hai caldo / freddo?
Would you like water, a blanket, a pillow, a urinal, a bed pan?	Acqua, una coperta, un cushino, un orinale, padella da letto?
Would you like to use the bathroom?	Hai bisogno del bagno?

Directions	Translation
Sign here.	Firma.
Left / Right.	Sinistra / Destra.
Up / Down.	Su / Giù.
Stand up.	In piedi.
Come toward me / Back up.	Vieni qui / Vai in dietro.
Turn around.	Gira.
Sit down / here / up.	Siedi / qui / su.
Let me help.	Hai bisogno.
Lay down on your back / on your stomach.	Soria ti sulla schiena / sullo stomaco.
Put your head on the pillow.	Metti giù la testa sull cushino.
Lift your knees / feet / head.	Alza le ginocchi / piedi / la testa.
Arms up / down.	Bracce su / giù.
Look straight up.	Guarda diritto.
Turn your head to the left / right.	Gira la testa a sinistra / destra.
Left / right arm over head.	Alza il braccia sinistra / destra sopra la testa.
Deep breath. Hold it. Let it out.	Respira profundo. Tiene lo. Lascia lo fuori.
Breathe normal.	Respira normale.
Do not move. Hold still.	Non muovere. Stai fermo.
We are taking a picture.	Facciamo le foto.
You are doing great.	Fa bene.
It will go faster soon.	Fa piu rapido subito.
Walk faster.	Camina piu rapido.
We are almost done.	Siamo quasi finiti.
You are almost / all done.	Stai quasi finito.
Wait here.	Aspetta qui.
You can go home now.	Puoi andare a casa adesso.
You are going back up to your room, now.	Adesso ritoni alla tua stanza.

Japanese

Introductions	Phonetics Only
Hello / Good-bye.	Ko-nee-she-wah or Moe-she moe-she / Sah-yo nara.
Excuse me.	Sue-me-mah-sin, koo-dah-sigh.
My name is	Wah-tock-she no nag-my wah . . . dess.
I am a technologist.	Wah-tock-she wa tek-no dess.
What is your name? / Is your name . . . ?	Oh-nah-my wah? / Oh-nah-tah wah? . . . -san dess kah?
How are you?	Ee-kaa-gaa dess kah?
Do you speak English?	Aa-ee-go gah han-nah-say-mah-sin?
I cannot speak Japanese.	Hee-hone-go gah han-nah-say-mah-sin.
Answer yes or no.	Hane-jee high / Ee-eh
Speak slowly.	Mot-toe yoo-koo-ree hah-nah-ssh-tay, koo-dah-sigh.

I do not understand.	Wah-kah-ree-mah-sin.
Do you understand?	Wah-kah-ree-mas ka?
Please.	Koo-dah-sigh.
Thank you / You're welcome.	Doe-moe ah-ree-gah-toe go-zee-mahss / Doe-ee-tah-she-mahsh-tay.
How do you say [—] in Japanese?	Nee-hon-go de [—] wah doe eye-mas kah?

Assessment ### Phonetics Only

What's the matter?	Doe she-mah-sshta kah?
Are you okay?	Die-joe-boo dess kah?
Good / Bad.	Ee-ee / Wah-roo-ee.
Do you have any pain?	Ee-tam-ee?
Where?	Doe-koe?
How long? 1–10 minutes / hours / days / weeks / months / years	Doe nah-gy? ee-chee, nee, san, she, go, roe-koo, she-chee, hachee, koo, juu. Poon / jie-kan / nichi / shah / gah-tsoo / toe-she.
Show me.	Oh-she-eh-mas.
Chest pain?	Ee-tah-mee moo-nay?
Are you hot / cold?	Aht-sue-ee / Sah-moo-ee dess kah?
Would you like water, a blanket, a pillow, a toilet?	Mee-zoo, moe-foo, mah-koo-rah, twa-ree?
Would you like to use the bathroom?	Oh-tay-ah-rie?

Directions ### Phonetics Only

Sign here.	Koe-koe day nah-my oh kite-tay, koo-dah-sigh.
Left / Right	Hee-dah-ree / mee-gee
Up / Down	Ooh-eh / Shrtah
Stand up.	Tat-te-pay, koo-dah-sigh.
Come towards me / Back up.	Ko-cheer-ah eh / ooh-sheer-oh eh
Turn around.	Mah-wat-the, koo-dah-sigh.
Sit down	Swat-tay, koo-dah-sigh.
May I help you?	Tat-soo-die mah-show kah?
Lay down on your back / on your stomach.	Say-nah-kah / oh-nah-kah nar-ee-tay.
Put your head on the pillow.	Mah-koo-rah ni oh ir-et-tay, koo-dah-sigh.
Lift your knees / feet / head.	He-zah / ah-she / ah-tah-mah oh.
Arms up / down.	Ooh-day ooh-eh / shrtah
Turn your head to the left / right.	Ah-tah-ma de hee-dah-ree / mee-gee ee mah-gah-roo no dess.
Deep breath. Hold it.	Foo-kah-yee koke-yoo / Ee-kee oh to-met-tay.
Breathe normal.	Foo-tsoo no koke-yoo
Do not move.	Chote-toe mot-tay.
We are taking a picture.	Wah-tock-she-tah-chee shah-sheen.
You are doing great.	Go-kuu-roe-sahn.
Wait here.	Koe-koe day mot-tay, koo-dah-sigh.

Polish

Introductions	Translation
Hello / Good-bye.	Dzień dobry / Do widzenia.
Excuse me.	Przepraszam.
My name is. . . .	Nazywam się. . . .
I am a technologist.	Jestem technologiem.
What is your name? / Is your name . . .?	Jak się pan (pani) nazy wał / Czy pan (pani) . . .?
How are you?	Jak się pan (pani) czuje?
Do you speak English?	Czy mówi pan (pani) po angielsku?
I speak very little Polish.	Ja mówię bardzo slabó po polsku.
Answer yes or no.	Proszę odpowiedzieć tak ubł nie.
Speak slowly.	Mów wolno proszę.
I do not understand.	Ja nie rozumię.
Do you understand?	Czy pan (pani) rozumię?
Please.	Proszę.
Thank you / You're welcome.	Dziękuję / Nie ma za co.
How do you say [—] in Polish?	Jak powiedzieć [—] po polsku?

Assessment	Translation
What's up? What's going on?	Co slychać? Co się dzieje?
Are you okay?	Czy wszystko z panią / panem dobrze?
Calm down, it's okay.	Proszę srę uspokoić, jest dobrze.
Good / Bad.	Dobrze / Źle.
Do you have any pain?	Czy ma pan (pani) jakiś ból?
Where?	Gdzie?
How long? 1–10 minutes / hours / days / weeks / months / years.	Jak dtugo? (1–10?) Minute / godziny / dni / tygodnie / miesią / lata.
Show me.	Proszę pokazać.
Chest pain?	Ból w klatce piersiowej?
Shortness of breath?	Krótki oddech?
Are you hot / cold?	Czy jest pan (pani) gorąco / zimno?
Would you like water, a blanket, a pillow, a urinal, a bed pan?	Czy chce pan (pani) wody, koc, poduszkę, kaczkę, kaczkę.
Would you like to use the bathroom?	Chce pan (pani) iść do łazienki?

Directions	Translation
Sign here.	Proszę tu podpisać.
Left / Right.	Lewa / Prawa.
Up / Down.	Góra / Doł.
Stand up.	Proszę wstać.

Come toward me / Back up.	Proszę iść do mnie / Do tyłu.
Turn around	Proszę obrócić się.
Sit down / here / up.	Proszę usiąść / tutaj / wstać.
Let me help.	Pomogę panu (pani).
Lay down on your back / on your stomach.	Proszę połuzyć się na plecach / na brzuchu.
Put your head on the pillow.	Proszę połuzyć głowę na poduszce.
Lift your knees / feet / head.	Proszę unieść kolana / stopy / głowę.
Arms up / down.	Ramiona do góry / do dołu.
Look straight up.	Proszę do góry (ppzed siebie).
Turn your head to the left / right.	Proszę obrócić głowę w lewa / prawo.
Left / right arm over head.	Lewa / prawe ramię nad głowę.
Deep breath. Hold it. Let it out.	Głęboki wdech. Zatrzymać. Wypuścić.
Breathe normal.	Oddychać normalnie.
Do not move. Hold still.	Proszę nie ruszać się. Się dzieć bez ruchu.
We are taking a picture.	Robimy zdjęcie.
You are doing great.	Spisuje się pan (pani) świetnie.
It will go faster soon.	To będzie prosać przyspieszyć nied?ugo.
Walk faster.	Proszę iść szybciej.
We are almost done.	Pranie skończyliśmy.
You are almost / all done.	Pranie wszystko zrobione.
Wait here.	Proszę poczekać tutaj.
You can go home now.	Moze pan (pani) iść do domu.
You are going back up to your room, now.	Teraz wraca pan (pani) do pokoju.

Portuguese

Introductions	Translation
Hello / Good-bye.	Alô / Adeus.
Excuse me.	Excuséme.
My name is. . . .	Meu nome é. . . .
I am a technologist.	Sou um tecnôlogo.
What is your name? / Is your name . . . ?	Qual é seu nome?
How are you?	Como vai?
Do you speak English?	Você fala Inglés?
I speak very little Portuguese.	Falo um poco Portugués.
Answer yes or no.	Responda sim o no.
Speak slowly.	Fale devagar.
I do not understand.	Näo entendo.
Do you understand?	Entende?
Please.	Por favor.
Thank you / You're welcome,	Obrigado / De nada,
How do you say [—] in Portuguese?	Como se diz [—] em Portugués?

Assessment	Translation
What's up? What's going on?	Que acontece?
Are you okay?	Esta bom?
Calm down, it's okay.	Seja calmo, tudo vai bem.
Good / Bad.	Bom / Mal.
Do you have any pain?	Sente dor?
Where?	Onde?
How long? 1–10 minutes / days / weeks / years	Quanto tempo? Um, dois, três, quatro, cinco, seis, sete, oito, nova, dez. Minutos / dias / semanas / anos.
Show me.	Me mostre.
Chest pain?	Dor do peito?
Shortness of breath?	Respiracão difícil?
Are you hot / cold?	Sente calor / frio?
Would you like water, a blanket, a pillow, a urinal, a bed pan?	Quer agua, um cobertor, uma almofada, urinol, panda de leito?
Would you like to use the bathroom?	Precisa do quarto de banho?

Directions	Translation
Sign here.	Firme aquí.
Left / Right.	Esquerdo / Direito.
Up / Down.	Arriba / Em baixo.
Stand up.	Esté em pé.
Come toward me / Back up	Venha aqui / Vai para atrás.
Turn around	Dei volta.
Sit down / here / up.	Sentese / aqui / Esté em pé.
Let me help.	Deixe ajudar-lhe.
Lay down on your back / on your stomach.	Deitese nas costas / no stômago.
Put your head on the pillow.	Ponha a testa na almofada.
Lift your knees / feet / head.	Levante os joelhos / pês / a testa.
Arms up / down.	Levante os braços / baixe os braços.
Look straight up.	Olhe arriba.
Turn your head to the left / right.	Volte a testa à esquerda / direita.
Left / right arm over head.	Ponha o braço esquerdo / direito sob a testa.
Deep breath. Hold it. Let it out.	Respire profundo. Tem ar e contenha. Respire.
Breathe normal.	Respire normalmente.
Do not move. Hold still.	Não mover, por favor.
We are taking a picture.	Estamos tirando uma imagem.
You are doing great.	Você está fazendo bem.
It will go faster.	Agora virá mais rápido.
Walk faster.	Caminhe mais rápido.
We are almost done.	Quase teminamos já.

You are almost / all done.	Você estará pronto já.
Wait here.	Espere aquí.
You can go home now.	Pôde ir à casa já.
You are going back up to your room, now.	Você vai para seu quarto agôra.

Russian

Note: Superscript y (X^yXX) pronounces as a "ye" within the word. Accented syllable of word is capitalized.

Introductions	**Phonetics Only**
Hello / Good-bye.	Pr^yee V^yEHT / Duh-sv^yee-DAHN^y-yuh.
Excuse me.	Eez-v^yee-N^YEE-t^yih.
My name is. . . .	Mah-YOH EE-m^yuh. . . .
I am a technologist.	Yah tecknico. . . .
What is your name? / Is your name . . . ?	Kahk vahs zah-VOOT?
How are you?	Kahk puh-zhi-VAH-yih-t^yih?
Do you speak English?	Vee guh-vah-R^yEE-t^yih pah-ahn-GL^yEE-sh^yee?
I speak very little Russian.	Yah n^yihm-NOH-guh guh-vah-R^yOO ROO-sk^yee.
Answer yes or no.	Aht-V^yEHT^y-t^yih dah EE-l^yee n^yeht.
Speak slowly.	Guh-vah-R^yEE-t^yih M^yEH-dl^yihn-n^yih-yih.
I do not understand.	Yah n^yih-puh-n^yee-MAH-yoo.
Do you understand?	Vee puh-n^yee-MAH-yih-t^yih-N^yAH?
Please.	Pah-ZHAH-lee-stuh.
Thank you / You're welcome.	Spah-S^yEE-buh / Pah-ZHAH-lee-stuh.
How do you say [—] in Russian?	Kahk skah-ZAHT^y pah-ROO-sk^yee [—]?

Assessment	**Phonetics Only**
What's up? What's going on?	Shtoh NOH-vuh-vuh?
Are you okay?	Khuh-rah-SHOH?
Calm down, it's okay.	Ee-Ge so-DAH.
Good / Bad.	DOH-bree-ee / plah-KHAH-yuh.
Do you have any pain?	Bah-L^YEET?
Where?	Gd^yeh?
How long? 1–10 minutes / hours / days / weeks / months / years.	Kahk DOHL-guh? Ah-D^yEEN, dvah, tr^yee, chih-TI-r^yih, p^yaht^y, shehst^y, s^yehm^y, VOH-s^yihm^y, D^yEH-v^yiht^y, D^YEH-s^yiht^y. M^yee-NOOT / chahs / d^yen^y / n^yih-D^YEH-l^yih / M^YEH-s^yih-tsi / goht.
Show me (please point).	Puh-kah-ZHI-t^yih, pah-ZHAH-lee-stuh.
Chest pain?	Groot^y bah-LYEET?
Shortness of breath?	Vey-ee-may, ta-BOLE grod^yee?
Are you hot / cold?	T^yih PLOH / KHOH-luhd-nuh?

Would you like water, a blanket, a pillow?	Vah-DAH, ah-d^yih-YAH-luh, pah-DOOSH-kuh?
Would you like to use the bathroom?	Tou-ah-L^yEHT?

Directions	Phonetics Only
Sign here.	Ruhs-p^yee-SHI-t^yihs^y zd^yehs^y.
Left / Right.	Nah-L^YEH-vuh / Nah-PRAH-vuh.
Up / Down.	Vv^yehrkh / Vn^yees.
Stand up.	V'STANT^yah.
Come toward me (come here).	Puh dah-ee-D^YEE-t^yih s^yoo-DAH.
Sit down / here.	Sah-D^yEE-t^yihs^y / Siz dis.
Let me help.	Mn^yeh pah-MOHCH.
On your back / on your stomach.	Sp^yee-NAH / zhee-LOO-duhk.
Lift your knees / feet / head.	Kah-L^YEH-nuh / nah-GAH / guh-lah-VAH.
Arms up / down.	Roo-KAH vv^yehrkh / vn^yees.
Turn your head to the left / right.	Guh-lah-VAH nah-L^YEH-vuh / nah-PRAH- vuh.
Left / right arm over head.	Nah-L^YEH-vuh / nah-PRAH-vuh roo-KAH guh-lah-VAH.
Deep breath.	V'dakneeti GROba core.
Breathe normal.	Dashet ^yeh namala.
Do not move. Hold still.	N^yih-DV^YEE-guh-ee-t^yih.
We are taking a picture.	Sfuh-tuh-grah-F^YEE-ruh.
Wait here.	Zd^yehs^y zhdaht^y.

Spanish

Introductions	Translation
Hello / Good-bye.	Hola / Adiós.
Excuse me.	Excuseme.
My name is. . . .	Me llamo. . . . or Mi nombre es. . . .
I am a technologist.	Yo soy un tecnólogo.
What is your name? / Is your name . . .?	Cómo se llama Usted?
How are you?	Cómo se siente Usted hoy? Cómo estás?
Do you speak English?	Habla inglés?
I speak very little Spanish.	Hablo un poco de español.
Answer yes or no.	Responda Sí o No.
Speak slowly.	Habla despacio.
I do not understand.	No comprendo, or No entiendo.
Do you understand?	Entiende?
Please.	Por favor.
Thank you / You're welcome.	Gracias / De nada.
How do you say [—] in Spanish?	Cómo se dice [—] en español?

Assessment	Translation
What's up? What's going on?	Qué pasa?
Are you okay?	Está bien?
Calm down, it's okay.	Cálmese, todo está bien.
Good / Bad.	Bueno / Malo.
Do you have any pain?	Siente dolor?
Where?	Dónde?
How long? 1-10 minutes / hours / days / weeks / months / years	Cuánto tiempo? Uno, dos, tres, cuatro, cinco, seis, siete, ocho, nueve, diez. Minutos / horas / días / semanas / meses / años.
Show me.	Muéstreme.
Chest pain?	Dolor en el pecho?
Shortness of breath?	Cortad de aliento? Respira difícil?
Are you hot / cold?	Siente calor? / Siente frío?
Would you like water, a blanket, a pillow, a urinal, a bed pan?	Quiere agua, una frazada, una almohada, un orinal, cuña?
Would you like to use the bathroom?	Quiere usar el baño?

Directions	Translation
Sign here.	Firme aquí.
Left / Right.	Izquierdo / Derecho.
Up / Down.	Arriba / Abajo.
Stand up.	Párese or Párate.
Come toward me / Back up.	Venga / Retroceda.
Turn around.	Dé la vuelta.
Sit down / here / up.	Siéntese / Siéntese aquí / Párese.
Let me help.	Déjeme ayudarle.
Lay down on your back / on your stomach.	Échese de espaldas / bocaabajo.
Put your head on the pillow.	Ponga la cabeza en la almohada.
Lift your knees / feet / head.	Levante las rodillas / los pies / la cabeza.
Arms up / down.	Levante los brazos / Baje los brazos.
Look straight up.	Mire hacia arriba.
Turn your head to the left / right.	Voltee la cabeza a la izquierda / derecha.
Left / right arm over head.	Ponga el brazo izquierdo / derecho sobre la cabeza.
Deep breath. Hold it. Let it out.	Respire profundo. Contenga la respiración. Expire.
Breathe normal.	Respire normalmente.
Do not move. Hold still.	No se mueva. Esté quieto.
We are taking a picture.	Estamos tomando una imagen.
You are doing great.	Usted está portándose muy bien.
It will go faster.	Ahora irá más rápido.
Walk faster.	Camine más rápido.

We are almost done.	Ya casi terminamos.
You are almost / all done.	Usted ya está listo / todo está listo.
Wait here.	Espere aquí.
You can go home now.	Ahora puede ir a casa.
You are going back up to your room, now.	Ahora quede ir a su cuarto.

Regulations

Misadministration

Radiation Safety

Misadministration

Current NRC Regulations

Note: The Nuclear Regulatory Commission (NRC) (and consequently agencies in agreement states, e.g., Bureau of Radiologic Control [BRC] in Florida) have, by issuance of their latest regulation changes, made it extremely difficult to cause a bona fide misadministration. The regulations concern *fission by-product material only*, e.g., ^{131}I, ^{125}I, ^{99}Mo, ^{99m}Tc, ^{133}Xe, ^{32}P, ^{51}Cr, etc. Most incidents fall under recordable events or reportable only within the individual department. Consult your radiation safety officer if there is any question or if the situation warrants it.

Misadministration

Diagnostic

- Only for doses > 30 μCi of ^{131}I NaI or ^{125}I NaI: wrong patient, or radiopharmaceutical, or dose difference $\geq 20\%$ and that difference is > 30 μCi.

- Other radiopharmaceuticals (including ^{99m}Tc): wrong patient, or radiopharmaceutical, or route, or dose amount, and the dose administered resulting in deep dose equivalent > 5 rem or total organ dose equivalent > 50 rem.

Therapeutic

- Wrong patient, or radiopharmaceutical, or route, and the dose difference $\pm > 20\%$.

Recordable Event

Diagnostic

- Only for doses > 30 μCi of ^{131}I NaI or ^{125}I NaI: No written directive for administration, and no record of directive, and the dose differs by 10% and that difference is > 15 μCi.

Therapeutic

- Any therapeutic radiopharmaceuticals: No written directive for administration, and no record of directive, and the dose differs by 10%.

Reportable Event

- All misadministrations are reportable.

Notification

- Within 24 hours: Telephone call to radiation safety officer, referring physician, and NRC or other regulatory agency (e.g., BRC).
- Within 15 days: Written report to NRC, referring physician, and patient or guardian.
- Records must be kept for 5 years.
- The department is to file a Quality Management Program with the NRC describing actions taken to prevent recurrence and its procedures for prescribing, calculating, dispensing, verifying, and administering radiopharmaceuticals, revised every 12 months.

All Other Incidents

- Spills, wrong patients, wrong radiopharmaceutical, wrong dose, wrong route, or by-product material that do not meet the above criteria and accelerator-produced radiopharmaceuticals should be brought to the attention of the supervisor and/or radiation safety officer along with a departmental incident report.

SUGGESTED READINGS

Early PJ, Sodee DB. Principles and Practice of Nuclear Medicine. 2nd ed. St. Louis: Mosby, 1995.

Lombardi M. Radiation Safety in Nuclear Medicine. Boca Raton, FL: CRC Press, 1999.

Wilson MA. Textbook of Nuclear Medicine. Philadelphia: Lippincott-Raven, 1998.

Notes

Radiation Safety

. . . .

This is intended only to serve as a limited review addressing some of the more common sources of confusion. Consult department policies and procedures for specific information concerning area surveys, spills, decontamination, and waste disposal. If there are any questions, contact your radiation safety officer.

Radiation

- Particles: alpha (α), beta$^+$ (β^+, positron), beta$^-$ (β^-, negatron), e$^-$ (electron), p$^+$ (proton), d$^+$ (deuteron), t$^+$ (triton), He^{2+} (helium ion beams), heavy nuclei (neutron beams).
- Photons (electromagnetic waves): cosmic energy, gamma (γ), x-ray, ultraviolet (UV), visible light, infrared (IR), radar (microwaves), radio, electric waves.

Modes of Decay

- Alpha (α): origin, nuclear; monoenergetic (discrete energies); soft-tissue penetration, 10–40 μm.
- Beta$^+$ (β^+, positron): origin, nuclear; continuum of energy, average energy = 1/3 E_{max}; > 1.02 MeV for annihilation radiation, produces two gamma emissions of 0.511 MeV at 180° (coincidence radiation) and neutrino.
- Beta$^-$ (β^-, negatron): origin, nuclear; continuum of energy, average energy = 1/3 E_{max}; antineutrino; soft-tissue penetration, 10 μm–1 cm.
- Gamma (γ): origin, nuclear; discrete energies, followed by prompt gamma emission or delayed gamma emission; soft-tissue penetration, infinite.
- Electron capture: usually K-electron capture; changes proton to neutron, releases gamma, neutrino, and x-ray.
- Isomeric transition: delayed gamma emission from metastable state.
- Internal conversion: gamma emission interacts with orbital electron; monoenergetic; conversion electron emitted, x-rays may do the same with auger electron emitted.
- Bremsstrahlung: braking radiation, secondary photon emission (x-ray) from negative acceleration of β particles passing closely to nucleus of atom. As it slows, the kinetic energy lost is released in the form of an x-ray. This is the source of most radiographic imaging.

Radiation Safety

- Time: reduce time spent near hot sources, e.g., patients, loaded syringes, open pigs, therapy doses (especially ^{131}I, even when shielded). Total exposure is directly and linearly related. Total millirems = millirems/hour × hours.
- Distance: step back from any hot source; the more distance, the less exposure. Inverse square law: $I_1 \times D_1^2 = I_2 \times D_2^2$, where I is intensity in milliroentgens per time, and D is distance.
- Shielding: use syringe shields, lead-lined carry cases, pigs, leaded glass shields, etc., when manipulating or transporting radiopharmaceuticals.

Units	Special Units	S.I. Units	Equivalents
Activity	curie	becquerel	1 mCi = 37 MBq
Exposure	roentgen	coulomb/kg air	C/kg air = 3876 R
Absorbed dose	rad	gray	1 Gy = 100 rad
Dose equivalent	rem	sievert	1 Sv = 100 rem

Biologic Effects

- Stochastic: chronic, low level, over long period. Measure of probability of linear and nonthreshold effect.

- Nonstochastic: acute, high level, short term. Measure of severity of effect. Linear with saturation level; reaching threshold results in degrees of radiation sickness.

- Hormesis: radiation-induced repair allowing resistance to future radiation damage on receiving minimal "triggering" dose. Existence is controversial.

Readings

- Lens (eye) dose equivalent (LDE): dose at 3 mm, taken from film badge.

- Shallow dose equivalent (SDE): whole-body dose (skin) at 70 μm, taken from film badge.

- Shallow dose equivalent (SDE): extremities (hands), taken from ring badge.

- Total organ dose equivalent (TODE): in nuclear medicine, also the same as deep dose equivalent (DDE) at 1 cm, taken from film badge.

- Total effective dose equivalent (TEDE): in nuclear medicine, also the same as DDE. Or, basically, in nuclear medicine, TODE = DDE = TEDE.

- Others: committed effective dose equivalent (CEDE), ingested radiation, not applicable; committed dose equivalent (CDE), organ radiation over 50 years, not applicable.

Annual Dose Limits

Occupational

Type of Reading	Measurement	Exposure
Whole-body TEDE (DDE)	5 rem	50 mSv/y
Whole-body SDE (skin)	50 rem	500 mSv/y
Internal TODE (organ)	50 rem	500 mSv/y
Extremity SDE	50 rem	500 mSv/y
Lens LDE (eye)	15 rem	150 mSv/y
Pregnant worker	500 mrem/9 months	5 mSv/9 months
	50 mrem/month	0.5 mSv/month
Minors, < 18 years old	10% of occupational limits	
Cumulative dose equivalent	Age of worker $\times$ 1 rem	

General Public

Whole body TEDE (DDE)	100 mrem/y	1 mSv/y
Unrestricted area	< 2 mrem/h and < 50 mrem/y	< 0.02 mSv/h and < 0.5 mSv/y
Embryo / fetus	500 mrem/9 months	5 mSv/9 months
Women of childbearing age	Physician approval, procedure at 10 days after menses	
Negligible dose	National Council on Radiation Protection (NCRP) has deemed 1 mrem (0.01 mSv) is negligible.	

A pregnant employee must declare her pregnancy in writing. At the time of declaration, if the estimated dose to the fetus is > 500 mrem, the dose for the remainder of the pregnancy must not exceed 50 mrem. If this is an infringement on her right to work, she can simply sign the appropriate paperwork to "undeclare" her pregnancy and continue working.

ALARA *(as low as reasonably achievable)*

- Level 1: Investigate and report. Quarterly reading (average for 3-month period), 10% of Nuclear Regulatory Commission (NRC) limit
  - whole body (organs), 125 mrem
  - whole body (skin), 1250 mrem
  - extremities, 1250 mrem
  - lens (eye), 375 mrem
- Level 2: Action level. Quarterly reading, 30% of NRC limit
  - whole body (organs), 375 mrem
  - whole body (skin), 3750 mrem
  - extremities, 3750 mrem
  - lens (eye), 1125 mrem

Packages

Label	Surface (mrem/h)	1 m (mrem/h)	Transportation Index[a]
White I	0.5	0	—
Yellow II	50	1	0.1 mrem/h (typically)
Yellow III nuclear medicine	100	3	1.2 mrem/h (typically)
Other industries	300	10	

[a](Applies to type II and III only. Actual exposure rate at 1 meter from surface of package at time of shipment.)

SUGGESTED READINGS

Early, PJ, Sodee DB. Principles and Practice of Nuclear Medicine. 2nd ed. St.Louis: Mosby, 1995.

Lombardi MH. Radiation Safety in Nuclear Medicine. Boca Raton, FL: CRC Press, 1999.

Wilson MA. Textbook of Nuclear Medicine. Philadelphia: Lippincott-Raven, 1998.

Notes

Patient Information for Thyroid Therapies

Ablation (> 30 mCi)

Hyperthyroid (< 30 mCi)

Patient Information for Thyroid Therapy (> 30 mCi)

1. You are not here because you are sick. The nursing staff will not be coming in to take daily vital signs like blood pressure and temperature.

2. This room is to keep you isolated during your therapy. Please confine yourself to the room.

3. The usual stay is about 3 days, depending on how much of the iodine is excreted as measured by a Geiger counter.

4. No visitors under the age of 18 or pregnant persons are allowed.

5. Visiting time permitted is no more than 20 minutes per visitor per day. The time increases slightly as the days progress.

6. Visitors must remain at the doorway (at least 10 feet from patient).

7. Iodine is released from the body in perspiration, as well as waste, so everything brought into the room and touched stays in the room. The clothes you wear and possessions handled will be bagged and stored for 3 months. Games and other items can be wrapped in plastic before being handled, then released once checked by the Geiger counter.

8. You will be given disposable plates and utensils. These must be stored for 3 months, then opened and surveyed with the Geiger counter. Please thoroughly rinse off dishes and rinse out cans and milk cartons before placing them in the storage bag.

9. Flush what you do not finish down the toilet (except for larger items like chicken bones, etc.) If you do not touch a meal at all, it can be surveyed and removed from the room.

10. When using the toilet, be careful not to contaminate the surrounding area, and, when done, flush three times to ensure dilution within the plumbing system. Wash hands often.

11. Questions: call the nuclear medicine department.

Patient Information for Hyperthyroid Therapy (< 30 mCi)

1. For at least 2 days, keep a distance of 3 feet or more between you and any people.

2. Do not hug or hold children close for 2 days.

3. Do not share utensils at home with anyone. Wash the ones you use thoroughly.

4. Keep your clothes and linen separate and wash them thoroughly. The iodine exits your body over time by bowel movements, urine, saliva, and perspiration.

5. Sleep alone for the first 2 nights.

6. When using the toilet, be careful not to contaminate the surrounding area and, when done, flush two times to ensure dilution within the plumbing system. Wash hands often.

7. You may feel a scratchy throat within a few days but that will subside.

8. It may take a couple of weeks to feel any benefit related to your condition from the capsules.

9. If you get sick and throw-up the capsule(s), try to do so in a toilet or sink or, at last resort, on the pavement. Call the nuclear medicine department so that they will know you no longer have the capsule(s) inside you. This is extremely rare and is usually caused by food or sickness unrelated to the iodine capsules.

10. Although any allergic reaction to the iodine capsules is extremely rare, if you feel you are having one, contact your doctor's office.

11. You have taken a capsule that contains radioactive iodine that emits beta and gamma rays. It is designed to do its therapeutic work on your thyroid and does not present a danger to anyone. These steps are taken only to reduce unnecessary exposure to people with whom you may come in contact.

12. Questions: call the nuclear medicine department.

Patient History Sheets

Adrenal Scans, mIBG, and NP59

Bone Scan

Brain Scan (SPECT)

Cardiac/MUGA Scan Rest/Stress/Redistribution

Gallium/Indium/Ceretec™ Scan

Gastric Empty Scan

GI Bleed/Meckel's

HIDA Scan

Lung Scan (Aerosol)

Lung Scan (Gas)

Liver/Spleen Scan

Miscellaneous Worksheet

Octreoscan®

OncoScint®/CEA-Scan®/Verluma™

ProstaScint®

Renal/Renogram Scan

Renal/Renogram/Captopril Scan

Scintimammography

Thyroid Uptake and Scan

Please feel free to copy these history sheets for department use.

History for Adrenal Scans, mIBG, and NP59

○ M   ○ F

. . . .

Date of exam _____   ❑ OP   ❑ ER   Room # _____

Patient name _____ Age _____   DOB ____ / ____ / _____

MR number _____ Height _____ Weight _____

Females: Pregnant _____ Physician: Dr. _____

Radiopharmaceutical: _____ Dose_____

Injection site _____ Time _____ Scans ____ /____ /____

Reason for scan _____

_____

Date symptoms began _____ Recent weight gain _____

Pain _____ Since when _____

Lugol or perchlorate (thyroid blocker) last night_____

Meds: list (both Rx and OTC) _____

Meds withheld for exam: how long _____

_____

Hx of CA (type) _____ When Dx _____

Allergy to iodine _____ Nausea and vomiting _____ Anxiety_____

Hyper- or hypotension _____ Oral contraceptives _____

Palpitations _____ Sweating _____ Headaches _____

Flushed face _____ Tingling in hands or feet _____

Radiation or chemo Tx _____ Diabetic _____

Hirsutism (abnormal hair growth) _____ Since when _____

Recent surgery _____

_____

♀Pt.: LMP____ /____ / ____   Hysterectomy _____ Menopause _____

Previous scans or related studies (type, when, where, Dx)

_____

_____

Other diagnosed diseases _____

Labs:_____ Date _____

Technologist _____

History for Bone Scan   ○ M   ○ F

....

Whole Body   Limited   3-Phase   (Circle One)

Date of exam _____ ❑ OP   ❑ ER   Room # _____

Patient name _____ Age _____ DOB ____/ ____/ _____

MR number _____ Height _____ Weight _____

Females: Pregnant _____ Physician: Dr. _____

Radiopharmaceutical:_____ Dose_____

Injection site _____ Time_____ Scan time_____

Reason for scan _____

_____

Bone Pain _____ Where _____ Radiating _____

_____

Broken bones _____ Recent trauma (falls, etc) _____

_____

Arthritis _____ Prosthesis _____

Infections _____ Swelling_____ Open sores _____

Hx of cancer (type, where, when Dx) _____

Chemo, radiation Tx _____ When _____

Recent surgery, related information _____

_____

_____

Previous scans or related studies (type, when, where, Dx) _____

_____

_____

Diabetic _____ Medications _____

Labs: _____ Date _____

Alk Phos _____ LDH _____ BUN _____ Creat _____

Ca^{2+}_____ PO_4 _____ PSA _____ Acid Phos _____

Comments _____

Technologist _____

History for Brain Scan (SPECT)

○ M ○ F

Date of exam _____ ❏ OP ❏ ER   Room # _____

Patient name _____ Age _____   DOB _____/_____/_____

MR number _____ Height _____ Weight _____

Females: Pregnant _____ Physician: Dr. _____

Radiopharmaceutical: _____ Dose_____

Injection site _____ Time _____ Scan time _____

Reason for scan _____

_____

Date symptoms began _____

Head pain (head aches, other area, pressure) _____

Since when _____ Where _____

Head trauma _____

CVA _____ When _____ What affected _____

Infection (e.g., meningitis, encephalitis) _____

Memory problems (short-term, long-term) _____

Since when _____

Seizures _____ Since when _____

Surgeries (any) _____

FHx of pain, CVA, memory loss _____

Shunt, metal plate _____ Location _____

Previous scans or related studies (EEG, MRI, CT, when, where, Dx) _____

_____

Diabetic _____ Medications _____

_____

Labs: _____ Date _____

Comments _____

Technologist _____

History for Cardiac/MUGA Scan Rest/Stress/Redistribution ○ M ○ F

Date of exam _____ ❏ OP ❏ ER Room # _____

Patient name _____ Age _____ DOB _____/ _____/ _____

MR number _____ Height _____ Weight _____

Females: Pregnant _____ Bra Size _____ Physician: Dr. _____

Radiopharmaceutical: _____ Dose _____

Radiopharmaceutical: _____ Dose _____

Drug interventions (type, amount) _____

Injection sites _____/_____   Times _____/_____   Scan times _____/_____

Reason for scan _____

Date symptoms began _____ Pain _____ How long _____

Where _____ SOB _____ How long _____

With exertion _____ Diet pills (type) _____

Hx of cancer _____ When Dx _____ Evaluation for chemo Tx _____

Hx of cardiac disease _____

What type (MI, CHF, CAD) _____

Family Hx of cardiac disease _____

Who, what type _____

Hypertension _____ When Dx _____ EtOH intake _____

Smoker (how much, how long) _____ Diabetic _____

Pacemaker _____ Nitro patch or meds _____ Asthma _____

Cardiac cath report (where, when) _____

Prior EKG _____ Results _____

Previous scans or related studies (type, when, where, Dx) _____

_____

Medications _____

_____

Labs: _____ Date _____

CPK _____ LDH _____ Chol _____ Troponin _____ Myoglobin _____

Comments _____

Technologist(s) _____ /_____

History for Gallium/Indium/Ceretec™ Scan   ○ M   ○ F

. . . .

Date of exam _____   ❑ OP   ❑ ER   Room # _____

Patient name _____ Age _____   DOB _____/_____/_____

MR number _____ Height _____ Weight _____

Females: Pregnant _____ Physician: Dr. _____

Radiopharmaceutical: _____ Dose _____

Injection site _____ Time _____ Scan time _____

Reason for scan _____

_____

Chief complaint _____

_____

Date symptoms began _____

Pain _____ Location _____

Fever _____ Since when _____ Frequency _____

Recent surgery _____ When _____

Where _____

Hx of cancer _____ What type _____

When Dx _____ Radiation or chemo Tx _____

Diabetes _____ Hx bowel disease _____

Biopsy or aspiration _____

Previous scans or related studies (type, when, where, Dx): _____

_____

_____

Diabetic _____ Medications _____

_____

Antibiotic therapy (what, when) _____

Labs: _____ Date _____

WBC _____ AST (SGOT) _____ ALT (SGPT) _____ GGTP_____

BUN _____ LDH _____ Alk Phos _____ Creat _____

Comments _____

Technologist _____

History for Gastric Empty Scan

○ M ○ F

Date of exam _____ ❏ OP ❏ ER Room # _____

Patient name _____ Age _____ DOB ____/ ____/ _____

MR number _____ Height _____ Weight _____

Females: Pregnant _____ Physician: Dr. _____

Radiopharmaceutical: _____ Dose _____

Injection site _____ Time _____ Scan time _____

Reason for scan _____

_____

Chief complaint _____

_____

Date symptoms began _____

Last solid meal _____ Feel full soon after eating _____

Abdominal pain _____ Where _____

Bloating _____ Acid burning _____ Ulcers _____

Diabetic _____ Nausea and vomiting _____

Hx of cancer _____ Where _____

Recent surgery (where, when) _____

Allergic to Reglan _____ Allergic to eggs _____

Previous scans or related studies (type, when, where, Dx) _____

_____

_____

Medications_____

_____

Labs:_____ Date _____

Intrinsic factor _____ Gastrin _____ Pepsin _____

Amylase _____

Comments _____

_____

_____

Technologist _____

History for GI Bleed/Meckel's   ○ M ○ F

. . . .

Date of exam _____ ❏ OP   ❏ ER   Room # _____

Patient name _____ Age _____   DOB _____ / _____ / _____

MR number _____ Height _____ Weight _____

Females: Pregnant _____ Physician: Dr. _____

Radiopharmaceutical:_____ Dose _____

Injection site _____ Time _____ Scan time _____

Reason for scan _____

_____

Chief complaint _____

_____

Date symptoms began _____

Abdominal pain _____ Where _____

Active bleeding _____ How long _____

Color of blood in stool (bright red, burgundy, dark) _____

Hx of cancer _____ Diverticulitis _____ Crohn's _____

Colostomy _____ Site _____ Surgery _____ Site _____

Recent transfusion _____ How many units _____

Receiving KCl IV fluids _____

Previous scans or related studies (type, when, where, Dx) _____

_____

_____

Diabetic _____ Medications _____

_____

Labs: _____ Date _____

RBC _____ Hematocrit _____ Hemoglobin _____

WBC _____ Guaiac Test _____

Comments _____

_____

_____

Technologist _____

History for HIDA Scan

O M   O F

. . . .

Date of exam _____   ❏ OP   ❏ ER   Room # _____

Patient name _____ Age _____   DOB _____/_____/_____

MR number _____ Height _____ Weight _____

Females: Pregnant _____ Physician: Dr. _____

Radiopharmaceutical: _____ Dose _____

Injection site _____ Time _____ Scan time _____

Reason for scan _____

_____

Chief complaint _____

_____

Date symptoms began _____

Last solid meal _____

Abdominal pain _____ Where _____

Nausea/vomiting _____ EtOH intake _____ Smoke _____

Jaundice _____ Intolerance to fatty food _____

Abnormal blood tests _____

Allergic to morphine _____

Hx of liver/GB disease or surgery (hepatitis, cancer, gallstones) _____

_____

_____

Recent sonogram _____ Results _____

Previous scans or related studies (type, when, where, Dx)

_____

Diabetic _____ Medications _____

_____

Labs: _____   Date _____

T. Bili _____ Alk. Phos _____ ALT (SGPT) _____ AST (SGOT) _____

GGTP _____ LDH _____ Amylase _____ CPK _____ WBC _____

Creat _____ BUN _____

Comments _____

Technologist _____

History for Lung Scan (Aerosol)   ◯ M   ◯ F

....

Date of exam _____   ❏ OP   ❏ ER   Room # _____

Patient name _____ Age _____   DOB _____/ _____/ _____

MR number _____ Height _____ Weight _____

Females: Pregnant _____ Physician: Dr. _____

Radiopharmaceutical: 99mTc-DTPA   Dose _____ Time _____

Radiopharmaceutical: 99mTc-MAA   Dose _____

Injection site _____ Time _____ Scan time _____

Reason for scan _____

_____

Date symptoms began _____ Oral contraceptives _____

Recent (within 24 hours) chest x-ray _____

Chest pain _____ Where _____ Syncopy _____

SOB _____ Fever _____ Hemoptysis _____

Smoker (how much) _____ Recent long trips _____

Recent or upcoming surgery _____

Hx of any lung disease (prior PE, emphysema, bronchitis, pneumonia, pleurisy) _____

_____

Hx of cancer, deep vein thrombosis, phlebitis, heart disease _____

_____

_____

Previous scans or related studies (type, when, where, Dx)? _____

_____

_____

Diabetic _____ Medications _____

_____

Heparin, Coumadin, Lovenox, Ticlid _____

Labs: _____ Date _____

$PaCO_2$_____ PaO_2_____ pH _____ O_2 Sat _____

Comments _____

Technologist _____

History for Lung Scan (Gas)

○ M   ○ F

. . . .

Date of exam _____   ❑ OP   ❑ ER   Room # _____

Patient name _____ Age _____   DOB ____/ ____/ _____

MR number _____ Height _____ Weight _____

Females: Pregnant _____   Physician: Dr. _____

Radiopharmaceutical: ^{133}Xe   Dose _____ Time _____

Radiopharmaceutical: ^{99m}Tc-MAA   Dose _____

Injection site _____ Time _____ Scan time _____

Reason for scan _____

_____

Recent (within 24 hours) chest x-ray _____

Date symptoms began _____   Oral contraceptives _____

Chest pain _____ Where _____   Syncopy _____

SOB _____ Fever _____   Hemoptysis _____

Smoker (how much) _____   Recent long trips _____

Recent or upcoming surgery _____

Hx of any lung disease (prior PE, emphysema, bronchitis, pneumonia, pleurisy)

_____

_____

Hx of cancer, deep vein thrombosis, phlebitis, heart disease

_____

_____

Previous scans or related studies (type, when, where, Dx)

_____

_____

Diabetic _____   Medications _____

_____

Heparin, Coumadin, Lovenox, Ticlid _____

Labs: _____   Date _____

PaCO$_2$ _____ PaO$_2$ _____ pH _____ O$_2$ Sat _____

Comments _____

Technologist _____

History for Liver/Spleen Scan   ○ M   ○ F

. . . .

Date of exam _____   ❑ OP   ❑ ER   Room # _____

Patient name _____ Age _____   DOB _____/ _____/ _____

MR number _____ Height _____ Weight _____

Females: Pregnant _____ Physician: Dr. _____

Radiopharmaceutical: _____ Dose _____

Injection site _____ Time _____ Scan time _____

Reason for scan _____

_____

Date symptoms began _____

Abdominal pain_____ Where _____

Nausea/vomiting _____ Jaundice _____

Hx of surgery or disease of liver, GB, spleen (hepatitis, cancer, abnormal blood tests)

_____

_____

Alcohol consumption_____ Smoking _____

Previous scans or related studies (type, when, where, Dx)

_____

_____

_____

Diabetic _____ Medications _____

_____

_____

Labs: _____   Date _____

T. Bili _____ Alk Phos _____ ALT(SGPT) _____ AST(SGOT) _____

GGTP _____ LDH _____ Hgb _____ HCT _____ Platelets _____

Comments _____

_____

_____

Technologist _____

Miscellaneous Worksheet   ○ M ○ F

. . . .

Scan _____

Date of exam _____ ❏ OP ❏ ER   Room # _____

Patient name _____ Age _____ DOB ____/ ____/ _____

MR number _____ Height _____ Weight _____

Females: Pregnant _____ Physician: Dr. _____

Radiopharmaceutical: _____ Dose _____

Injection site _____ Time _____ Scan time _____

Clinical and scan data _____

_____

_____

_____

_____

_____

_____

_____

_____

_____

_____

_____

_____

_____

_____

_____

_____

_____

_____

_____

_____

_____

_____

_____

Technologist _____

History for Octreoscan®

○ M ○ F

Date of exam _____ ❑ OP ❑ ER Room # _____

Patient name _____ Age _____ DOB ____/ ____/ _____

MR number _____ Height _____ Weight _____

Females: Pregnant _____ Physician: Dr. _____

Radiopharmaceutical: _____ Dose _____

Injection site _____ Time _____ Scan time _____

Reason for scan _____

_____

Date symptoms began _____

Pain _____ Since when _____

Hx of CA (type) _____ When Dx _____

Tx of octreotide acetate _____ Since when _____

Other Tx _____

Hx of insulinoma _____ Since when _____

Hx of impaired renal function _____ Since when _____

Pt. on total parenteral nutrition _____ Since when _____

Recent surgery _____

_____

_____

♀Pt.: LMP ___/ ___/ ___ Hysterectomy _____ Menopause _____

Previous scans or related studies (type, when, where, Dx)

_____

_____

_____

Diabetic _____ Medications _____

_____

Labs: _____ Date _____

Comments _____

_____

_____

Patient needs to purchase 4 cans of magnesium citrate.

Technologist _____

History for OncoScint®/CEA-Scan®/Verluma™   ○ M   ○ F

. . . .

Date of exam _____   ❏ OP   ❏ ER   Room # _____

Patient name _____ Age _____   DOB _____/ _____/ _____

MR number _____ Height _____ Weight _____

Females: Pregnant _____ Physician: Dr. _____

Radiopharmaceutical: _____ Dose _____

Injection site _____ Time _____ Scan time _____

Reason for scan _____

_____

Any known allergies (murine products, indium, etc.) _____

Previous MoAb tests _____

Pain (where, since when) _____

Hx of CA (type, when Dx) _____

Surgery (type, when) _____

_____

Radiation Tx _____Chemo _____

Related scans (previous, pending, e.g., bone scan, bone marrow, MRI, CT, US, x-ray, biopsy)

_____

_____

Abnormal lab reports (CEA, CA-125, HAMA, other) _____

_____

Diabetic _____ Medications _____

_____

Laxative/enema ordered _____

Injection monitoring

Time	HR	BP	Resp. Rate	Comments
Baseline				
5 min				
15 min				
30 min				
60 min				

RN _____Technologist _____

History for ProstaScint®   ○ M   ○ F

Date of exam _____   ❑ OP   ❑ ER   Room # _____

Patient name _____ Age _____   DOB _____ / _____ / _____

MR number _____ Height _____ Weight _____

Females: Pregnant _____ N/A _____ Physician: Dr. _____

Radiopharmaceutical: _____ Dose _____

Injection site _____ Time _____

Scan days/time _____ / _____ / _____

Reason for scan _____

Any known allergies (murine products, indium, etc.) _____

Biopsy _____ Previous MoAb tests _____

Pain (where, since when) _____

Hx/FHx of CA (type, when Dx) _____

Surgery (type, when) _____

_____

Radiation Tx _____ Chemo _____

Related scans (previous, pending, e.g., bone, MRI, CT, US, x-ray)

_____

Labs: Date: _____ PSA _____ HAMA _____ BUN _____ Creat _____ Ca²⁺ _____

Acid Phos _____ Phosphorus _____ T. Bili _____ T. Protein _____

Albumin _____ AST _____ ALT _____ Glucose _____ CEA _____

Diabetic _____ Medications _____

_____

Laxative/enema ordered _____

Injection monitoring

Time	HR	BP	Resp. Rate	Comments
Baseline				
5 min				
15 min				
30 min				
60 min				

RN _____ Technologist _____

History for Renal/Renogram Scan   ○ M   ○ F

....

Date of exam_____   ❑ OP   ❑ ER   Room #_____

Patient name_____ Age_____ DOB_____/_____/_____

MR number_____ Height_____ Weight_____

Females: Pregnant_____ Physician: Dr. _____

Radiopharmaceutical:_____ Dose _____

Injection site_____ Time _____ Scan time _____

Reason for scan_____

_____

Date symptoms began _____

Pain _____ Hematuria _____

Nausea and vomiting _____ Allergy to IVP dye _____

Hx of cancer _____ When Dx _____

Hx of stones, infections (bladder or kidneys), obstructions, surgery _____

_____

Urinary frequency _____ Urgency _____

Hypertension _____ Diabetes _____

Dialysis _____ CHF or cardiac disease _____

Previous scans or related studies (type, when, where, Dx)

_____

_____

_____

Medications _____

_____

Captopril: BP _____   _____   _____   _____   _____   _____

Labs: Date _____ Furosemide_____ mg   Time _____

BUN _____ Protein/albumin _____ Creat _____

Comments _____

_____

                                        Technologist _____

History for Renal/Renogram/Captopril Scan   ○ M ○ F

. . . .

Date of exam _____ ❏ OP ❏ ER   Room # _____

Patient name _____ Age _____   DOB ____/____/_____

MR number _____ Height _____ Weight _____

Females: Pregnant _____ Physician: Dr. _____

Radiopharmaceutical: _____ Dose 1st _____ 2nd _____

Injection site _____ Time _____ Time _____

Reason for scan _____

_____

Date symptoms began _____ Pain _____

Hematuria _____ Nausea and vomiting _____ Dialysis_____

Hx of cancer _____ When Dx _____ Allergy to IVP dye _____

Hx of stones, infections (bladder or kidneys), obstructions, surgery _____

_____

Hypertension _____ Meds _____ Diabetes _____

Urinary frequency _____ Urgency _____ CHF, cardiac disease _____

Previous scans or related studies (type, when, where, Dx)

_____

_____

Medications_____

_____

Labs: Date _____ Furosemide_____ mg Time _____

BUN _____ Protein/albumin _____ Creat _____

Comments_____

_____

Captopril _____ mg   Time _____

Time	HR	BP	Resp. Rate	Comments
Baseline				
5 min				
15 min				
30 min				
60 min				

RN _____ Technologist _____

History for Scintimammography   ○ M   ○ F

....

Date of exam_____   ❑ OP   ❑ ER   Room #_____

Patient name_____ Age_____ DOB_____/_____/_____

MR number_____ Height_____ Weight_____

Females: Pregnant_____ Bra Size_____ Physician: Dr._____

Radiopharmaceutical:_____ Dose_____

Injection site_____ Time_____ Scan time_____

Reason for scan_____

_____

Date symptoms began_____

Palpable nodules_____ When_____

Pain or tenderness in breasts (where, how often)_____

_____ Discharge (side, how often)_____

Implants_____ Type_____ Side(s)_____

Recent surgery or mastectomy_____

Where_____ When_____

Recent trauma to chest (type, when, where)_____

Hx of CA (type, when Dx)_____

FHx of CA (type, who)_____

Radiation or chemo Tx_____

Recent or previous scans (mammogram, MRI, CT, x-rays, biopsy, date, where, Dx)_____

_____

_____

Diabetic_____ Medications_____

_____

Labs:_____ Date_____

Comments_____

_____

Technologist_____

History for Thyroid Uptake and Scan   ○ M   ○ F

Date of exam _____   ❏ OP   ❏ ER   Room # _____

Patient name _____ Age _____   DOB ____/ ____/ _____

MR number _____ Height _____ Weight _____

Females: Pregnant _____ Physician: Dr. _____

Radiopharmaceutical: $^{99m}Tc\ O_4^-$ Dose _____ mCi _____

Injection site _____ Time _____ Scan time _____

^{123}I Dose _____ μCi   Time _____ Standard count _____

4- to 6-h uptake _____ %   Normal range _____   to _____ %

24-h uptake   _____ %   Normal range _____   to _____ %

Reason for uptake and scan _____

_____ Date symptoms began _____

Lumps or swelling in neck _____ Tenderness _____

Exactly where _____

Difficulty swallowing _____ Nervous _____ Tired _____

Weight gain/loss _____ How much _____ Since when _____

Appetite good/bad _____ Perspire more _____ Fevers _____

Heat/cold bother _____ Heart palpitations _____

Menstrual problems (irregular, infrequent, heavy) _____

Past Hx of thyroid disease _____ When _____ Type _____

Treatment _____ When _____ Type _____

Hx goiter _____ Hx nodules _____ Hx surgery _____

Hx thyroid CA _____ When _____ Type _____

FHx of thyroid disease _____ Type _____

Recent iodine contrast, dye studies (CT, IVP, GB, arteriogram, venogram, when, where, Dx)

_____

_____

Previous scans, studies, biopsy (type, when, where, Dx)

_____

_____

Palpate patient's thyroid

Draw (anterior view) position of lump(s) or tenderness if found

Check list questions for patient (circle those that apply)

Hyperthyroid	Hypothyroid
Neck swelling	Lethargy
Increased nervousness	Increased tiredness
Weight loss (amount)	Weight gain (amount)
Increased appetite	Decreased appetite
Heat intolerance	Cold intolerance
Diarrhea	Constipation
Increased irritability	Drowsiness
Hand tremors	Edema
Warm, moist skin	Dry skin
Hair loss	Dry, coarse hair
Hoarseness	Weakness
Sore throat	
Difficulty swallowing	
Heart palpitations	
Exophthalmus (bulging eyes, do a visual check)	

Thyroid medications _____

When taken off _____

(Synthroid 3 wk, Cytomel 2 wk, PTU 2 wk, thyroid grains 6 wk)

Other meds, vitamins, antiarrhythmics _____

Labs:_____ Date _____

RT_3U _____ T_4 _____ T_7 _____ TSH _____

Parathyroid disease (↑Ca, ↑PTH, Surgery, +FH) _____

Sensitive to pain _____ Ca _____ PTH _____

Diabetic _____ Comments _____

Technologist _____

Abbreviations Commonly Used in Nuclear Medicine

Acc or accel	accelerator
ACD	citric acid, sodium citrate, dextrose—blood thinner
ACE	adrenal cortical extract, angiotensin-converting enzyme
ACF	antecubital fossa
ACTH	adrenocorticotropic hormone
A-fib	atrial fibrillation
AFP	α-fetoprotein
AIDS	acquired immune deficiency syndrome
Al	aluminum
Alk	alkaline
ALT	alanine amino transferase (SGPT)
ANT	anterior
APUD	amine precursor uptake in decarboxylation
ARDS	adult respiratory distress syndrome
AST	aspartate amino transferase (SGOT)
AtOH	alcohol
AVM	arteriovenous malformation
BBB	blood–brain barrier
BE	barium enema
b.i.d.	*bis in die,* twice daily
Bkg	background
b.m.	bone marrow
BP	blood pressure
BUN	blood urea nitrogen
CA	cancer
CAD	coronary artery disease
CBC	complete blood count
CBD	common bile duct
cc	cubic centimeter
CCK	cholecystokinin
CEA	carcinoembryonic antigen
chemo	chemotherapy
CHF	congestive heart failure
Chol	cholesterol
Cl	chloride

cm	centimeters		**FDG**	floro deoxyglucose
Co	cobalt		**EtOH**	alcohol (ethanol)
COPD	chronic obstructive pulmonary disease		**FDG**	fluorodeoxyglucose
COR	center of rotation		**FHx**	family history
CPK	creatine phosphokinase		**fib**	fibula
cpm	counts per minute		**FN**	false negative
Creat	creatinine		**FNA**	fine needle aspiration
CSF	cerebrospinal fluid		**FOV**	field of view
CT	computerized tomography, cat scan		**FP**	false positive
cts.	counts		**Ga**	gallium
CVA	cerebrovascular accident		**GFR**	glomerular filtration rate
CYT	conjugate of antibody 7E11-C5.3-gly-cyl-tyrosyl-(N,e-diethylenetriamine pentaacetic acid)-lysine		**GGTP**	γ-glutamyl transpeptidase
			GH	glucoheptonate
			GI	gastrointestinal
DEXA	dual energy x-ray absorptiometry		**H/A**	headache
DMSA	2,3-dimercaptosuccinic acid		**HAM**	human albumin microspheres
DOB	date of birth		**HAMA**	human anti-mouse antibodies
DTPA	diethylene triamine pentaacetic acid		**HBP**	high blood pressure
dopa	3,4-dihydroxyphenylalanine		**HCT**	hematocrit
DPA	dual photon absorptiometry of gamma rays		**HDP**	hydroxyethylene diphosphonate
			Hgb	hemoglobin
DPM	disintegrations per minute		**HIDA**	*N*-(2,6-dimethylphenylcarbamoyl-methyl)iminodiacetic acid
DTPA	diethylenetriaminepentaacetic acid			
DVT	deep vein thrombosis		**HMPAO**	D,L-hexamethylpropyleneamine oxime
Dx	diagnosis			
EC	electron capture		**HTN**	hypertension
ECG/EKG	electrocardiogram		**Hx**	history
ED	end diastole		**I**	iodine
EDTMP	ethylenediamine-tetramethylene phosphonate		**IDA**	iminodiacetic acid
			IF	intrinsic factor
EDV	end-diastolic volume		**IHD**	intrahepatic duct
EF	ejection fraction		**IM**	intramuscular
E/F	evaluate for		**IMP**	iodoamphetamine
ER	emergency room		**In**	indium
ERPF	effective renal plasma flow		**IP**	in-patient
ES	end systole		**IT**	isomeric transition
ESV	end-systolic volume		**ITLC**	instant thin-layer chromatography
F	fluorine			

IV	intravenous	NPO	*non per os*, nothing by mouth
k	kilo	N/V/D	nausea, vomiting and diarrhea
keV	kiloelectrovolts	MUGA	multi-gated acquisition
kg	kilogram	MUGA-X	stress MUGA
KUB	kidney-ureter-bladder x-ray	NM	nuclear medicine
LAT	left anterior oblique	OIH	orthoiodohippurate
LATS	long-acting thyroid stimulator	OP	out-patient
LDH	lactic dehydrogenase	PE	pulmonary embolism
LEAP	low-energy, all-purpose	ped(s)	pediatric (children)
LEHR	low-energy, high-resolution	PET	positron emission tomography
LEM	low-energy, mobile	phos	phosphatase
LEHS	low-energy, high-sensitivity	PI	post-injection
LFOV	large field of view	PRN	*pro re nata*, as necessary
LLAT or LL	left lateral	PO	*per os*, by mouth
LMP	last menstrual period	PSA	prostate-specific antigen
LPO	left posterior oblique	p-scope	persistence scope
LSC	liquid scintillation counter	pyp	pyrophosphate
LVEF	left ventricular ejection fraction	QC	quality control
MAA	macroaggregated albumin	q.i.d.	*quater in die*, four times daily
MAG$_3$	mercaptoacetyltriglycine	RAIU	radioactive iodine uptake
MBq	megabecquerels	RAO	right anterior oblique
μCi	microcuries	RBC	red blood cell
μg	microgram	RDS	respiratory distress syndrome, reflex dystrophy syndrome
mCi	millicuries	RES	reticuloendothelial system
MDP	methylene diphosphonate	RLAT or RL	right lateral
MEAP	medium-energy, all-purpose	R/O	rule out
meds	medications	RIS	radioimmunoscintigraphy
mg	milligrams	ROI	region of interest
MEGP	medium-energy, general-purpose	RP	radiopharmaceutical
MI	myocardial infarction	RPO	right posterior oblique
mL	milliliter	RSO	radiation safety officer
mIBG	*meta*-iodobenzylguanidine	RVEF	right ventricular ejection fraction
MoAb	monoclonal antibody	sal.	saline
MRI	magnetic resonance imaging	SC	sulfur colloid
msec	millisecond(s)	SEXA	single energy x-ray absorptiometry
Na	sodium	SGOT	(AST) serum glutamic-oxaloacetate transaminase
ng	nanogram(s)		

SGPT	(ALT) serum glutamic-oxaloacetate transaminase		**TIA (position)**	tail in the air
SOB	short(ness) of breath		**tib**	tibia
SPA	single photon absorptiometry		**t.i.d.**	*ter in die,* three times a day
SPECT	single photon emission computer tomography		**Tl**	thallium
			TN	true negative
SPEM	single photon emission mammograph		**TOD**	tail on detector
SSKI	saturated solution potassium iodide		**TP**	true positive
SSN	suprasternal notch		**TPN**	total parenteral nutrition
STAT	order to be done immediately		**TRH**	thyrotropin-releasing hormone
$t_{1/2}$	radioactive half-life		**TSH**	thyroid-stimulating hormone, thyrotropin
TAG	tumor-associated glycoprotein		**Tx**	therapy
t_b	biological half-life		**US**	ultrasound
t_e	effective half-life		**UTI**	urinary tract infection
T. Bili	total bilirubin		**v-fib**	ventricular fibrillation
Tc	technetium		**vit.**	vitamin
TER	tubular excretion rate		**WBC**	white blood cell
TIA (brain)	transient ischemic attack		**Xe**	Xenon

REFERENCES

Alazraki NP, Mishkin FS, eds. Fundamentals of Nuclear Medicine. 2nd ed. New York: Society of Nuclear Medicine, 1988.

Bernier DR et al., eds. Nuclear Medicine: Technology and Techniques. 2nd ed. St. Louis: Mosby, 1989.

Bernier DR, Christian PE, Langan JK, eds. Nuclear Medicine: Technology and Techniques. 3rd ed. St. Louis: Mosby, 1994.

Chohan N, ed. Nursing 99 Drug Handbook. Springhouse, PA: Springhouse, 1999.

Datz FL. Handbook of Nuclear Medicine. 2nd ed. St. Louis: Mosby, 1993.

Diatide, Inc. AcuTect Image Atlas. Londonderry, NH, 1998.

Duffy MA, ed. Physicians' Desk Reference. 46th ed. Montvale, NJ: Medical Economics Company, 1992.

Duncan K. Radiopharmaceuticals in PET imaging. Pamphlet. J Nucl Med Technol 1998;26:228-234.

Du Pont Pharma Radiopharmaccuticals. Introduction to Nuclear Cardiology. 3rd ed. Du Pont Pharma, 1993.

Early PJ, Sodee DB. Principles and Practice of Nuclear Medicine. 2nd ed. St. Louis: Mosby, 1995.

Genzyme Therapeutics. Thyrogen®, thyrotropin alfa for injection. Pamphlet. Cambridge: Genzyme and Knoll, 1999.

Gilbert S, ed. Journal of Nuclear Medicine Technology. Reston, VA: The Society of Nuclear Medicine, 1997.

Goldsmith SJ, ed. Journal of Nuclear Medicine. Reston, VA: The Society of Nuclear Medicine, 1997.

Hacker C. Radiation Decay: Emissions Tables and Spectra. 3.5-inch floppy disk program, Rockville, MD: Grove Engineering, 1995.

Harruff RC. Pathology Facts. Philadelphia: JB Lippincott, 1994.

Klingensmith W, Eshima D, Goddard J. Nuclear Medicine Procedure Manual 1992-93. Englewood, CO: Wick, 1993.

Klingensmith W, Eshima D, Goddard J. Nuclear Medicine Procedure Manual 1997-98. Englewood, CO: Wick, 1998.

Loeb S, ed. Nursing 94 Drug Handbook. Springhouse, PA: Springhouse, 1994.

Lombardi MH. Radiation Safety in Nuclear Medicine. Boca Raton, FL: CRC Press LLC, 1999.

Marieb EN. Human Anatomy and Physiology. 2nd ed. Redwood City, CA: Benjamin/Cummings, 1992.

Murray IPC, Ell PJ, eds. Nuclear Medicine in Clinical Diagnosis and Treatment. Vols. 1 and 2. New York: Churchill Livingstone, 1994.

O'Connor MK. The Mayo Clinic Manual of Nuclear Medicine. New York: Churchill Livingstone, 1996.

Smeltzer SC, Bare BG. Brunner and Suddarth's Textbook of Medical-Surgical Nursing. 8th ed. Philadelphia: Lippincott-Raven, 1996.

Sorenson JA, Phelps ME. Physics in Nuclear Medicine. 2nd ed. Philadelphia: WB Saunders, 1987.

Squibb. Nuclear Medicine Handbook. Princeton: ER Squibb & Sons, 1990.

Thomas C, ed. Taber's Cyclopedic Medical Dictionary. 17th ed. Philadelphia: FA Davis, 1993.

Travis EL. Primer of Medical Radiobiology. 2nd ed. Chicago: Year Book, 1989.

Van De Graaff KM, Fox SI. Concepts of Human Anatomy and Physiology. Dubuque, IA: Brown, 1986.

Wilson MA. Textbook of Nuclear Medicine. Philadelphia: Lippincott-Raven, 1998.

Unpublished Resources

- Information from the Nuclear Medicine curriculum at
  - Hillsborough Community College, Tampa, FL. Dr. Max Lombardi, Director (retired)
- Information from courses at
  - Plymouth State College of the University of New Hampshire, Plymouth, NH
  - St. Petersburg Junior College, St. Petersburg, FL
- Information from Nuclear Medicine Department manuals at
  - Bayfront Medical Center, St. Petersburg, FL
  - Columbia Doctor's Hospital, Sarasota, FL
  - Columbia South Bay Hospital, Sun City, FL
  - H. Lee Moffitt Cancer Center, Tampa, FL
  - James A. Haley Veterans Hospital, Tampa, FL
  - Morton Plant Hospital, Clearwater, FL
  - Palms of Pasadena Hospital, St. Petersburg, FL
  - St. Joseph's Hospital, Tampa, FL

Considerations and thanks given to the many physicians, technologists, and nursing staff at these various institutions for their instruction, suggestions, observations, and insight. Thanks also to the following for their language expertise:

Patrick DelMastro—Italian
Ania Lipska—Polish
Max Lombardi—Spanish, Portuguese, Italian
Joe Vuu—Mandarin Chinese
Shimzen Young—Japanese

AcuTect™ is a trademark of Diatide, Inc., Londonderry, NH.

Adalat® is a registered trademark of Miles, Inc., West Haven, CT.

Ativan® is a registered trademark of Wyeth-Ayerst Laboratories, Philadelphia, PA.

Axid® is a registered trademark of Whitehall-Robins Laboratories, New York, NY.

Benadryl® is a registered trademark with Parke-Davis, Morris Plains, NJ.

Betadine® is a registered trademark of Purdue Fredrick Co., Norwalk, CT.

Blocadren® is a registered trademark of Merck, Sharp, & Dohme, West Point, PA.

Brevibloc® is a registered trademark of Du Pont Pharmaceuticals, Wilmington, DE.

Calan® is a registered trademark of GD Searle & Co., Chicago, IL.

Capoten® is a registered trademark of ER Squibb & Sons, Inc., Princeton, NJ.

Cardene® is a registered trademark of Syntex Laboratories, Inc., Palo Alto, CA.

Cardiolite® is a registered trademark of DuPont Pharmaceuticals, Wilmington, DE.

Cardizem® is a registered trademark of Marion Merrell Dow Inc., Kansas City, MO.

Cartrol® is a registered trademark of Abbott Laboratories, North Chicago, IL.

CEA-Scan® is a registered trademark of Immunomedics, Inc., Morris Plains, NJ.

Centrax® is a registered trademark of Parke-Davis, Morris Plains, NJ.

Ceretec™ is a trademark of Amersham International Plc, Amersham, UK.

Choletec® is a registered trademark of Bracco Diagnostics, Inc., Princeton, NJ.

CLOtest® is a registered trademark of Tri-Med Specialties, Inc., Lenexa, KS.

Conray® is a registered trademark of Mallinckrodt Medical, Inc., St. Louis, MO.

Corgard® is a registered trademark of Bristol Laboratories, Evansville, IN.

Dalmane® is a registered trademark of Roche Laboratories, Nutley, NJ.

Demerol® is a registered trademark of Sanofi Winthrop Pharmaceuticals, New York, NY.

Diamox® is a registered trademark of Lederle Laboratories, Wayne, NJ.

Dilaudid® is a registered trademark of Knoll Pharmaceuticals, Whippany, NJ.

Doral® is a registered trademark of Wallace Laboratories, Cranbury, NJ.

Dulcolax® is a registered trademark of CIBA Consumer Pharmaceuticals, Edison, NJ.

DynaCirc® is a registered trademark of Sandoz Pharmaceuticals, East Hanover, NJ.

Elixophyllin® is a registered trademark of Forest Pharmaceuticals, Inc., St. Louis, MO.

Fleet® Kit is a registered trademark of CB Fleet Co., Inc., Lynchburg, VA.

Fosamax® is a registered trademark of Merke and Co., Inc., Fort Washington, PA.

Gelusil® is a registered trademark of Warner-Lambert Co., Morris Plains, NJ.

Halcyon® is a registered trademark of The Upjohn Company, Kalamazoo, MI.

Inderal® is a registered trademark of Wyeth-Ayerst Laboratories, Philadelphia, PA.

Inderide® is a registered trademark of Wyeth-Ayerst Laboratories, Philadelphia, PA.

Isoptin® is a registered trademark of Knoll Pharmaceuticals, Whippany, NJ.

Kerlone® is a registered trademark of GD Searle & Co., Chicago, IL.

Kinevac® is a registered trademark of Bracco Diagnostics, Inc., Princeton, NJ.

Klonopin® is a registered trademark of Roche Laboratories, Nutley, NJ.

Lasix® is a registered trademark of Hoechst-Roussel Pharmaceuticals, Inc., Somerville, NJ.

Levatol® is a registered trademark of Reed & Carnrick, Jersey City, NJ.

Librium® is a registered trademark of Roche Laboratories, Nutley, NJ.

Lopressor® is a registered trademark of Geigy Pharmaceuticals, Ardsley, NY.

Maalox® is a registered trademark of CIBA Consumer Pharmaceuticals, Edison, NJ.

MAG$_3$® is a registered trademark of Mallinckrodt Medical, Inc., St. Louis, MO.

Metastron® is a registered trademark of Amersham International Plc, Amersham, UK.

Microlite® is a registered trademark of DuPont Merck, Wilmington, DE.

Miraluma™ is a trademark of DuPont Merck, Wilmington, DE.

Monopril® is a registered trademark of Mead Johnson Pharmaceuticals, Evansville, IN.

Mylanta® is a registered trademark of Merck & Co., Inc., Fort Washington, PA.

Myoview® is a registered trademark of Amersham International Plc, Amersham, UK.

NeoTect™ is a trademark of Diatide, Inc., Londonberry, NH.

Neurolite™ is a trademark of DuPont Merck, Wilmington, DE.

Nimotop® is a registered trademark of Miles, Inc., West Haven, CT.

Normozide® is a registered trademark of Schering Corporation, Kenilworth, NJ.

OctreoScan® is a registered trademark of Mallinckrodt Medical, Inc., St. Louis, MO.

OncoScint® is a registered trademark of Cytogen Corporation, Princeton, NJ.

Osteolite® is a registered trademark of DuPont Merck, Wilmington, DE.

Paxipam® is a registered trademark of Schering Corporation, Kenilworth, NJ.

PDR® is a registered trademark of Medical Economics Company, Montvale, NJ.

Pepcid® is a registered trademark of Merck & Co., Inc., Fort Washington, PA.
Peptavlon® is a registered trademark of Wyeth-Ayerst Laboratories, Philadelphia, PA.
Pepto-Bismol® is a registered trademark of Proctor & Gamble, Cincinnati, OH.
Persantine® is a registered trademark of Boehringer Ingelheim Pharmaceuticals, Inc., Ridgefield, CT.
Plendil® is a registered trademark of Merck, Sharp, & Dohme, West Point, PA.
Prevacid® is a registered trademark of TAP, Deerfield, IL.
Prilosec® is a registered trademark of Merck, Sharp, & Dohme, West Point, PA.
Prinivil® is a registered trademark of Merck, Sharp, & Dohme, West Point, PA.
Prinzide® is a registered trademark of Merck, Sharp, & Dohme, West Point, PA.
Procardia® is a registered trademark of Pfizer Labs Division, New York, NY.
ProstaScint® is a registered trademark of Cytogen Corporation, Princeton, NJ.
Proventil® is a registered trademark of Schering Corporation, Kenilworth, NJ.
Pulmocare® is a registered trademark of Ross Laboratories, Columbus, OH.
Pulmolite® is a registered trademark of DuPont Merck, Wilmington, DE.
Pulmonex® is a registered trademark of Atomic Products, Center Moriches, NY.
Pyrolite® is a registered trademark of DuPont Merck, Wilmington, DE.
Pytest® is a registered trademark of Tri-Med Specialties, Inc., Lenexa, KS.
Quadramet® is a registered trademark of Cytogen Corporation, Princeton, NJ.
Quibron® is a registered trademark of Bristol Laboratories, Evansville, IN.
Reglan® is a registered trademark of AH Robbins Company, Richmond, VA.
Restoril® is a registered trademark of Sandoz Pharmaceuticals, East Hanover, NJ.
Rolaids® is a registered trademark of Warner-Lambert Co., Morris Plains, NJ.
Sectral® is a registered trademark of Wyeth-Ayerst Laboratories, Philadelphia, PA.
Serax® is a registered trademark of Wyeth-Ayerst Laboratories, Philadelphia, PA.
Slo-phyllin® is a registered trademark of Rhône-Poulenc Rorer Pharmaceuticals, Inc., Collegeville, PA.
Synthroid® is a registered trademark of Boots Laboratories, Lincolnshire, IL.
Tagamet® is a registered trademark of SmithKline Beecham Pharmaceuticals, Pittsburg, PA.
Tenoretic Tablets® is a registered trademark of ICI Pharma, Wilmington, DE.
Tenormin® is a registered trademark of ICI Pharma, Wilmington, DE.
Theo-Dur® is a registered trademark of Key Pharmaceuticals, Inc., Kenilworth, NJ.
Thyrogen® is a registered trademark of Genzyme Therapeutics, Cambridge, MA.
Timolide Tablets® is a registered trademark of Merck, Sharp, & Dohme, West Point, PA.
Tums® is a registered trademark of SmithKline Beecham Pharmaceuticals, Pittsburg, PA.
UltraTag® is a registered trademark of Mallinckrodt Medical, Inc., St. Louis, MO.
Valium® is a registered trademark of Roche Laboratories, Nutley, NJ.
Vascor® is a registered trademark of Wallace Laboratories, Cranbury, NJ.
Vaseretic® is a registered trademark of Merck, Sharp, & Dohme, West Point, PA.
Vasotec® is a registered trademark of Merck, Sharp, & Dohme, West Point, PA.
Verluma™ is a trademark of DuPont Merck, Wilmington, DE.
Visken® is a registered trademark of Sandoz Pharmaceuticals, East Hanover, NJ.
Xanax® is a registered trademark of The Upjohn Company, Kalamazoo, MI.
Zantac® is a registered trademark of Glaxo Wellcome, Inc., Morris Plains, NJ.
Zestoretic® is a registered trademark of Stuart Pharmaceuticals, Wilmington, DE.
Zestril® is a registered trademark of Stuart Pharmaceuticals, Wilmington, DE.

Abbreviations, 459–462
ACE inhibitors, renal scans and, 227
Acetazolamide (Diamox)
    for brain SPECT, 40, 43
    dosage and administration of, 395
ACTH-augmented adrenocortical scan, 7
Activity, equation for, 348
AcuTect study, for deep vein thrombosis, 96–100
Adenoma, toxic, radioiodine for, 298–303
    dosage for, 346
    patient information sheet for, 436–437
Adenosine
    in cardiac stress test, 76, 77
    dosage and administration of, 394, 397
Adrenal cortex, structure and function of, 8
Adrenal hormones, 8
Adrenal medulla, structure of, 8
Adrenergics, side effects of, 401
Adrenocortical scan, 3–8
    with ACTH augmentation, 7
    dosages for, 345
    patient history sheet for, 439
    with suppression, 6
Adrenocortical steroids, side effects of, 401
ALARA, 434
Angiography, 16–20
Angiotensin-converting enzyme (ACE) inhibitors, renal
    scans and, 227
Annual dose limits, 434
Antacids, side effects of, 401
Antianginals, side effects of, 401
Antiarrhythmics, side effects of, 401
Antibiotics, side effects of, 401
Anticholinergics, side effects of, 402
Anticoagulants, side effects of, 402
Anticonvulsants, side effects of, 402
Antidepressants, side effects of, 402
Antihistamine, for iodine sensitivity, 5
Ascites, shunt patency scan and, 141–144
^{198}Au, for synovectomy, 272

Benzodiazepines, withholding of, for brain SPECT, 44
Beta blockers
    for cardiac resting test, 71
    for cardiac stress test, 79
Bicisate
    for brain scan, 38
    for brain SPECT, 40

Biliary dyskinesia, HIDA scan and, 139
Biologic half-lives, equation for, 348
Bleeding, gastrointestinal. See Gastrointestinal bleed
    scan
Body surface area nomogram, 351
Bone density assessment, 21–26
Bone marrow scan, dosage for, 345
Bone mineral content assessment, 26
Bone pain, palliative treatment for, 262–267
Bone scan, 27–32
    dosages for, 345
    patient history sheet for, 440
Bowel preparation, for adrenocortical scan, 5
Brain scan/death, 34–38
    dosages for, 345
Brain scan–PET, 206–207
Brain scan–SPECT, 40–44
    with Diamox, 43
    dosage for, 345
    patient history sheet for, 441
Breath test, for ulcers, 46–50

^{11}C-1-butanol, 209
C-14 urea breath test, 46–50
^{11}C-acetate, 209
Calcium-channel blockers
    for cardiac resting test, 71
    for cardiac stress test, 79
Cancer
    lung, NeoTect scan for, 183–187
    lung, Verluma scan for, 323–327
    PET for, 207–210
    whole-body study for, 317–320
Captopril study
    dosage and administration in, 395
    for glomerular filtration rate, 225, 226
    patient history sheet for, 455
    for renal tubular function, 232, 233
Carcinoembryonic antigen (CEA) scan.
    See CEA-Scan
Cardiac function, equations for, 342, 348
Cardiac imaging
    dosages for, 345
    gated first-pass study, 51–55
    MUGA/MUGA-X, 56–61
    myocardial infarction (MI) scan, 62–66
    patient history sheet for, 442
    PET, 207

resting test (perfusion), 67–71
    with stress test, 71, 73–79
  stress-rest tests, 71
  stress test, 71, 73–79
Cardiac output, equation for, 348
Cardiac SPECT, 256
Cardiolite. *See* ^{99m}Tc-sestamibi
Cariporide, 65–66
Catheters, urinary, for children, 95
CEA-Scan, 81–84
  dosage for, 345
  patient history sheet for, 452
Centimeters-inches conversion
  equation for, 348
  table for, 340
Ceretec
  for brain scan, 34, 38
  for brain-SPECT, 40
  patient history sheet for, 443
  for white blood cell scan, 329, 334
    dosage of, 346
^{11}C-glucose, 209
Children
  dosages for, 351–355
    calculation of, 348, 351–352
  urinary catheters for, 95
Chinese, phonetic translations for, 415–416
Cholecystokinin (CCK)
  actions of, 139
  dosage and administration of, 393
  for HIDA scan, 138, 139
Chromatography, kit preparation for, 349–350
Cimetidine, for Meckel's diverticulum scan, 180, 181
Cisternography, 86–90
  dosage for, 345
^{11}C-*N*-methylspiperone, 209
^{57}Co, decay table for, 384
^{57}Co cookie sheet
  in lung transmission scan, 164
  in lymphoscintigraphy, 175, 176
^{57}Co-cyanocobalamin, for Schilling test, 240
  dosage of, 346
Committed dose equivalent (CDE), 433
Committed effective dose equivalent (CEDE), 433
Computed tomography (CT)
  for deep vein thrombosis, 107
  in single/dual photon absorptiometry, 26
Concentrations
  doses from, 348
  equations for, 348
Conversion tables
  inches-centimeters, 340
  millicuries-megabecquerels, 343
  pounds-kilograms, 340
  target heart rates, 342
Corticosteroids, side effects of, 401
^{11}C-palmitate, 209
^{137}Cs, decay table for, 383

Cystography, 91–95
  dosage for, 345

Decay. *See* Radionuclide decay
Deep venous thrombosis (DVT)
  AcuTect study for, 96–100
  venography for, 102–108
Densitometry, 21–26
Denver shunt patency, 141–144
DEXA (dual energy x-ray absorptiometry), 25, 26
Diamox (acetazolamide)
  for brain SPECT, 40, 43
  dosage and administration of, 396
Dilaudid (hydromorphone), for HIDA scan, 138
Dipyridamole (Persantine)
  in cardiac stress test, 76, 77
  dosage and administration of, 394
Disofenin (DISIDA), for HIDA scan, 134
Diverticulum, Meckel's, 178–181
Dobutamine
  in cardiac stress test, 76, 77
  dosage and administration of, 394, 398
Dosages
  adult, 345–346
    calculation of, 348
  pediatric, 351–355
    calculation of, 348, 351–352, 393
Dose equivalents, 433
Dose limits, annual, 434
DPA (dual photon absorptiometry), 25, 26
Drip conversions, 393
Drugs. *See also* Radiopharmaceuticals
  dosage and administration of, 393–395
  infusion tables for, 397–400
  side effects of, 401–403
Drug withholding
  for brain SPECT, 44
  for cardiac resting test, 68
  for glomerular filtration rate, 224, 227
  for ^{123}I, 403
  for pheochromocytoma scan, 14
  for renal tubular function scan, 231, 234
Dual energy x-ray absorptiometry (DEXA), 25, 26
Dual photon absorptiometry (DPA), 25, 26
Duodenal ulcers, breath test for, 46–50
DVT. *See* Deep venous thrombosis (DVT)
^{165}Dy-FHMA (ferric hydroxide macroaggregates), for synovectomy, 272
^{90}DY-FHMA (ferric hydroxide macroaggregates), for synovectomy, 272

Ectopic thyroid tissue scan, 292–296
  dosage for, 346
Edge sign, in lung perfusion scan, 158
Effective half-lives, equation for, 348
Effective renal plasma flow, calculation of, 233–234
Ejection fraction, equation for, 348

Enalaprilat (Vasotec), dosage and administration of, 395

Enzymes, production sites, substrates, and actions of, 409

Epinephrine, in pheochromocytoma, 14

Equations, 348

Erythrocytes, tagged. *See* Tagged red blood cells

Esophageal transit time, 109–112

^{18}F-16α-fluoro-17β-estradiol, 210

Fab fragments, for OncoScint, 197

Fatty meal, for HIDA scan, 138, 139

Fentanyl citrate, for HIDA scan, 138

^{18}F-FDG, 210

Fissure sign, in lung perfusion scan, 158

Foreign language translations, 415–429

French, translations for, 417–418

^{18}F-spiperone, 210

Furosemide (Lasix), dosage and administration of, 395

^{67}Ga, decay table for, 385

^{68}Ga-citrate/transferrin, 210

Gallbladder scan with ejection fraction (HIDA), 134–140

    dosage for, 345

    patient history sheet for, 456

Gallium scan, 114–117

    brain, 38

    dosage for, 345

    patient history sheet for, 443

Gastric empty scan, 119–123

    dosage for, 345

    patient history sheet for, 444

Gastric ulcers, breath test for, 46–50

Gastroesophageal reflux scan, 125–128

Gastrointestinal bleed scan, 129–132

    dosage for, 345

    patient history sheet for, 445

Gated first-pass cardiac study, 51–55

Gates method, for glomerular filtration rate, 226–227

German, translations for, 418–420

Glomerular filtration rate, 222–227

Glucagon, for Meckel's diverticulum scan, 181

Goiter, toxic nodular, radioiodine for, 298–303

    dosage for, 346

    patient history sheet for, 436–437

Graves' disease, radioiodine for, 298–303

    dosage for, 346

    patient information sheet for, 436–437

Half-lives

    for commonly used radionuclides, 347

    equation for, 348

HAMA titer, 197

Heart rates

    conversion table for, 342

    equation for, 348

Helicobacter pylori, breath test for, 46–50

Hemangioma, hepatic, SPECT for, 145–148

Hepatic hemangioma, SPECT for, 145–148

Hepatobiliary scan with ejection fraction (HIDA). *See* HIDA (hepatobiliary/gallbladder) scan

HIDA (hepatobiliary/gallbladder) scan, 134–140

    dosage for, 345

    patient history sheet for, 446

Hormesis, 433

Hormones, production sites, targets, and actions of, 410–414

Hot pyp, for myocardial infarction scan, 62

    dosage of, 345

Human albumin microspheres. *See* ^{99m}Tc-HAM; ^{99m}Tc-HAMM

Hydromorphone (Dilaudid), for HIDA scan, 138

Hyperthyroidism, radioiodine for, 298–303

    dosage for, 346

    patient information sheet for, 436–437

^{123}I

    decay table for, 387

    drugs/studies affecting, 403

    for ectopic thyroid tissue scan, 292, 293, 295, 296

        dosage of, 346

    for thyroid scan, 304–309

    for thyroid uptake, 310, 311

^{131}I

    decay table for, 388

    for ectopic thyroid tissue scan, 292, 293, 295, 296

        dosage of, 346

    for hyperthyroidism, 298–303

        dosage of, 346

    for thyroid ablation, 284–290

        dosage of, 346

    for thyroid scan, 304–309

    for thyroid uptake, 310, 311

        dosage of, 346

    for whole-body cancer study, 317–320

        dosage of, 346

    with rTSH augmentation, 320–321

^{123}-mIBG (-*meta*-iodobenzylguanidine), for pheochromocytoma scan, 9–14

    dosage for, 345

    patient history sheet for, 449

^{131}-mIBG (-*meta*-iodobenzylguanidine)

    for pheochromocytoma scan, 9–14

        dosage for, 345

        patient history sheet for, 439

    for whole-body cancer study, 321

IDA (iminodiacetic acid), for HIDA scan, 134

^{131}I-diphosphonate, for bone pain palliation, 267

^{125}I-fibrinogen, for deep vein thrombosis, 107

^{123}I-iodoamphetamine, for brain scan, 38

^{131}I-6β iodomethylnorcholesterol (NP-59), for adrenocortical scan, 3

    dosage of, 345

Iminodiacetic acid (IDA), for HIDA scan, 134

^{111}In, decay table for, 386

^{111}In-capromab pendetide, for ProstaScint scan, 212

Inches-centimeters conversion
    equation for, 348
    table for, 341

^{111}In chloride satumomab pendetide, for OncoScint
    scan, 194

Incident reports, 431

^{111}In-CYT-356, for ProstaScint scan, 212
    dosage of, 346

Indium scan, patient history sheet for, 443

^{111}In-DTPA (diethylenetriaminepentaacetic acid)
    for cisternography, 86
        dosage of, 345
    for gastric empty scan, 119

Infusion tables, 397–400

^{111}In-oxine (oxyquinoline), for white blood cell scan,
    329–335

^{111}In-pentetreotide, for lung scan, 188
    dosage of, 345

^{125}In-platelets, for deep vein thrombosis, 107

^{111}In-satumomab pendetide, for OncoScint scan, 194
    dosage of, 345

Intracavitary infusion, 273–277

Inverse square law, 348

Iodine sensitivity, antihistamine for, 5

^{131}I-OIH (orthoiodohippurate)
    for cystography, 91
    for glomerular filtration rate, 222, 226
        dosage for, 346

Isotopes, PET, 209–210

Italian, translations for, 420–421

Japanese, phonetic translations for, 421–422

Kidney depth calculation, Tonnesen method for, 234

Kilograms-pounds conversion
    equation for, 348
    table for, 340

Kinevac (sincalide), dosage and administration of, 394

Kit preparation, 349–350

Labels, package, 435

Laboratory tests, normal ranges for, 405–408

Language translations, 415–429

Lasix (furosemide), dosage and administration of, 394

Lens dose equivalent (LDE), 433, 434

LeVeen shunt patency, 141–144

Liver SPECT, 145–148
    dosage for, 345

Liver/spleen scan, 149–153
    dosage for, 149–153
    patient history sheet for, 449

Lung cancer, NeoTect scan for, 183–187

Lung cancer, Verluma scan for, 323–327

Lung perfusion scan, 154–159

dosage for, 345

lung ventilation scan and, 165–170

quantitation in, 158

Lung scan, patient history sheets for, 447, 448

Lung transmission scan, 161–164

Lung ventilation scan, 165–170
    dosage for, 345

Lymphangiogram, 171–177

Lymphoscintigraphy, 171–177
    dosage for, 345

Magnesium citrate, for OctreoScan, 190

Magnetic resonance imaging (MRI), for deep vein
    thrombosis, 107

Mebrofenin, for HIDA scan, 134
    dosage of, 345

Meckel's diverticulum scan, 178–181
    dosage for, 345
    patient history sheet for, 445

Megabecquerels-millicuries conversion table, 343

Meperidine (Demerol), for HIDA scan, 138

Metastasis, whole-body study for, 317–320
    I^{131} and bone scan, 27–32

6-Methoxyisobutyl isonitrile. See 99mTc-sestamibi

Metoclopramide (Reglan)
    dosage and administration of, 395
    for gastric empty scan, 119

mIBG scan, for pheochromocytoma, 9–14
    dosage for, 345
    patient history sheet for, 449

Microlite, for cystography, 91

Millicuries-megabecquerels conversion table, 343

Miraluma. See ^{99m}Tc-sestamibi

Misadministration, 430–431

^{99}Mo, decay table for, 389

Monoclonal antibodies, for OncoScint, 197

Morphine sulfate
    dosage and administration of, 394
    for HIDA scan, 138

MUGA/MUGA-X scan, 56–61
    dosage for, 345
    patient history sheet for, 442

Myocardial infarction (MI) scan, 62–66
    dosage for, 345

Myoview. See ^{99m}Tc-tetrofosmin

Na^{99m}TcO$_4$$^{-}$. See ^{99m}Tc-pertechnetate

NeoTect scan, 183–187

Neurolite
    for brain scan, 38
    for brain-SPECT, 40

^{13}N-NH$_3$, 210

Nonstochastic effects, 433

Norepinephrine, in pheochromocytoma, 14

NP-59 (^{131}I-6β iodomethylnorcholesterol), for adreno-
    cortical scan, 3
    dosage of, 345

Occupational dose limits, 434
^{15}O-CO, 210
OctreoScan, 188-192
   dosage for, 345
   patient history sheet for, 451
^{15}O-H$_2$O, 210
OncoScint, 194-198
   dosage for, 345
   patient history sheet for, 452
^{15}O-O$_2$, 210
Osteopenia, densitometry for, 21-26
Osteoporosis, densitometry for, 21-26

Package labels, 435
Pain, bone, palliative treatment for, 262-267
Palliation
    for bone pain, 262-267
    intracavitary infusion for, 273-277
Parathyroid scan, 199-204
   dosage for, 346
   dual-isotope subtraction technique for, 202
   single-isotope two-phase, 202-203
Patient history sheets, 439-458
Patient information sheet, for thyroid therapies,
   436-437
^{32}P-chromic phosphate
   for intracavitary infusion, 273
   for synovectomy, 268
Pediatric dosages, 351-355
   calculation of, 348, 351-352, 393
Pediatric urinary catheters, 95
Pentagastrin (Peptavlon)
   dosage and administration of, 395
   for Meckel's diverticulum scan, 180
Pentazocine, for HIDA scan, 138
Peptic ulcers, breath test for, 46-50
Perchlorate, for angiography, 18
Peritoneovenous shunt patency scan, 141-144
Persantine (dipyridamole)
   in cardiac stress test, 76, 77
   dosage and administration of, 394, 399
PET. *See* Positron emission tomography (PET)
Pheochromocytoma scan, 9-14
   dosage for, 345
   with renal and skeletal imaging, 14
Plethysmography, for deep vein thrombosis, 107
Plummer's disease, radioiodine for, 298-303
   dosage for, 346
   patient information sheet for, 436-437
Polish, translations for, 423-424
Polycythemia vera, ^{32}P-sodium phosphate for,
   279-283
^{32}P-orthophosphate, for bone pain palliation,
   267
Portuguese, translations for, 424-426
Positron emission tomography (PET), 205-211

brain, 206-207
cardiac, 207
isotopes for, 209-210
oncologic, 207
Positrons, 210
Potassium perchlorate, for Meckel's diverticulum scan,
   181
Pounds-kilograms conversion
   equation for, 348
   table for, 340
Pregnancy, annual dose limits and, 434
ProstaScint scan, 212-216
   dosage for, 346
   patient history sheet for, 453
^{32}P-sodium phosphate, for polycythemia vera,
   279-283
Pulmonary embolism, 108
Pyrophosphate (pyp; Pyrolite)
   dosage and administration of, 395
   for liver SPECT, 51, 52
   for myocardial infarction scan, 62
     dosage of, 345
PYtest C-14 urea breath test, 46-50

Radiation
   biologic effects of, 433
   properties of, 432
Radiation safety, 432-433
Radioimmunoscintigraphy (RIS)
   CEA-Scan, 81-84
     dosage for, 345
     patient history sheet for, 443
   OncoScint, 194-198
     patient history sheet for, 443
   ProstaScint, 212-216
   Verluma, 323-327
     patient history sheet for, 323-327
Radioiodine therapy
   dosage for, 346
   for hyperthyroidism, 298-303
   for thyroid ablation, 284-290
Radionuclide(s). *See also specific radionuclides*
   activity of, equation for, 348
   concentrations of, equation for, 348
   misadministration of, 430-431
   properties and medical uses of, 347
   properties of, 356-381
Radionuclide decay
   equation for, 348
   modes of, 432
   tables for, 382-392
Radiopharmaceuticals. *See also specific compounds*
   blood-brain penetrating, 38
   dosages for, 345-346
   medical applications of, 209-210
   misadministration of, 430-431

non-blood-brain penetrating, 38
    for PET, 209-210
^{82}Rb-RB$^+$, 210
Recordable events, 430-431
Red blood cells, tagged. *See* Tagged red blood cells
^{186}Re-etidronate (hydroxyethylidene diphosphonate),
    for bone pain palliation, 267
Reflux, gastroesophageal, 125-128
Reglan (metoclopramide), for gastric empty scan, 119
Renal depth calculation, Tonnesen method for, 234
Renal scan
    cortical imaging, 217-221
    dosage for, 346
    glomerular filtration rate, 222-227
    patient history sheet for, 454, 455
    tubular function, 229-234
Renography, 222-227
    dosage for, 346
    patient history sheet for, 454, 455
^{188}Re-phosphonate, for bone pain palliation, 267
Reportable events, 431
Resting test, cardiac (perfusion), 67-71
Rule of two's, for Meckel's diverticulum, 181
Russian, phonetic translations for, 426-427

Safety measures, 432-433
    in PET, 210-211
Salivary gland imaging, 236-239
Schegel method, 233-234
Schilling test, 240-245
    dosage for, 346
Scintimammography, 246-251
    dosage for, 346
    patient history sheet for, 456
Serosal intracavitary infusion, 273-277
SEXA (single energy x-ray absorptiometry), 24, 26
Shallow dose equivalent (SDE), 433, 434
Shielding
    equations for, 348
    methods of, 433
Shunt patency, for LeVeen/Denver shunt, 141-144
Sincalide (Kinevac), 139
    dosage and administration of, 393
Single energy x-ray absorptiometry (SEXA), 24, 26
Single photon absorptiometry (SPA), 24, 26
Single photon emission computed tomography. *See*
    SPECT
Skeletal imaging, 27-32
Small cell lung cancer, Verluma scan for, 323-327
^{153}Sm-lexidronam, for bone pain palliation, 262
^{90}Sn-chelate, for bone pain palliation, 267
Sodium ^{99m}TcO$_4^-$. *See* ^{99m}Tc-pertechnetate
Sodium iodide thyroid ablation, 284-290
Somatostatin, OctreoScan and, 192
SPA (single photon absorptiometry), 24, 26
Spanish, translations for, 427-429

SPECT, 249, 252-257
    in bone scan, 30
    brain, 40-44
    cardiac, 256
        in cardiac resting test, 70
        in cardiac stress test, 76, 77
    in CEA-scan, 83
    in gallium scan, 116
    liver, 145-148
    in liver/spleen scan, 151, 152
    in myocardial infarction scan, 64
    in NeoTect scan, 185, 186
    in OctreoScan, 190
    in OncoScint, 197
    in parathyroid scan, 201, 203
    in ProstaScint scan, 215
    in scintimammography, 249
    in Verluma scan, 323-327
Sphincter of Oddi spasm, HIDA scan and, 139
Spleen scan, 149-153
    dosage for, 345
    patient history sheet for, 449
^{89}Sr-chloride, for bone pain palliation, 262
Steroids, side effects of, 401
Stochastic effects, 433
Stress MUGA (or MUGA-X), 56-61
Stress test, cardiac (perfusion), 71, 73-79
Stroke volume, equation for, 348
Substernal thyroid scan, 292-296
    dosage for, 346
Super Scan, in bone scanning, 31
Synovectomy, 268-272

Tagged red blood cells
    angiography, 16-20
    for gastrointestinal bleed scan, 102, 105-106
        dosage of, 345
    for liver SPECT, 145, 147, 148
        dosage of, 345
    for MUGA/MUGA-X scan, 56-61
        dosage of, 345
    for venography, 102, 105-106
Talbot's nomogram (modified), 351
Target heart rates
    conversion table for, 342
    equation for, 348
^{99m}Tc, decay table for, 390
^{99m}Tc-albumin colloid, for gastric empty scan, 119
^{99m}Tc-apcitide (AcuTect), for deep vein thrombosis,
    96
^{99m}Tc-arcitumomab, for CEA-scan, 81
    dosage of, 81
^{99m}Tc-depreotide (NeoTect), for lung mass, 183
^{99m}Tc-DMSA (dimercaptosuccinic acid), for renal corti-
    cal imaging, 217, 219
    dosage of, 346

^{99m}Tc-DTPA (diethylenetriaminepentaacetic acid)
  for adrenocortical scan, 6
  for angiography, 16
  for brain scan, 34, 38
    dosage of, 345
  for cisternography, 86
  for cystography, 91
  for gastric empty scan, 119
  for glomerular filtration rate, 222, 226
    dosage of, 346
  for lung ventilation scan, 165, 168, 169
    dosage of, 345
^{99m}Tc-ECD (ethyl cysteinate dimer)
  for brain scan, 38
  for brain SPECT, 40
^{99m}Tc-GH (glucoheptonate), for brain scan,
34, 38
  dosage of, 345
^{99m}Tc-HAM (human albumin microspheres)
  for LeVeen/Denver shunt patency scan, 141
  for lung perfusion scan, 154
^{99m}Tc-HAMM (human albumin mini-microspheres), for
lung ventilation scan, 165
^{99m}Tc-HDP (hydroxyethylene diphosphonate)
  for bone scan, 27
    dosage of, 345
  for brain scan, 38
^{99m}Tc-HMPAO (hexamethylpropyleneamine oxine)
  for brain scan, 34, 38
  for brain SPECT, 40
  patient history sheet for, 453
  for white blood cell scan, 329, 334
    dosage of, 346
^{99m}Tc-HMPAO (hexamethylpropyleneamine oxine)
platelets, for deep vein thrombosis, 107
^{99m}Tc-MAA (macroaggregated albumin)
  for LeVeen/Denver shunt patency scan, 141, 143,
144
  for lung perfusion scan, 154, 159
    dosage of, 345
  for venography, 102
^{99m}Tc-MAG$_3$ (mercaptoacetyltriglycine)
  for cystography, 91
  for glomerular filtration rate, 222, 226
    dosage of, 346
^{99m}Tc-MDP (methylene diphosphonate)
  for bone scan, 27
    dosage of, 345
  for brain scan, 38
^{99m}Tc-nofetumomab merpentan, for small cell lung
cancer scan, 323–327
^{99m}TcO$_4$$^-$. *See* ^{99m}Tc-pertechnetate
^{99m}Tc-pertechnetate
  for angiography, 16, 18
  for brain scan, 34, 38
    dosage of, 345

for cystography, 91
  dosage of, 345
for ectopic thyroid tissue scan, 292, 293, 295–296
for gastrointestinal bleed scan, 129
for gated first-pass cardiac study, 51
kit preparation for, 349–350
for liver SPECT, 14518
for lung transmission scan, 161
for Meckel's diverticulum scan, 178
  dosage of, 345
for MUGA/MUGA-X scan, 56
for parathyroid scan, 199
  dosage of, 161
for salivary gland imaging, 236
for testicular scan, 258
  dosage of, 346
for thyroid scan, 304, 305, 307
  dosage of, 346
for thyroid uptake, 310, 311
for venography, 102
^{99m}Tc-pyp
  for liver SPECT, 51, 52
  for myocardial infarction scan, 62
    dosage of, 345
^{99m}Tc-SC (sulfur colloid)
  for cystography, 91
    dosage of, 345
  for esophageal transit time, 109
  for gastric empty scan, 119
    dosage of, 345
  for gastroesophageal reflux assessment, 125
  for gastrointestinal bleed scan, 129, 130,
131–132
  for intracavitary infusion, 273
  for LeVeen/Denver shunt patency scan, 141, 143,
144
  for liver/spleen scan, 149
    dosage of, 345
  for lymphoscintigraphy, 171
    dosage of, 345
  for synovectomy, 268
^{99m}Tc-sestamibi
  for cardiac resting test, 67, 71
  for cardiac stress test, 71, 73, 78, 79
  for gated first-pass cardiac study, 51
  for parathyroid scan, 199
  for scintimammography, 246
^{99m}Tc-stannous pyrophosphate
  for myocardial infarction scan, 62
^{99m}Tc-T$_2$G$_1$ antifibrin, for brain SPECT, 40
^{99m}Tc-tetrofosmin
  for cardiac resting test, 67, 71
  for cardiac stress test, 71, 73, 78, 79
  for gated first-pass cardiac study, 51
  for parathyroid scan, 199
  for scintimammography, 246

Testicular scan, 258–261
  dosage for, 346
Thrombosis, venous. *See* Deep venous thrombosis
  (DVT)
Thyroid ablation, 284–291
  dosage for, 346
Thyroid hyperactivity, radioiodine for, 298–303
  dosage for, 346
  patient information sheet for, 437
Thyroid scan, 304–309
  dosage for, 346
  patient history sheet for, 457–458
  substernal, 292–296
    dosage for, 346
  whole-body, 317–320
    with rTSH augmentation, 320–321
Thyroid uptake, 310–316
  dosage for, 346
  patient history sheet for, 457–458
Thyrotropin alfa (Thyrogen), for whole-body scan
  with rTSH augmentation, 320–321
^{201}Tl
  for cardiac resting test, 67, 71
  for cardiac stress test, 71, 73, 78, 79
  decay table for, 391
  for parathyroid scan, 199, 200
    dosage of, 346
  for whole-body scan cancer study, 321
^{201}Tl-chloride
  for brain scan, 38
  for cardiac resting test, 67, 71
  for cardiac stress test, 71, 73–78, 79
Tonnesen method, for kidney depth calculation, 234
Total effective dose equivalent (TEDE), 433, 434
Total organ dose equivalent (TODE), 433, 434
Toxic nodular goiter/adenoma, radioiodine for,
  298–303
  dosage for, 346
  patient information sheet for, 436–437
Translations, language, 415–429
Treadmill test, 73–79

Ulcers, breath test for, 46–50
Ultrasonography, for deep vein thrombosis, 107
UltraTag
  dosage and administration of, 395

for angiography, 16–20
  for gastrointestinal bleed, 129–132
  for liver SPECT, 145–148
  for MUGA scan, 59
  for venography, 102–108
Urea breath test, 46–50
Urinary catheters, for children, 95
Urokinase, infusion table for, 400

Vasotec (enalaprilat), dosage and administration of,
  395
Venography
  AcuTect study and, 100
  for deep vein thrombosis, 102–108
Venous thrombosis. *See* Deep venous thrombosis
  (DVT)
Ventilation scan, 165–170
Verluma scan, 323–327
  patient history sheet for, 452
Vitamin B-12, for Schilling test, 240
  dosage of, 346
Voiding cystourethrogram, 91–95

Webster's rule, for pediatric dosage, 352
Weight/metabolic rule, for pediatric dosage,
  352
Wellman's rule, for pediatric dosage, 352
White blood cell scan, 329–335
  dosage for, 346
Whole-body cancer study, 317–320
  dosage for, 346

^{133}Xe (xenon)
  for brain scan, 38
  decay table for, 392
  for lung ventilation scan, 165, 168, 169
    dosage of, 345

^{90}Y-calcium oxalate, for synovectomy,
  272
^{90}Y-citrate, for bone pain palliation, 267
Young's rule, for pediatric dosage, 352

Zona fasciculata, 8
Zona glomerulosa, 8
Zona reticularis, 8